Plant Protein

GIGI GRASSIA

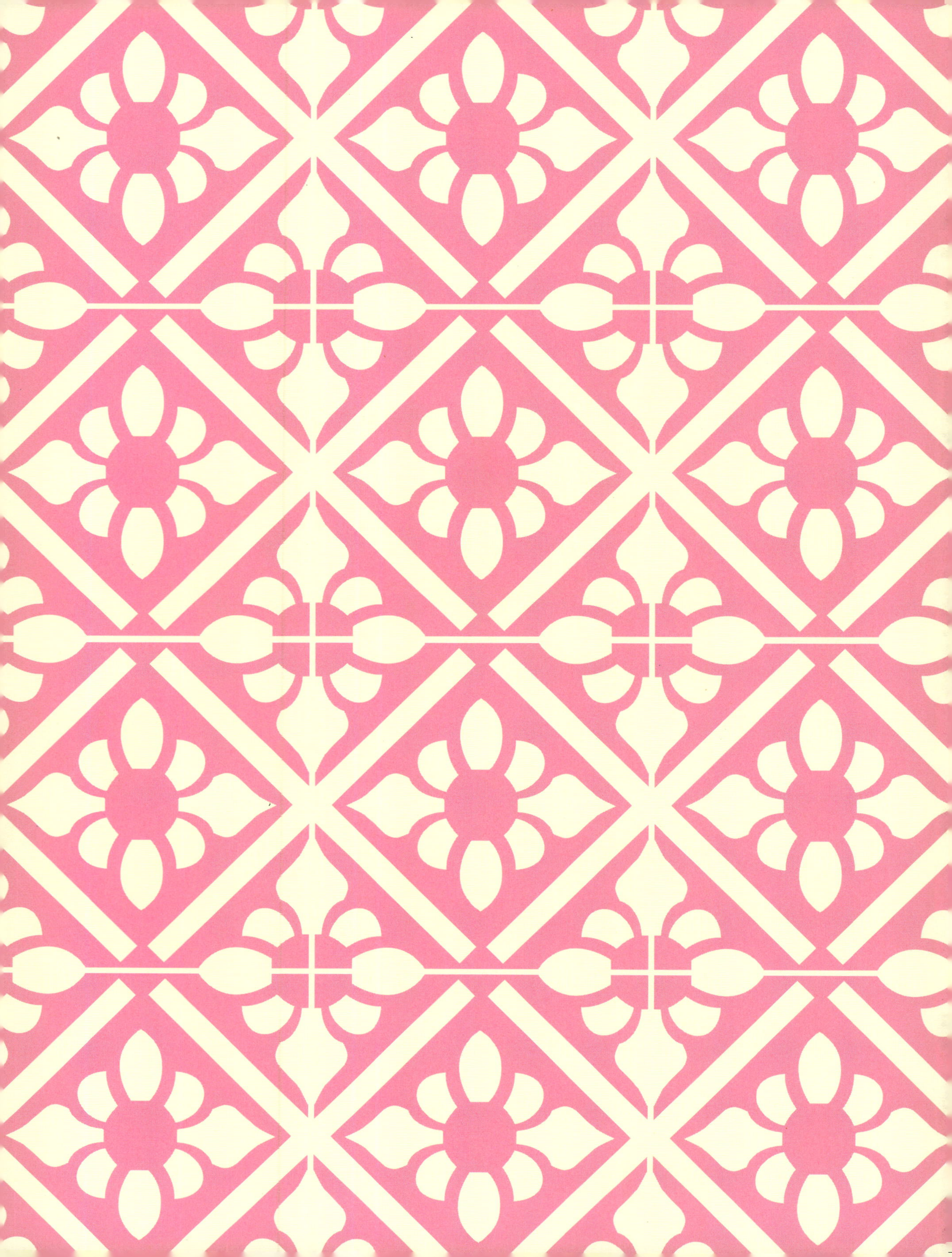

Plant Protein

80 HEALTHY & DELICIOUS HIGH-PROTEIN VEGAN RECIPES

GIGI GRASSIA

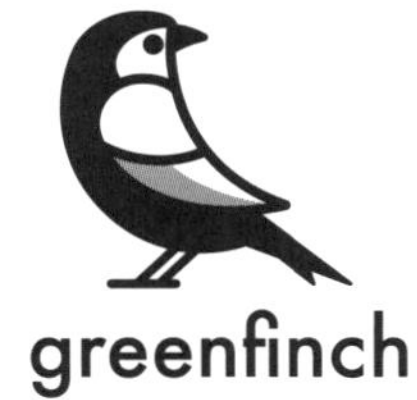

greenfinch

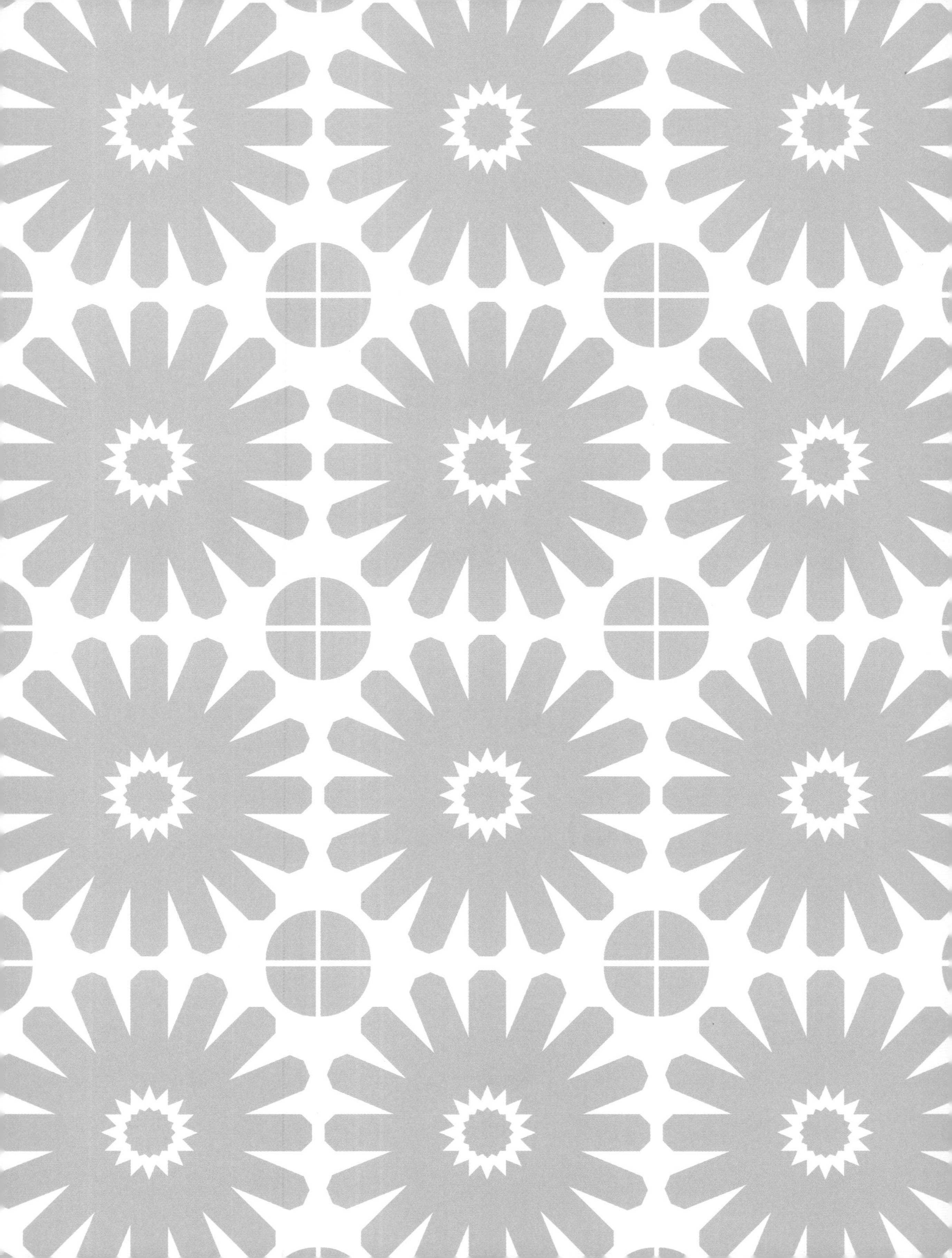

CONTENTS

INTRODUCTION

This book is a love story. Don't worry, you didn't accidentally pick up the wrong book – it is a cookbook, but it is really about love. My love of food. My love of fitness. And my love of animals.

My food journey began in my Italian childhood home, surrounded by family and the delicious aroma of homemade meals. Food has always been a love language in my family, a way to show care and create lasting memories. Inspired by my mamma and nonna's traditional cooking in Italy, I developed a deep appreciation for high-quality, whole foods that are minimally processed.

Later in life, I moved abroad, first to Germany and then to China, Hong Kong and finally to London. In addition to learning their cultures and becoming fluent in five languages, these travels taught me the wonder of international cuisine. I learned that all cultures love food almost as much as Italians and, like an art collector, I began to pick up new and exciting tastes and flavour combinations.

Like any good love story, though, my relationship with food has had its ups and downs. There were times as a young adult when I did not love myself or the way my body looked and, as a result, my relationship with food suffered. However, I eventually discovered a love for fitness – whether it's working out in the gym, running ultra-marathons in the hills outside London or simply doing some calming yoga or stretching at the end of a long day, I love the feeling of balance I get from moving my body. And that passion also benefited my relationship with food. I started to learn about the importance of a healthy and sustainable diet with the right balance of macronutrients (and protein in particular). It was a desire to help others make the same transition, from insecure and food-negative to confident and strong, that eventually led me to become a qualified nutrition coach and personal trainer.

But wait, what about veganism? Where does that fit in? Well for that I have to give credit to my lovely cocker spaniel, Manuka. His loving, caring and sweet presence made me truly realize that all meat or animal products require the sacrifice of another animal. And those animals all have personalities of their own. I am not a militant vegan who thinks meat-eaters are evil, but ever since I made that connection – between animal and meat – I haven't looked back.

Along the way, I created an Instagram page to document my vegan journey, and it quickly started to form a community of more than half a million followers! One recurring theme I notice is the concern about maintaining a balanced diet after switching to veganism. Many people are in the process of reducing dairy and meat, but struggle with figuring out how to get enough protein to sustain their active lifestyles. There is a common belief that plants do not have enough protein, which I knew from my nutrition and fitness knowledge isn't true. This realization inspired me

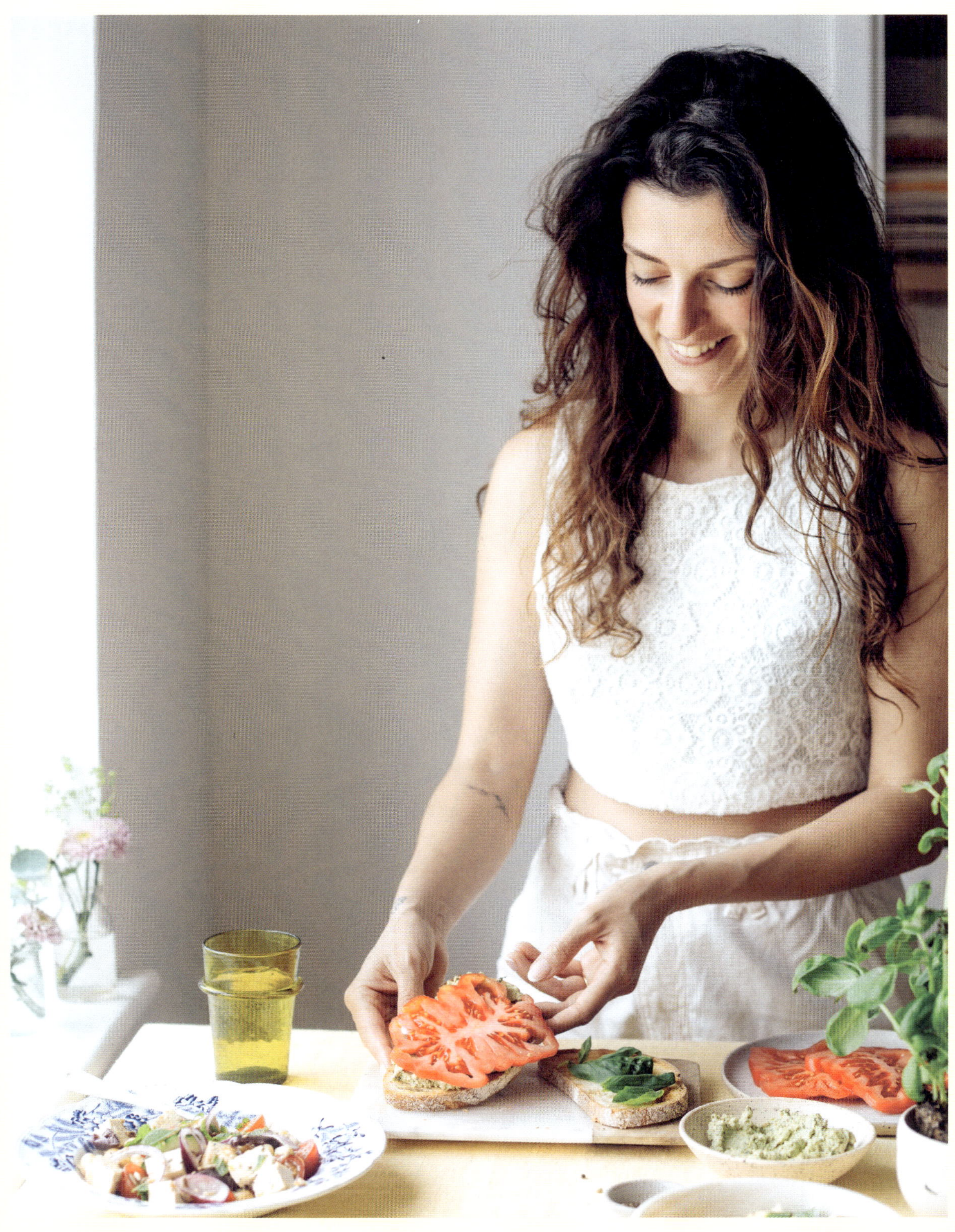

to combine my loves and focus on high-protein recipes to demonstrate that a high-protein diet can be deliciously plant-based.

This mission led here, to this cookbook filled with vegan recipes that are rich in protein and fibre and which are designed to support your active lifestyle while bringing joy to your meals. I wrote the book to share my love story with food and hopefully inspire others to try the journey for themselves. Each dish is crafted to bring joy to your meals while ensuring you get the nutrients you need. These recipes are my very own creations, inspired by my Italian roots and my travels and seasoned with my passion for veganism and fitness. In my kitchen, there are no limitations – it's about engaging with a feeling and cooking with no rules.

I hope this book helps you as much as writing it has helped me, proving that a high-protein, plant-based diet is not only possible but also incredibly delicious. Let these recipes support your journey, help you create lasting memories, and bring love to your meals.

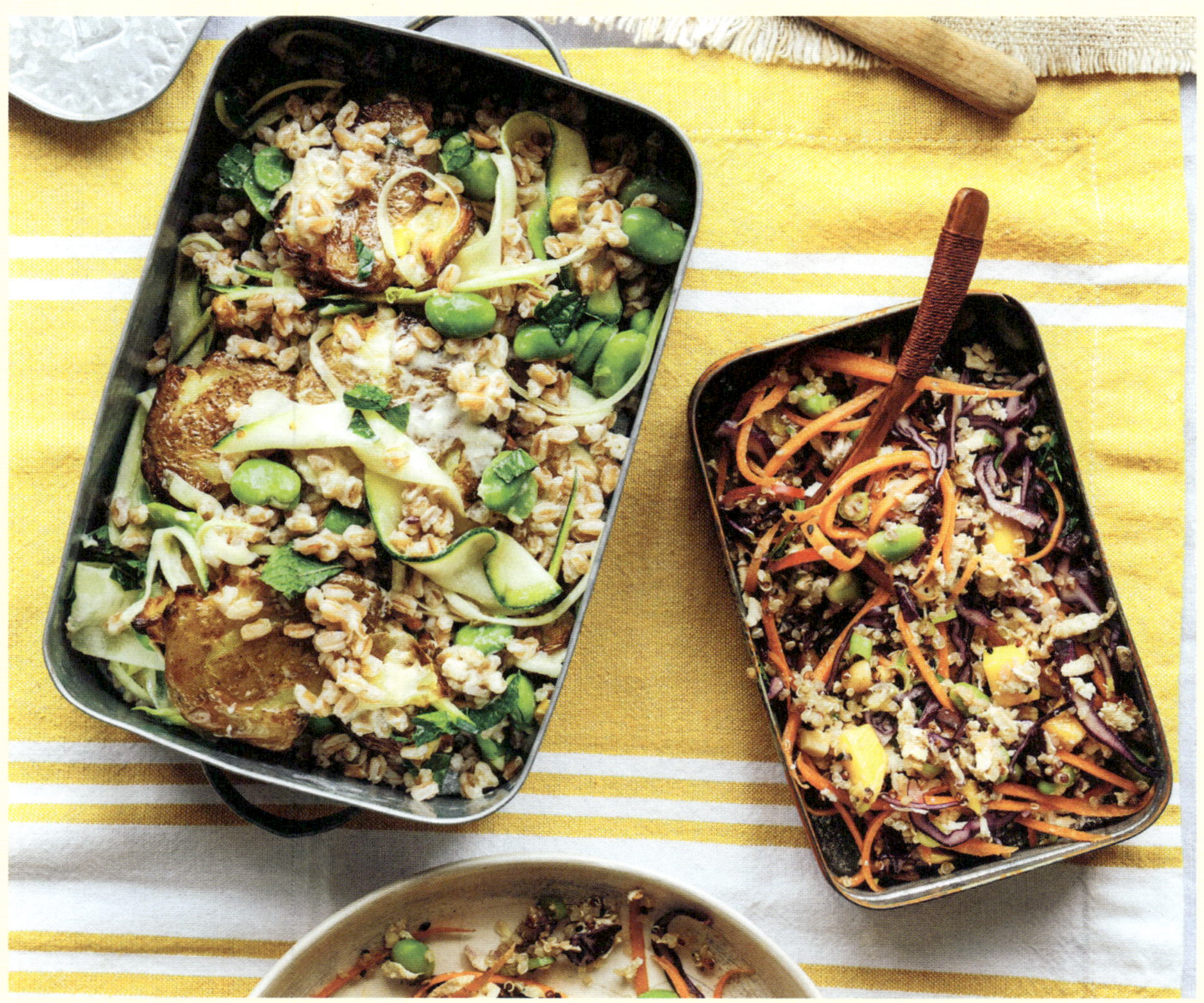

COOK'S NOTES

All fruits and vegetables are assumed to be medium-sized (unless stated otherwise) and washed. Garlic and onions are assumed peeled.

Herbs are assumed to be fresh unless stated otherwise.

All salt is fine salt unless stated otherwise.

Protein powder is always plant-based.

RECIPE ICONS

The recipes are marked with the following helpful dietary and timing icons.

 High in fibre

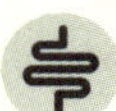 Good for gut health

 Source of iron

 Gluten-free

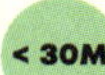 Takes less than 30 minutes to make

 Takes less than 1 hour to make

 Takes more than 1 hour to make

The timing icons refer to active cooking time, not including resting, marinating or cooling times. Please read all recipes carefully before you begin cooking.

BUT WHAT ABOUT PROTEIN?

If I had a coin for every time I've been asked, 'Can you really get enough protein on a vegan diet?' I'd be rolling in riches by now. We've all heard it a million times, and the answer is a resounding yes. It's been proven over and over again that not only can you get enough protein on a vegan diet, you can also support a highly active lifestyle with it.

MACRONUTRIENTS – WHERE DOES PROTEIN FIT?

Think of your body as a garden. **Calories** are like the sunlight that fuels the garden. Just as plants need sunlight to grow and thrive, your body needs calories to perform all its functions. Without enough sunlight, the plants in the garden will wither and die; similarly, without enough calories, your body can't function properly. The impact of calories on our weight and health depends on the source of these calories – the macronutrients and how they're processed by our body.

- **Macronutrients** are like the different types of nutrients in the soil that help the plants grow.

- **Proteins** are like the nitrogen in the soil. Nitrogen is essential for the growth and repair of plants, helping them develop strong stems and leaves. In your body, proteins are crucial for building and repairing tissues, making enzymes and supporting immune function.

- **Carbohydrates** are like the water that nourishes the plants. Water is vital for plants' immediate needs, helping them absorb nutrients and grow. In your body, carbs are broken down into glucose, which fuels your brain, muscles and other tissues.

- **Fats** are like the phosphorus and potassium in the soil. These nutrients support the long-term health of the plants, helping them store energy, produce flowers and withstand harsh conditions. In your body, fats are used for long-term energy storage, hormone production and protecting vital organs.

The efficiency of calorie absorption can vary slightly depending on the source of the macronutrient. While for carbohydrates and fats the rate of calorie absorption is around 80–100 per cent, it varies slightly for protein. When you consume protein, not all of it is absorbed into the body, and the quantity varies depending on the source of the protein. For example, when you eat 100 calories of chicken, about 70–80 calories are actually absorbed and usable by your body. For a plant-based alternative, such as tofu, the absorption rate is slightly lower, around 60–70 per cent. Therefore, you would get approximately 60–70 usable calories from 100 calories of tofu.

But don't panic! This just means that someone following a plant-based diet and trying to build muscle mass might need to consume slightly more protein (roughly 10 per cent) to ensure they are meeting their body's needs.

WHY PROTEIN IS KING

Why does everyone seem to be raving about protein?

Protein is like the Swiss Army knife of nutrients. It's essential for building and repairing tissues, making enzymes and hormones, and supporting a healthy immune system by creating antibodies that help fight infections. Unlike carbohydrates and fats, which are primarily a fuel source, protein is structurally essential for building and repairing muscle. For active vegans, protein is therefore crucial for ensuring you stay strong and energized.

Protein also has a significant impact on satiety, which is the feeling of fullness after eating. High-protein foods can help reduce hunger and increase feelings of fullness, making it easier to manage your weight. By keeping you fuller for longer, protein helps prevent overeating and reduces the likelihood of reaching for unhealthy snacks between meals.

Protein is made up of smaller units called amino acids, which are the building blocks of life. There are 20 different amino acids, nine of which are essential because our bodies can't produce them on their own. This means we need to get them from our diet.

When we consume protein, our bodies break it down into these amino acids, which are then used for the jobs mentioned above. The amino acids also play a critical role in producing enzymes that speed up chemical reactions in the body, aiding in digestion, energy production and muscle contractions. The hormones they help to produce, such as insulin and glucagon, help regulate metabolism, blood sugar levels and other critical processes.

For active individuals, getting enough protein is especially important. It helps with muscle recovery and growth after workouts, keeps energy levels steady and supports overall health and performance. Building and maintaining muscle is essential not just for performance but also for health and longevity. Having more muscle mass is linked to a lower risk of developing metabolic syndrome and cardiovascular diseases. In fact, studies show that higher muscle mass is associated with a decreased risk of death from any cause, meaning that muscle plays a significant role in leading a longer, healthier life. A recent study has also shown how plant protein had the most significant positive association with healthy ageing. Each 3 per cent energy increment from plant protein was associated with a 38 per cent higher likelihood of healthy ageing (vs 14 per cent higher odds for dairy protein and 7 per cent higher odds for animal protein). So, understanding the role of protein and making sure you get enough of it is key to thriving on a vegan diet.

It is true that things like chicken, fish and eggs are classic high-protein foods that non-vegans will point to when they say a vegan diet cannot be high in protein. But there are a bunch of high-protein vegan ingredients that can match animal-based protein sources when it comes to protein content (see pages 21–29 for more on this).

A QUICK NOTE ON MICRONUTRIENTS

For active individuals on a plant-based diet, ensuring adequate intake of essential micronutrients like vitamin B12, iron, calcium, iodine and vitamin D is crucial for optimal performance. Including these micronutrients in your diet is necessary to avoid energy pitfalls. There are common misconceptions that vegans do not get enough of these micronutrients due to the nature of their diet. However, with a little planning, it's entirely possible to meet your nutritional needs and keep your performance and energy levels top-notch.

- **Vitamin B12:** Vitamin B12 is essential for red blood cell production and energy metabolism. Since it's primarily found in animal products, vegans need to look for fortified foods like plant-based milks and cereals or take a B12 supplement. Without enough B12, you might feel sluggish and see a dip in your endurance, making it harder to power through workouts.

- **Iron:** Iron is crucial for transporting oxygen in the blood and supporting energy production. While plant-based iron sources like lentils, beans and fortified cereals are plentiful sources of iron, pairing these foods with vitamin C-rich items like (bell) peppers or oranges can boost absorption. A lack of iron can lead to anaemia, leaving you feeling tired and decreasing your stamina.

- **Calcium:** Calcium is important for strong bones and proper muscle function. You can find it in leafy greens, fortified plant-based milks and tofu. Missing out on calcium can result in muscle cramps and weakness, so load up on those greens and fortified goodies to keep your muscles and bones in tip-top shape.

- **Iodine:** Iodine supports thyroid function, which regulates your metabolism and energy levels. Seaweed and iodized salt are great sources for those on a plant-based diet. Not getting enough iodine can leave you feeling fatigued, so sprinkle a little iodized salt on your meals or enjoy some seaweed snacks.

- **Vitamin D:** Vitamin D aids in calcium absorption and muscle function. While you can get some from sun exposure, fortified foods like plant-based milks and orange juice are good dietary sources. Without enough vitamin D, you might experience muscle weakness and a higher risk of injuries. Don't forget to soak up some sun and check those labels for fortified options.

By including these key micronutrients in your plant-based diet, you can avoid energy pitfalls. With a bit of careful planning and a focus on nutrient-dense foods, vegans can meet their nutritional needs and keep their bodies performing at their best.

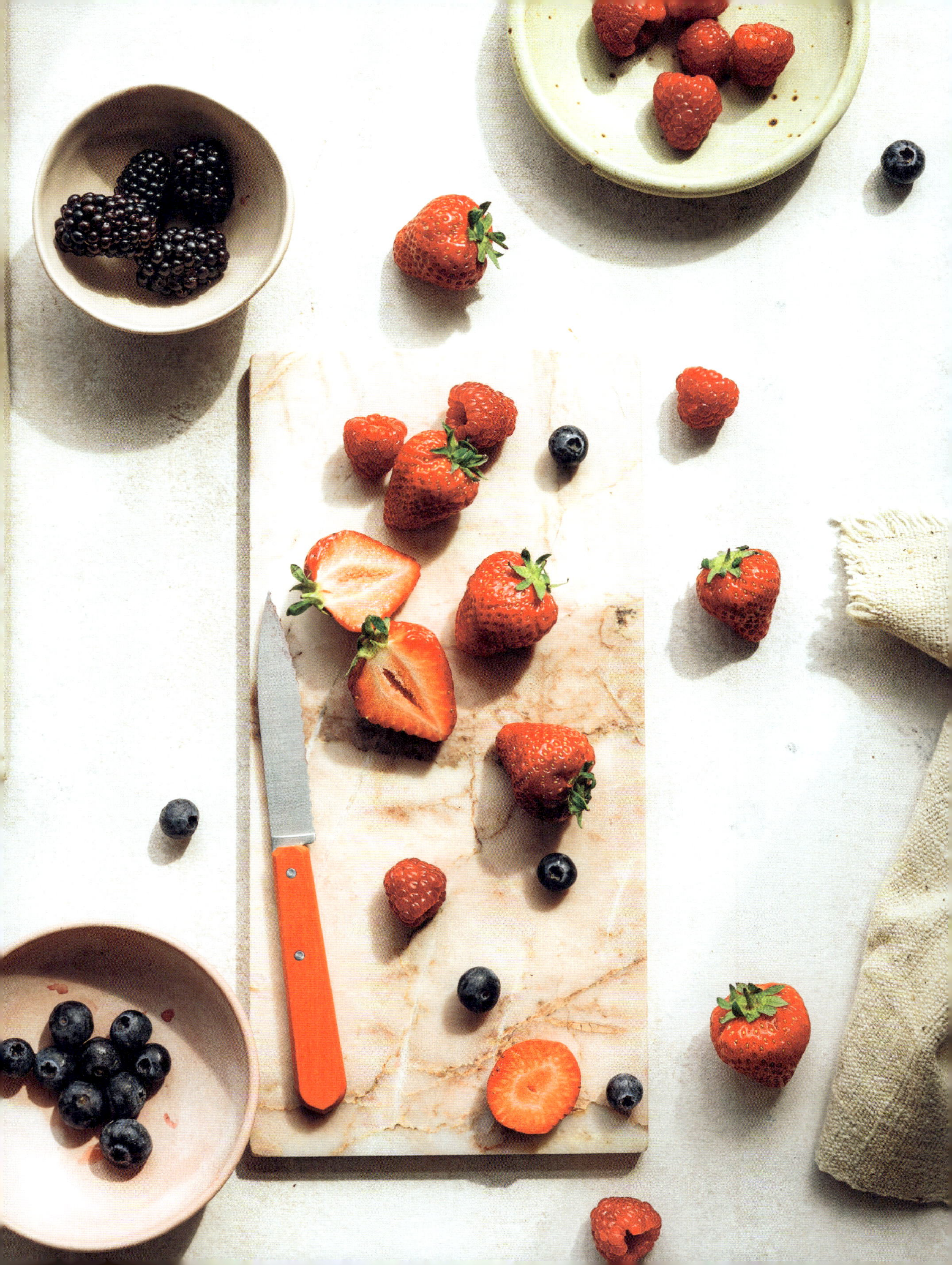

HOW MUCH PROTEIN DO I NEED?

OK, so protein is clearly super important, but how much do I need? The short answer is: it depends. Protein needs vary based on age, sex, activity level and fitness goals. While counting calories and tracking macronutrients and protein can be helpful and avoid underfuelling, it's also important to listen to your body. Focus on overall dietary patterns, such as how are you feeling, how your energy levels are, how your performance is and how your body is reacting, rather than obsessing over numbers.

The EAR (estimated average requirement) of protein for adults is 0.66g/kg of body weight, and the RDA (recommended dietary allowance) is 0.8g/kg. However, updated research shows that active adults (both women and men) who engage in regular physical exercise and aim to build lean muscle and improve strength should aim for 1.6–2.2g/kg of body weight, depending on the intensity of activity. For example, individuals engaging in endurance exercises such as running, swimming or cycling will have a protein need varying from 1.0 to 1.6g/kg/day. Strength exercises, such as weightlifting or crossfit, require 1.6 to 2.0g/kg/day. Intermittent sports like football (soccer) or hockey are in the range of 1.4 to 1.7g/kg/day. Individuals following a plant-based diet and aiming to build muscle mass should consider consuming slightly more protein (due to plant protein's slightly lower absorption rate) to ensure they meet their body's needs. Practically, it really comes down to the individual needs. Remember, these are guidelines, not hard and fast rules. The key is to ensure you're consuming a balanced diet with a variety of protein sources.

PROTEIN DENSITY CHART

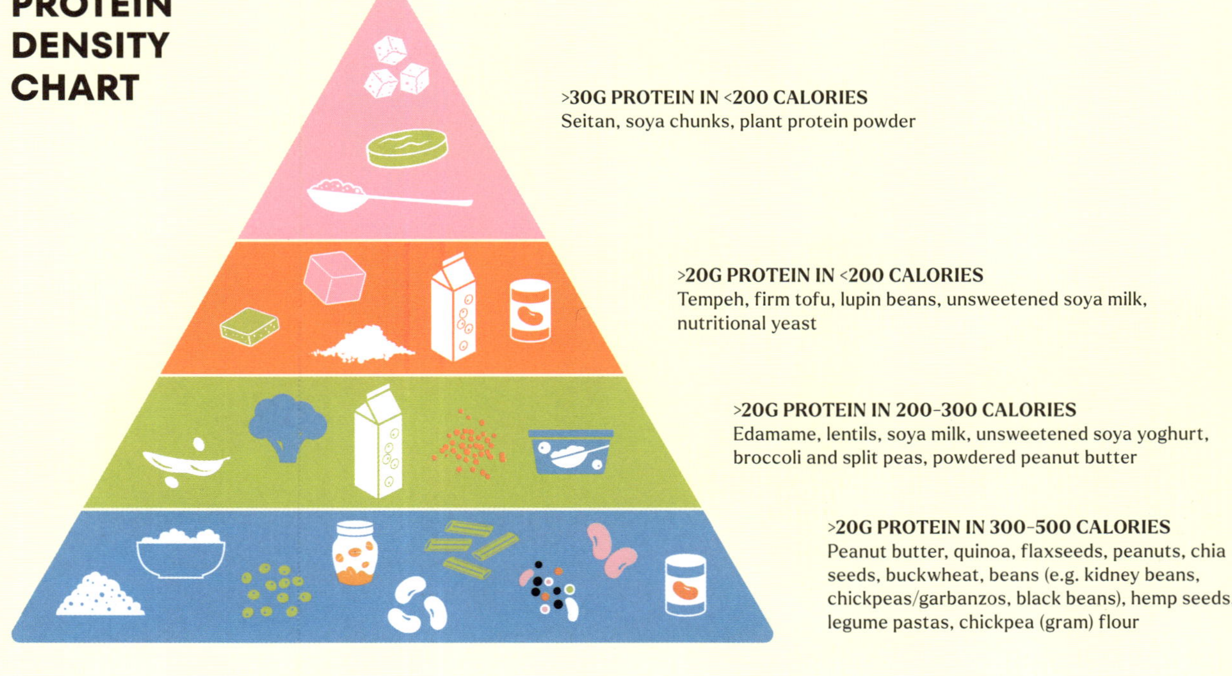

The importance of protein for women

Most of the existing information on nutrition and exercise performance is based on male needs because men have historically dominated participation in these studies. As a result, women have often received the same nutritional and exercise advice as men, despite significant physiological differences.

Recognizing the physiological sex differences is crucial when planning nutrition. Women's bodies experience unique hormonal changes that impact nutritional needs as well as exercise performance.

Menstruation is one of the main examples of this. The menstrual cycle is characterized by fluctuations in the levels of two key hormones, oestrogen and progesterone, which affect metabolism and protein breakdown in the body. For example, after ovulation and during the luteal phase (when hormone levels are high), progesterone increases and breaks down proteins, carbs and fats to support the formation of the uterine lining. During these phases, women need a bit more protein to help preserve muscle mass.

Recent studies have proven that women's daily protein intake should fall within the mid- to upper ranges of current guidelines (1.8–2.2g/kg / day). During the luteal phase, eumenorrheic (regularly menstruating) active women should consider increasing their protein intake by about 12 per cent to counteract the increased protein catabolism effects of progesterone. Peri- and post-menopausal women, regardless of sport, should aim for the upper end of the range.

Timing matters

Timing your meals to ensure an even distribution of protein throughout the day can make a significant difference in maintaining a good nitrogen balance, stimulating a correct MPS (muscular protein synthesis) and reducing muscle protein breakdown. Putting this another way: you can't eat all your protein at dinner time. By making sure you're taking in regular doses of protein throughout the day, and especially soon after exercise, you'll improve your recovery, reduce post-exercise soreness and lower your risk of injury. This approach helps in maintaining overall health and supporting an active lifestyle.

THE RULE OF THE PLATE

Beyond protein, your overall caloric intake is also important. Instead of being scared of the scale going up, you should be thinking that too little fuel will result in low energy levels and difficulty getting fitter and building muscle. Your target for daily calories will vary depending on your age, sex and level of exercise, but your caloric intake levels should also align with your goals. If you aim to pack on muscle, consume slightly more calories than your body utilizes (roughly 300–500 above your base caloric need a day). In contrast, if you are looking to lose weight or cut body fat, aim for slightly fewer calories.

Ensuring you consume enough calories throughout your day doesn't have to be complicated. One effective method for main meals is the 'rule of the plate', which provides a simple visual guideline to help you balance your meals:

- **Fill half the plate with vegetables and fruits:** These provide essential vitamins, minerals and fibre, keeping your meals nutrient-dense and filling. Aim to include at least five portions a day and always aim for variety. Remember the saying 'eat the rainbow'? Well, this is because different colours mean you'll provide your body with a wide range of vitamins, minerals and phytonutrients.

- **Fill a quarter of the plate with protein-rich foods:** For plant-based eaters, this includes foods like legumes, tofu, tempeh and seitan. Don't forget that many of these protein sources are also excellent sources of fibre, magnesium, zinc, iron and (if fortified) calcium. This ensures you're getting enough protein to support muscle maintenance and growth.

- **Fill a quarter of the plate with carbohydrates:** The remaining quarter of your plate should include whole grains or starchy vegetables like brown rice, quinoa, whole grain pasta, potatoes or sweet potatoes. These provide the energy needed to fuel your activities. If you're struggling to reach your protein goal, a good idea can be to bulk up your protein with carbs that are also rich in protein. An example could be to swap white rice for brown rice or quinoa. Don't forget variety. Try to include as many different types as possible to make sure you stock up on fibre and micronutrients like vitamins and iron.

- **Include healthy fats:** Don't forget to add a source of healthy fats, such as avocado, nuts, seeds or olive oil. Be mindful to also include sources of Omega-3 fatty acids, which are crucial for optimal cell function, hormone production and overall health and can help reduce inflammation and promote recovery after exercising.

This rule applies even in recipes where the sections of the plate doesn't quite look so obvious. When building all of my recipes – whether a pasta or a breakfast burrito – I try to use the above as a formula for balancing ingredients and quantities to ensure the right balance of macro- and micronutrients.

While 'one ring to rule them all' might be true in *The Lord of the Rings*, it doesn't apply to nutrition, especially not every day. Why? Because your days vary, with rest days, moderate exercise days and intense training days. It's essential to know how to adapt your nutrition rules to meet your needs.

The chart below is designed for light training days, which involve low-intensity activities like yoga, walking or light jogging. On these days, your need for carbohydrates is relatively low.

For days with roughly 1 hour of high-intensity exercise, such as running, swimming or cycling, you will need more carbohydrates to maintain glycogen stores and prevent performance drops due to early fatigue. On these days, divide your plate into three equal sections: one third protein, one third carbs and one-third fruits and vegetables. Don't forget to include healthy fats!

On days with more intense activity, your need for carbs is even higher. For these days, aim to fill half the plate with carbs. Divide the remaining half between protein and veggies/fruits. On these days, you may also need to get a bigger plate to ensure you are meeting your calorie needs!

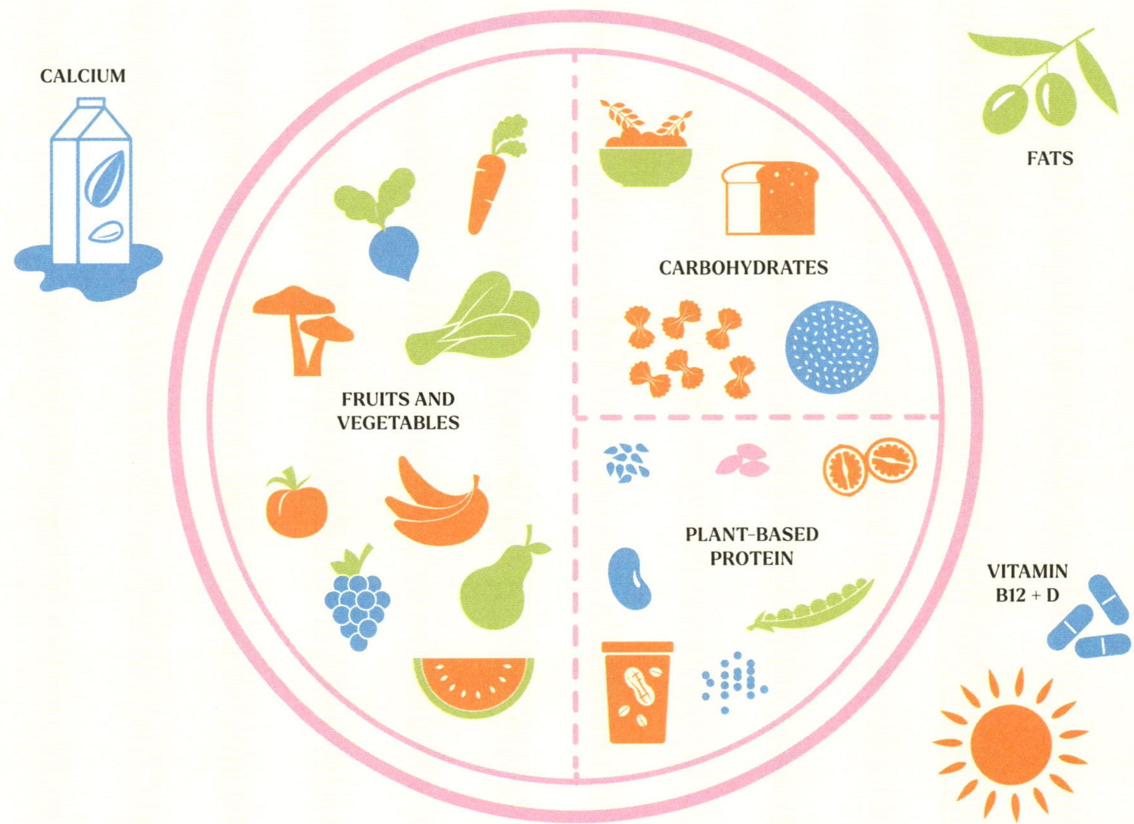

Energy availability (EA) is like the leftover pizza in your fridge – it's the energy your body has left for basic functions and health after you burn off calories during physical activity. For those who love numbers, it's roughly 45kcal/kg of fat-free mass.

If you burn too much energy exercising and not eating enough, your body won't have enough juice for things like maintaining muscle, bone health and overall wellbeing. This is called low energy availability (LEA). This happens when there's not enough energy intake to support the energy expenditure required for health, daily living and exercise. Think of your body as a smartphone. To work well, it needs a full battery (energy). LEA is like using your phone for video streaming (exercise and daily activities) without charging it enough (eating sufficient calories). Over time, the battery drains, and your phone starts lagging, losing signal and eventually shuts down. Not cool, right? On a more technical level, it means your hypothalamus – the command centre in your brain – tells your thyroid to slow down various body processes to save energy.

Several factors can lead to LEA, such as not knowing how much food you need to support your activity levels, having an extremely active job and lifestyle combined with intense training, low appetite due to certain medications or health conditions, climate, poor food timing around workouts and a high-fibre/low-calorie diet. Signs of LEA can include fatigue, poor recovery, poor sleep, digestive issues (like bloating and constipation), irritability, mood swings, training plateaus and frequent illnesses and injuries.

Some people report feeling low on energy when switching from an omnivore diet to a vegan diet. But don't blame the plants! If energy levels drop, it's likely due to a poorly planned plant-based diet that lacks adequate replacements for meat and dairy. In reality, research shows that eliminating animal products allows for a higher intake of whole foods rich in vitamins, minerals, antioxidants and phytonutrients. These nutrients enhance glycogen storage, reduce oxidative stress and inflammation, and improve blood flow, thereby strengthening your overall health.

How to avoid LEA on a plant-based diet

Plant-based diets often have more filling but lower-calorie foods, which can leave you feeling full without meeting your body's energy needs. Here are some tips to avoid LEA:

- **Plan your meals**: Make sure you're eating enough, especially on days that you will be exercising. Check out the 'rule of the plate' on pages 16–17.

- **Focus on carbs and protein**: Carbs help restore glycogen stores and protein repairs muscle tissue.

- **Stock up on snacks**: If larger portions are a challenge, keep snacks handy that include both protein and healthy fats. Try my Chewy Granola Bars (see page 179), Sweet Potato Oat Protein Bars (see page 177) or Tomato Bruschetta with Tofu Ricotta (see page 172).

Protein combining – incomplete and complete protein

The myth of protein pairing stems from the premise, popularized in the 1970s, that vegetarian and vegan diets provide insufficient content of essential amino acids, making it necessary to combine plant-based proteins to get the same 'complete' protein you'd get from an animal. Protein combining has since been discredited by the medical community, but there are still people who adhere to this practice, and even more people who still believe plant-based protein is incomplete. Starting from the premise that all plants contain all essential amino acids, there's a distinction that can be made:

- **Complete proteins:** These are proteins that contain all nine essential amino acids in the proper proportions that our bodies need. While it's true that animal products are typically complete proteins, several plant-based foods also fit the bill. Quinoa, soya and buckwheat are all examples of plant-based complete proteins.

- **Incomplete proteins:** These proteins lack one or more of the nine essential amino acids in sufficient amounts that our body needs. However, this doesn't mean they are inadequate or inferior. Historically, there was a belief that you had to combine proteins across different ingredients to reach a complete protein profile in every meal. However, this viewpoint is outdated and no longer recognized as good science. Our bodies are incredibly adept at combining amino acids from different foods consumed throughout the day to create complete proteins. It is therefore super easy to form complete proteins over the course of a day out of various ingredients which, by themselves, are incomplete protein sources. Teamwork makes the dreamwork!

For those arguing about plants having a lower availability of leucine (a key amino acid for promoting muscular protein synthesis), recent studies conducted on bodybuilders suggests that completely plant-based diets, when scaled to meet energy requirements for bodybuilders, can provide sufficient total protein and key amino acids like leucine.

The key takeaway is that you don't need to stress about consuming complete proteins in every meal. By enjoying a varied diet rich in different plant foods, your body will naturally gather all the essential amino acids it needs over the course of the day.

Is it OK to eat soya?

Soya consumption is a hotly contested topic, with conflicting information circulating about its health implications. Is soya healthy? Is it dangerous? If it's safe to eat, why do some people argue otherwise?

Soya is a versatile legume native to East Asia. It serves as a staple in many diets worldwide, especially for those following plant-based diets. Common soya products include tofu, tempeh, soya milk edamame and soya-protein isolates.

Among other nutritional benefits, soya foods are particularly valued for their high protein content, making them a nutritious ally for those following a plant-based diet and aiming to increase lean muscle mass. Soya has a high protein digestibility and contains all essential amino acids, similar to animal proteins.

The most distinctive, and debated, aspect of the soya bean is its high isoflavone content. Isoflavones are often believed to mimic the hormone oestrogen due to their similar chemical structure. However, research indicates significant differences in their action and effects. While isoflavones can bind to oestrogen receptors in the body, they do so much more weakly than oestrogen.

Concerns that soya might cause cancer, specifically breast and prostate cancer, stem from its oestrogen-like properties. However, recent studies find no negative effects but instead have demonstrated, in some instances, that isoflavones can actually provide protective effects, particularly when consumed early in life. Soya has also been linked to thyroid issues, mainly due to animal studies suggesting potential interference with thyroid function. Human studies, however, have consistently shown that soya-based foods do not adversely affect thyroid function in people with normal thyroids. Lastly, the myth of soya causing feminization in men (such as reduced testosterone levels, development of breast tissue and changes in sexual function or physical appearance) arises from isolated cases of extreme soya consumption, where individuals consumed amounts far exceeding typical dietary levels at the cost of a more balanced, nutrient-rich diet.

In summary, while soya isoflavones have sparked concerns due to their (weak) oestrogen-like effects, extensive research supports the safety and health benefits of soya-based foods. Soya can be a valuable component of a balanced diet, offering high-quality protein and potential protective effects against certain cancers without the feared adverse impacts on thyroid function or male hormone levels.

Protein powder: friend or foe?

Protein powders have a bit of a bad reputation for some people, but I don't think they should. Protein powders can be a convenient addition to your diet, especially if you're active and need an extra protein boost. Choosing a high-quality protein powder means there's no need for concern. Just be sure not to rely solely on protein powders for your entire protein intake. When used as part of a balanced diet, protein powder is perfectly safe and can be a regular part of your routine.

Look for protein powders that include a blend of different plant proteins, such as pea, soya, rice or hemp to provide a complete amino acid profile, that contain at least 20g of protein per serving, and that include at least 2g of leucine per serving.

STAPLES FOR ACTIVE VEGANS

'Oh cool, you're a vegan! But how do you get any protein?'

Have you heard that one before? I have. I think one of the main reasons that people think that veganism = all carbs and no protein is that they don't know how to properly stock their kitchen.

Whether you've been a vegan for some time or are just exploring veganism but have asked yourself the above question about protein, this book will seriously help you. I will set out the hero ingredients that will become your best friends when building protein-rich (but also super yummy) meals. By filling your cupboards, refrigerator and freezer with all the goodies in this chapter, your mid-week dinners, weekend brunches and post-workout snacks will never feel like a chore and you will have no worries meeting your protein (and other nutritional) needs!

'Oh cool, you're a vegan! Does that mean you only eat tofu?'

Here's another myth I hear all the time. Veganism doesn't mean you have to restrict your variety of foods. Instead, this lifestyle blesses you with so many options provided by Mother Nature herself. I think people just aren't aware of all the unique and wonderful ingredients and flavours that vegan cuisine has to offer. And that doesn't mean combining hard to find or unpronounceable ingredients; it actually just means stocking up on good-quality staples that can be used to create any dish under the sun.

So, instead of complaining about the lack of choices or thinking there's no protein to be found in vegan foods, keep reading for an extensive list of ingredients that you can rely on. Let's dive in!

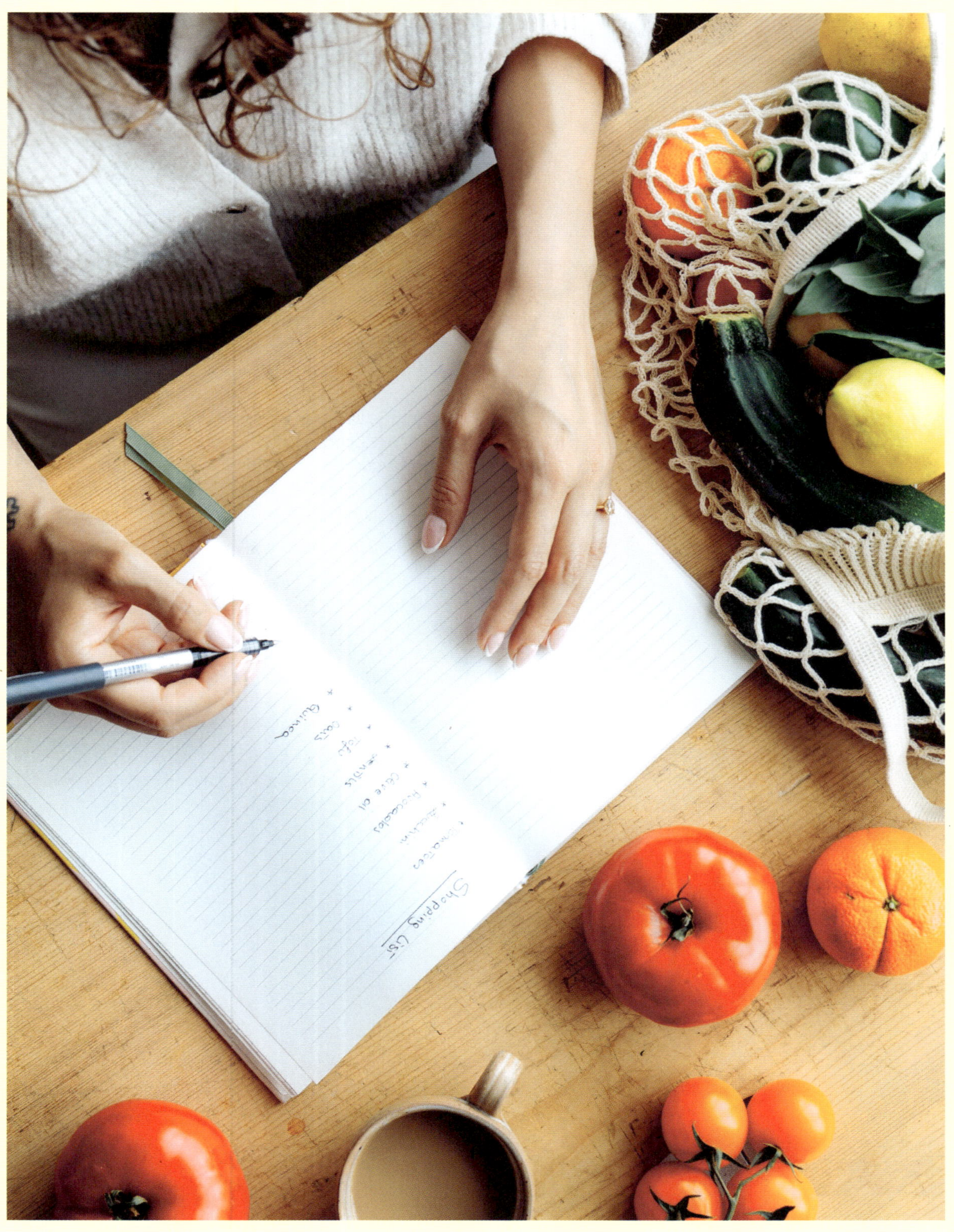

Tofu

Tofu is a blank canvas and you're the painter. From obvious uses like stir-fries or curries to forming the bases of creamy pasta sauces or even chocolate cakes and mousses (see page 188), its versatility will astonish you if you learn the tricks to get the best out of it! Among its many benefits, tofu is a vegan high-protein source that provides all essential amino acids and around 20g of protein per 100g (3½oz). Its nutrients include vitamins and minerals such as iron, calcium, manganese, vitamin A, isoflavones and flavonoids. There are a loads of different types of tofu, so the first rule is to get the right kind for the flavour and texture you need. I usually have at least four types: extra-firm, firm, smoked and silken. Just a note on silken tofu: you can buy both refrigerated silken tofu and shelf-stable silken tofu. Be sure to read the recipe to see which one you need because they can turn out differently.

Tempeh

Tempeh is a traditional Indonesian product made from fermented soya beans. It is super easy to cook and is known for its firm texture and unique nutty flavour. I often use it with stronger sauces or marinades and its texture makes it perfect to crumble over salads or to use in tacos (see pages 69 and 150).

Tempeh is a lean protein, serving approximately 21g of protein per 100g (3½oz). It also contains probiotics (especially if homemade), vitamin B6, magnesium and calcium.

Seitan

Seitan is a less well known, but no less awesome, alternative plant protein source. It is a little harder to find than tempeh or tofu but is perfect for stir-fries and has a really unique texture and flavour that I love. It's worth hunting for it and substituting it into your diet for some variety.

The other great thing about seitan is that it provides approximately 25g of protein per 100g (3½oz), making it the highest protein option for active individuals who want to follow a vegan lifestyle. It provides an array of minerals, including selenium, iron, calcium and phosphorus.

High-protein dairy alternatives

You won't find a vegan refrigerator without a plant-based milk alternative. As well as being a staple for your morning coffee, it is also a great protein booster if you know which ones to go for. Soya milk, pea milk and hemp milk in particular are real protein powerhouses, which can supercharge your smoothies and even savoury recipes. While I love the flavour, some other plant-based milks (for example, almond milk or oat milk) have pretty much no protein.

I wouldn't get far with my recipes without high-protein plant-based yoghurt. It can be made with soya, almond, cashew, coconut or oat milk and is rich in proteins, probiotics and beneficial nutrients. Soya yoghurt is the highest-protein option, providing up to 10g per serving. Greek-style plant-based yoghurt is something I use almost every day across a variety of dishes – on my granola, as a base for dips and with my curries.

Edamame

I'm addicted to edamame. When I go to Japanese restaurants, I will happily eat a bowl (or maybe even two) by myself. Without sharing (this is a no-judgement zone).

Edamame beans are young soya beans that are harvested before they are fully ripe and they are packed full of protein and nutrients. They have approximately 11g of protein per 100g (3½oz) which is great if you need to quickly pump up your macros on a particular dish. They also contain a bunch of other good stuff essential to any diet (fibre, calcium, iron, folate, magnesium, phosphorus, potassium, zinc, vitamins C and K and antioxidants – thanks for bearing with me!). Because they freeze well, you can buy in bulk, pre-cook and freeze for reuse later. High-protein, tasty and convenient – what's not to love?

Peas

Everyone has a forgotten half bag of peas at the back of the freezer. But forget soggy microwaved misery, what you don't know is that peas are actually relatively high-protein additions that can be added to a whole bunch of dishes to give them an extra pop of colour, texture and nutrients! So, fish them out from behind the ice-cube trays and let them work their magic.

Dried and tinned pulses

Pulses are un-bean-lievable when it comes to nutrition (sorry). Pulses – including pretty much any bean, lentil, chickpea (garbanzo) or other legume – are superstars due to their high protein and fibre content and they are a staple ingredient in many cuisines around the world and even throughout history. You know the saying, 'Do as the Romans do'? Well, their diet was heavy on pulses, so you can't argue with that! We all know they work well in stews, pasta sauces and curries, but you can actually use them pretty much anywhere! Have you tried baking chickpeas to make a crunchy movie-night snack? What about making blondies out of butter (lima) beans or cookies out of kidney beans (see pages 186 and 180)? Given their flexibility and nutritional value, I always have a good mix of the following in my cupboards: chickpeas, lentils (brown, green and split red lentils), yellow split peas, butter beans, broad (fava) beans, cannellini beans, kidney beans, black beans and borlotti (cranberry) beans, So go out and grab a selection – either dried or tinned – and get experimenting!

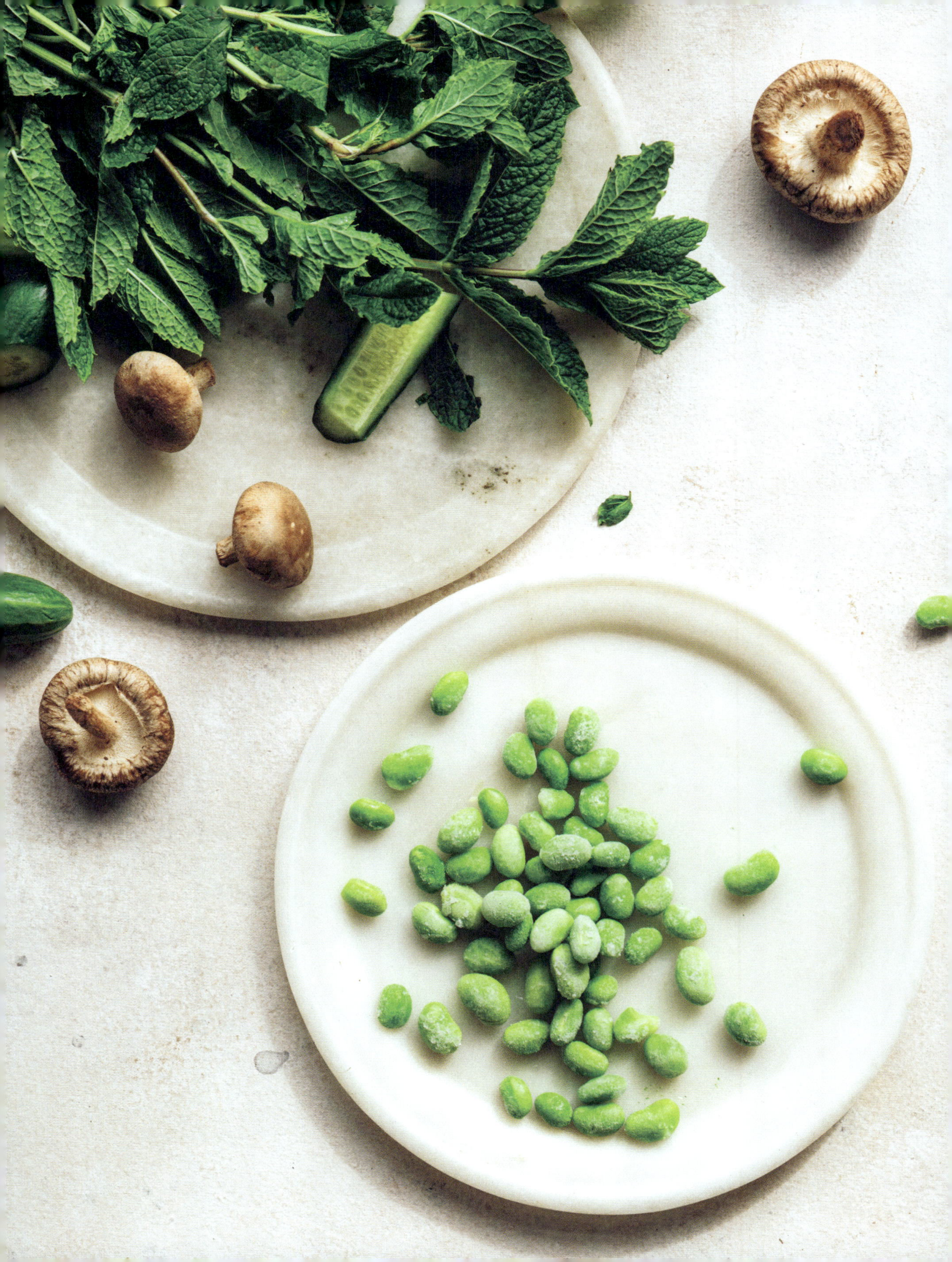

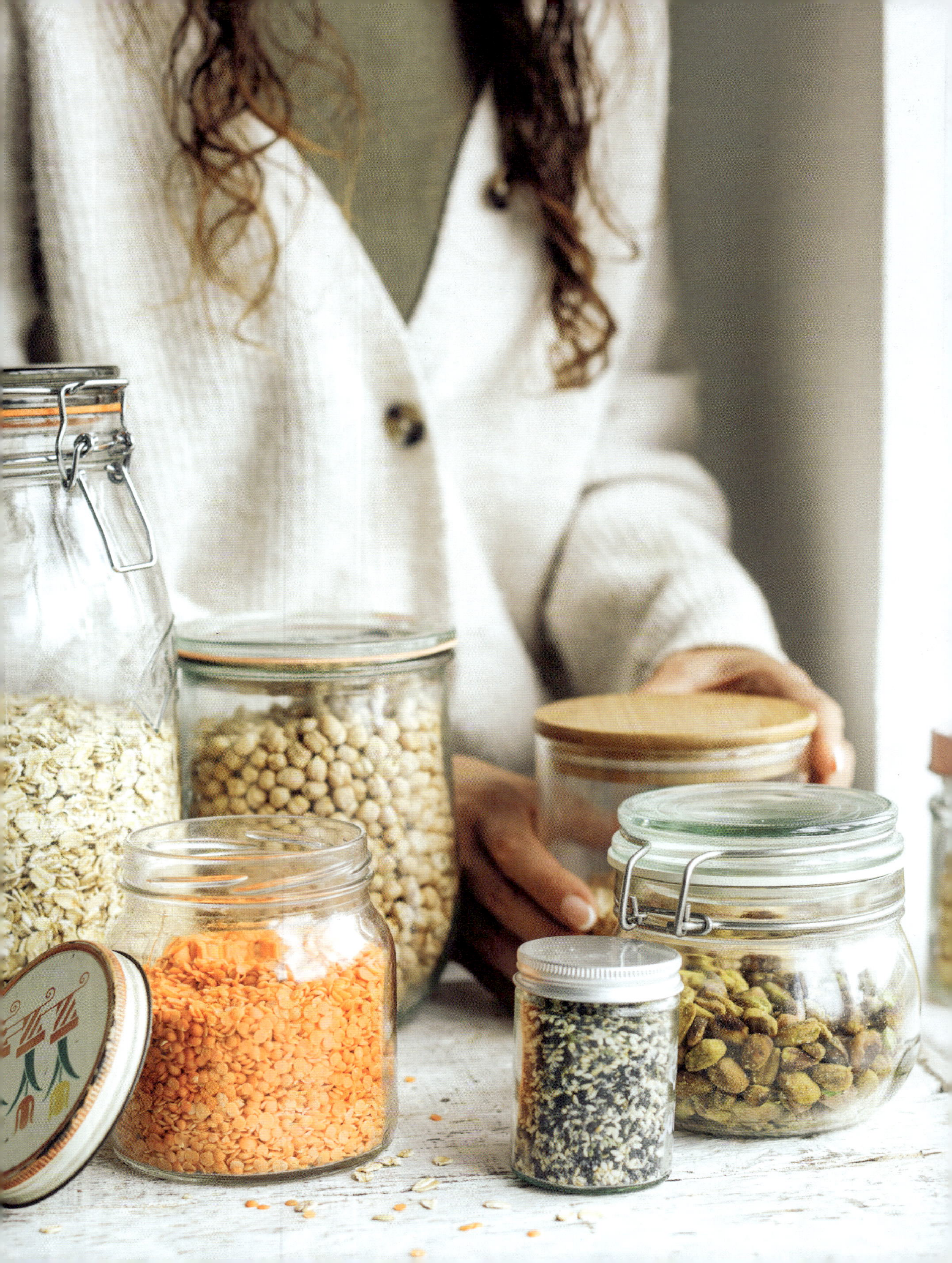

Whole grains

Who doesn't love a good life hack? You can increase a dish's protein value by simply using the right whole grain. By choosing high-protein grains like quinoa, buckwheat, kamut or millet you can get between 10–15g of protein per 100g (3½oz) serving (uncooked). Even humble oats, which you can use for quick breakfasts or in smoothies, will give you around 12g of protein per 100g (3½oz). This is one where a little bit of thought and creativity as to what carb can accompany a meal goes a long way. Rice has its place (and I love it) but give some other grains a chance too – you won't regret it and neither will your body!

Seeds

Seeds like chia, flax, hemp, sesame, sunflower and pumpkin are not just tasty additions to your diet, they're also packed with health benefits. Seeds contain high amounts of unsaturated fatty acids, also known as 'good fats', which keep your cholesterol levels low and your heart healthy. They're also a surprising source of protein. For example, hemp seeds contain about 25g of protein per 100g (3½oz). You heard that right – 25 per cent protein content! Other seeds, like pumpkin seeds, chia seeds and flaxseeds, also pack in a respectable 22–30g of protein per 100g (3½oz)! But how can you incorporate them into your diet? Well, some of them are a great snack by themselves, but I also use them as a base for many of my snack recipes (e.g. homemade granola bars, see page 179). They're also a good finishing touch to salads and curries to add extra flavour, texture and nutrients.

Nuts and nut butters

Nuts (like seeds) are a great source of protein and healthy fats but are also high in vitamin E and B6 and contain loads of micronutrients like calcium, copper, zinc, potassium, iron and folate. Just like seeds, they can be used in a variety of recipes to add flavour, crunch and texture and elevate any meal. I usually have a good mix of nuts to hand, including peanuts, almonds, walnuts, pistachios, cashews and hazelnuts. You'd be surprised at the benefits of including nuts – even where you wouldn't expect them. For example, walnuts in a ragù sauce – absolutely delicious!

Don't forget about nut butters. I mean, come on – who doesn't LOVE peanut butter? My dog certainly does! Nut butters are essential for many sweet recipes and smoothies and carry all the same nutritional benefits as nuts. So load up on peanut butter, but also keep an eye out for other kinds, too – I personally love almond butter and pistachio cream (if you can find a vegan one!).

Nutritional yeast

Nutritional yeast, also known as 'nooch', is a vegan must-have, cherished for its cheesy, umami flavour. It may look like fish-food, but I promise it is like gold dust! Packed with nutrients, it's a powerhouse, boasting B vitamins and folate, plus a whopping 50g of protein per 100g (3½oz), making it a go-to for active vegans looking to boost their intake. I use it all the time in sauces, but also as a substitute for Parmesan on pasta dishes.

Pasta

There is an ancient saying in Italy that goes: 'Eat spaghetti to forgetti your regretti'. The idea behind this is that comfort food can provide relief and even cure a broken heart. I think this is absolutely true, but what if I also told you that with a few careful choices, your favourite pasta dishes could also be protein-rich? Instead of any old pasta, try to opt for durum wheat pasta or keep an eye out for legume pasta like lentil or pea pasta. Being a little bit conscious about this will increase the protein content of your pasta dishes and also bring additional health benefits through increased fibre and other nutrients.

Flours

I won't say too much about flour, but it is an important part of a few recipes in this book so is worth a quick mention. Like pasta, being considerate about which flour to use can reap rewards – both in terms of texture and flavour but also nutritionally. I generally keep regular wholemeal (whole-wheat) flour in the house alongside a few others like chickpea (gram) flour, quinoa flour and almond flour, which are not only high in protein but gluten-free, too. A word of warning, though – all flours do not behave the same. Please use the flour I've recommended if you don't want to end up with a disaster in the kitchen!

Soya chunks

Soya chunks (or TVP, meaning 'textured vegetable protein') are a meat substitute made from defatted soya flour. The problem with some meat replacements is that they are ultra-processed and contain loads of salt and other additives, but soya chunks don't have this problem as they are more or less additive-free! The secret to enhancing their flavour lies in soaking them in vegetable stock rather than plain water and then adding flavouring as you would to tofu or tempeh. One final tip: they act like a sponge, so be sure to squeeze out the excess moisture after soaking (but before flavouring) to let them absorb all the deliciousness from your marinade or sauce.

Protein powder

This is a book about protein, so I couldn't not include something on protein powders. Despite many beliefs, it is OK to use protein powder on a daily basis and can, in fact, be essential if you are active or trying to build lean muscle mass and therefore need an above average amount of protein. It can be overwhelming when you're confronted with the range of powders available. The key considerations for me are to look for blends that combine multiple plant protein sources for an optimal amino acid profile, that whatever I choose should have at least 20g of protein per serving and that each serving should contain at least 2g of leucine (one of the essential amino acids). If you find a powder that ticks those boxes, you'll be good to go!

FLAVOUR HEROES

I am not going to list all the spices, herbs and sauces you should keep in your pantry to make delicious vegan meals. This chapter is focused on high protein must-haves in your kitchen as an active vegan – I haven't sought to include everything you'll need to make super yummy dishes. Having said that, I thought it would be helpful to include a quick note on two of the more unusual ingredients I use that are real flavour heroes!

Kala namak (black salt)

Kala namak (black salt) is a type of rock salt that is primarily used in South Asian cuisine, particularly in India, Pakistan and Bangladesh. Despite its name, its actually pinkish/grey or purple! Its superpower is its sulfuric aroma, which may not sound great, but is vital when seeking to replicate an egg-like flavour in vegan cuisine. Be careful not to use too much, but in the right quantities this will blow your mind. It can be a little tricky to find in supermarkets, but is easily obtainable online or in Asian speciality shops.

Liquid smoke

This sauce is, believe it or not, really made by condensing smoke from burning wood chips! It sounds like magic and I can tell you it tastes like magic, too! I use it in dishes when I want to replicate a punchy BBQ-like flavour or to give depth and an interesting twist to sauces and marinades. Give it a go and experience the magic for yourself.

BATCH COOKING TIPS: GETTING ORGANIZED FOR A BUSY WEEK

Alright, let's talk about batch cooking. Being an active vegan with a jam-packed schedule can feel like you're juggling flaming tofu blocks. But with a little bit of organization and a few hours of prep, you can lay the groundwork for easy and nutritious meals all week long.

I think most people already understand the benefits of meal prep and batch cooking. It's like pairing your socks – you know that you should do it, but sometimes you just can't be bothered! Imagine saving time, reducing stress and cutting down on food waste, all while enjoying homemade, nutrient-dense dishes that keep you fuelled. Plus, you'll save money and avoid the unhealthy temptation of takeaways.

Now stop imagining, because anyone can do it. And it isn't actually that hard! The tips I have included below are just some of the discoveries I have made over the past few years that have been game-changers for me. So, let's roll up our sleeves and get started!

PREPARE YOUR BREAKFAST

Let's face it, starting your day with a nutritious breakfast is like giving your morning a high-five. But mornings are always a challenge. Whether you are rushing to get to work, scrambling to get the kids ready for school or running late to your morning gym class, it never feels like there is enough time before 10 a.m., which is why we all so often make sacrifices when it comes to breakfast, skipping it entirely or grabbing something on the go. Breakfast is the meal that should set us up for the day but is often the one that lets us down! For us active folks, prepping breakfast ahead of time is revolutionary. Here's why it's awesome:

HIGH-PROTEIN: kick off your day with a protein punch that helps your muscles repair and grow. You'll feel like a superhero before you even leave the house.

NUTRIENT-DENSE: pack your breakfast with all the vitamins and minerals you need to jump-start your day. It's like a multivitamin, but tastier.

CONVENIENT: with a refrigerator full of pre-made tasty breakfasts ready to go, you'll breeze through your mornings without the frantic cereal scramble. Prep ahead, and mornings will become your favourite time of day.

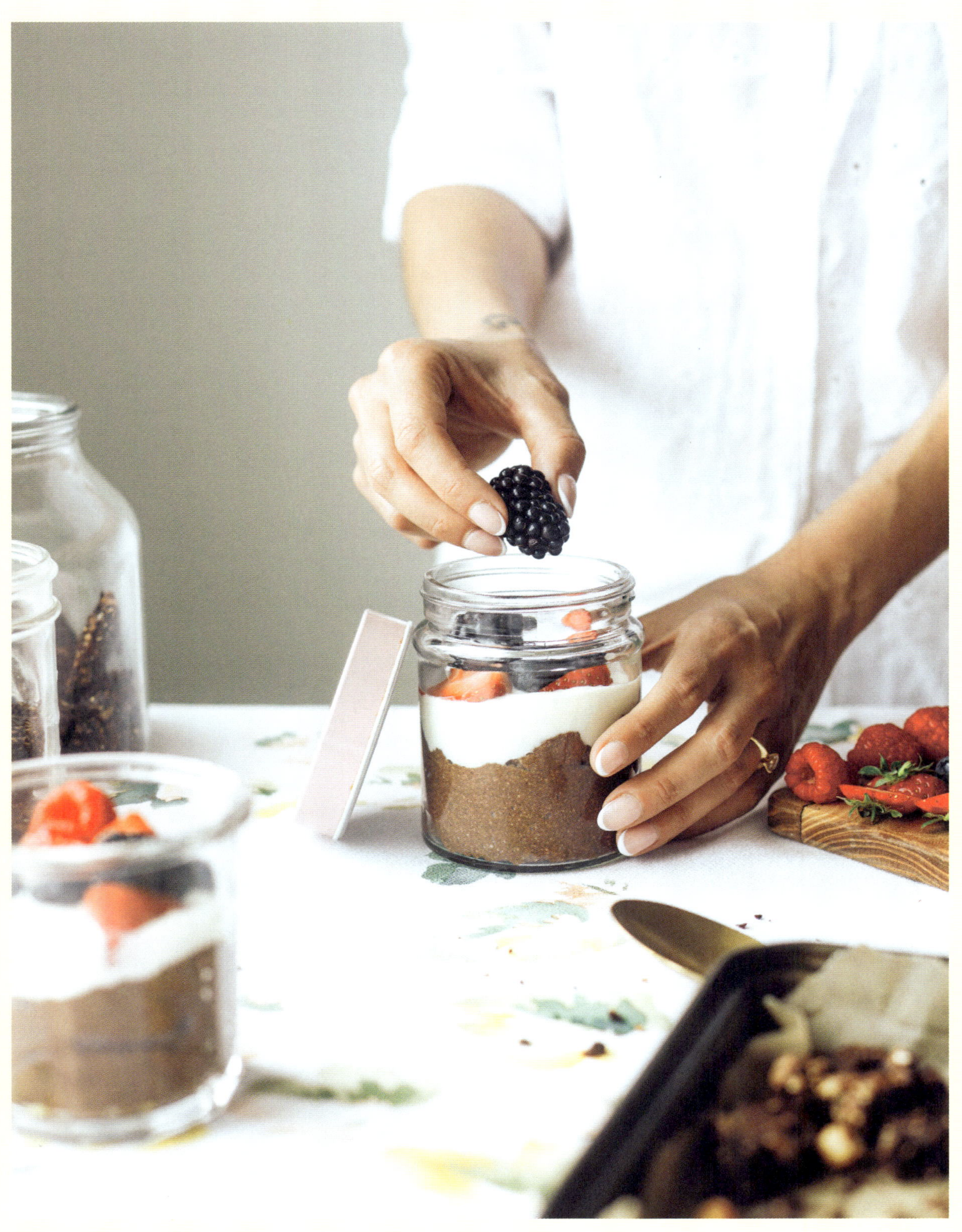

BUDGET-FRIENDLY: save money! No need for pricey café breakfasts when you've got a way better alternative already in your bag.

PORTION CONTROL: keep those calories in check with perfectly portioned breakfasts. Your future self will thank you.

OPTIMAL FUEL AFTER A WORKOUT: just crushed a morning workout? Refuel with a breakfast that gives your body exactly what it needs to recover and thrive.

In the breakfast chapter (see pages 38–59), you'll find a bunch of ideas to try, many of which are perfect for batch cooking. For a sweet start, whip up a week's worth of brownie baked oats (see page 43) or Snickers-inspired overnight oats (see page 42). Not a fan of sweets in the morning? No problem! Whip up a batch of savoury breakfast burritos (see page 56), which keep perfectly in the refrigerator or can even be frozen! Prepping these meals in advance means you'll have a nutritious, delicious start to your day, no matter how crazy your schedule gets.

PREPARE YOUR SNACKS

Let's talk about the dreaded mid-afternoon slump. You know, that time of day when your energy levels nose-dive and you start eyeing that vending machine like it's an oasis in the desert. But why does this energy dip happen in the first place? Blame it on your circadian rhythm – a natural, internal process that regulates the sleep-wake cycle and repeats roughly every 24 hours. This rhythm can cause a dip in alertness and energy in the mid-afternoon, often leading to those pesky snack cravings.

But fear not, snack-savvy vegan, you do not need to be a slave to the slump because prepping your snacks in advance is your secret weapon to powering through the afternoon with ease.

Just like with breakfast, any time you are feeling snackish can lead you down the wrong path nutritionally. So rather than hovering near the biscuit (cookie) tin or demolishing a bag of crisps (chips), why not pre-make your snacks so they are ready when hunger strikes? We all get snackish and being prepared helps you maintain steady protein intake, ensures you'll go for nutrient-dense options rather than empty calories, provides convenience and saves money.

In my snack chapter (see page 160), there are plenty of batch-cooking friendly ideas for you to try. Have a serving of chocolate crispy chickpeas (see page 176) or sweet potato and oat protein bars (see page 177). Or why not opt for some soy-free lentil tofu bites (see page 170), polenta chips (see page 174), or harissa-roasted crunchy butter (lima) beans (see page 166)?

Prep some of these snacks in advance and pop them in a container in the refrigerator or cupboard and be sure to take them to work or when you are out and about so you're not caught snackless when you need them most! Having a few nutritious and satisfying snacks around when your energy levels start to flag will ensure you are able to power through the day.

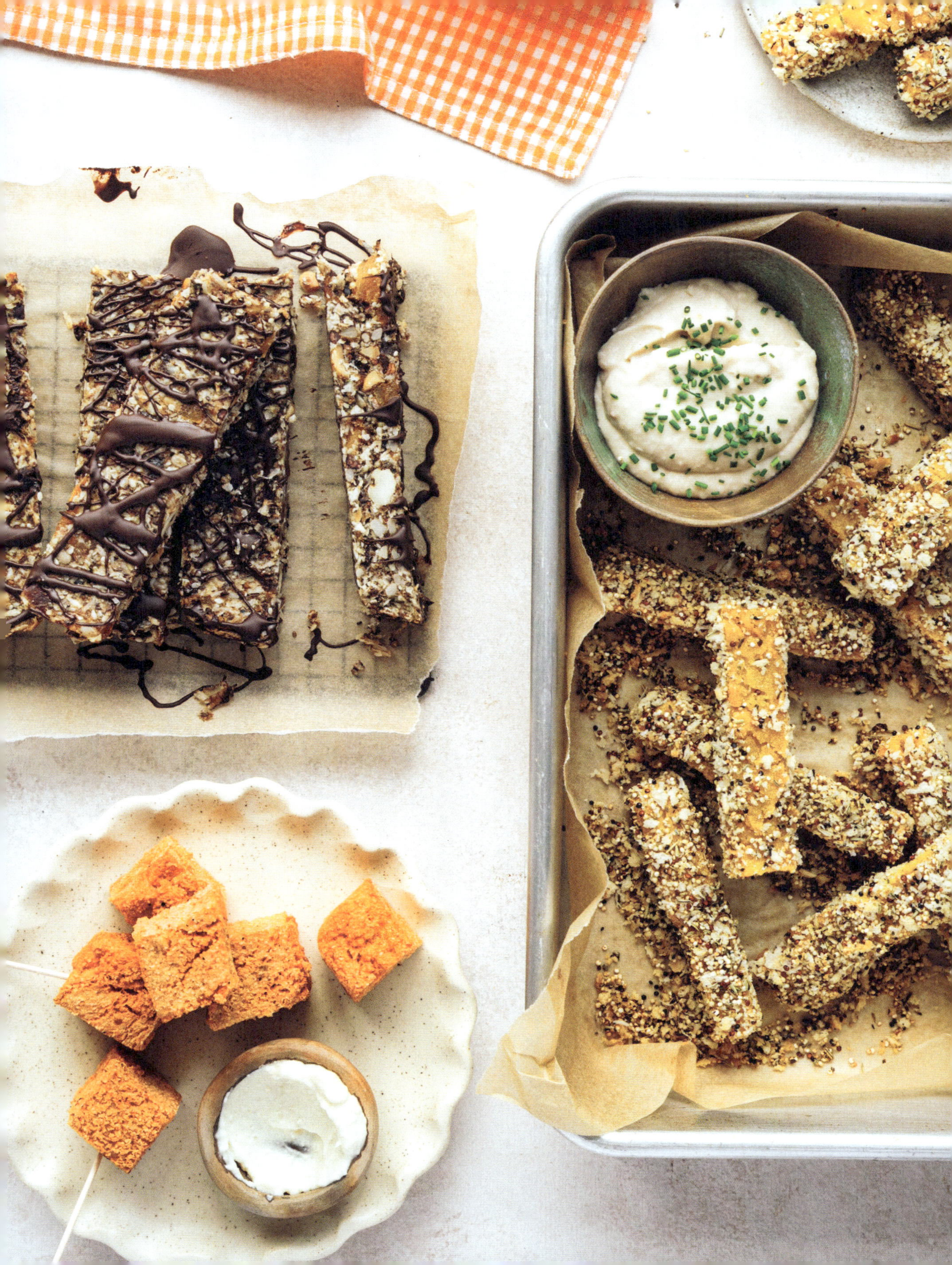

COOK SOME MORE AND FREEZE!

It may sound obvious, but cooking double and freezing half is a smart tactic to save money and ensure you have nutrient-rich lunches or dinners ready to go. Future-you will thank present-you for being so thoughtful!

So many of the recipes in this book are great to freeze and reheat the next day. So when you try one of the pasta sauces, curries or stews, why not double the portion size and freeze the extra? You'll then have a delicious, home-cooked meal at your fingertips for when you need it – whether it is on a 'can't be bothered to cook Wednesday' or for quick lunches! No more stressing about what's for dinner – just heat, eat and enjoy!

THE POWER OF PREPPING YOUR BASES

Let's get one thing straight – food prep does not mean spending an entire day cooking identical meals for the whole week like those gym bros who swear by chicken, broccoli and rice. With a few clever tricks and a bit of organization, you can make your weeknight dinners easier, more varied and way more exciting. When it comes to meal prep, the little things can make a big difference. Prepping the bases for your dishes can save you tons of time during the week, especially when there's a lot of chopping involved.

SOFFRITTO
3 portions

Let's talk about *soffritto*. A staple of Italian cooking, soffritto is a mix of finely chopped carrots, celery, onions and garlic. It's the flavourful base for many sauces, soups and stews (including many of my recipes) and gives recipes depth. But starting from scratch can feel like a nightmare – I won't lie, I have looked at a recipe requiring me to peel and chop onions and garlic and immediately given up! But what if I told you that you could make your soffritto in advance? It's super easy to do and can be frozen for later use. Prepping your soffritto will save you at least 15 minutes of chopping!

2 carrots (peeled if not organic)
2 celery sticks
1½ onions
4–5 garlic cloves
High-quality olive oil

Put the vegetables into a food processor and pulse until finely chopped.

Scrape into ice-cube trays, then pour in the oil, but don't let it overflow.

Freeze. When you need a cube, simply add it to your pan and let it melt over a low-medium heat, breaking it up with a fork.

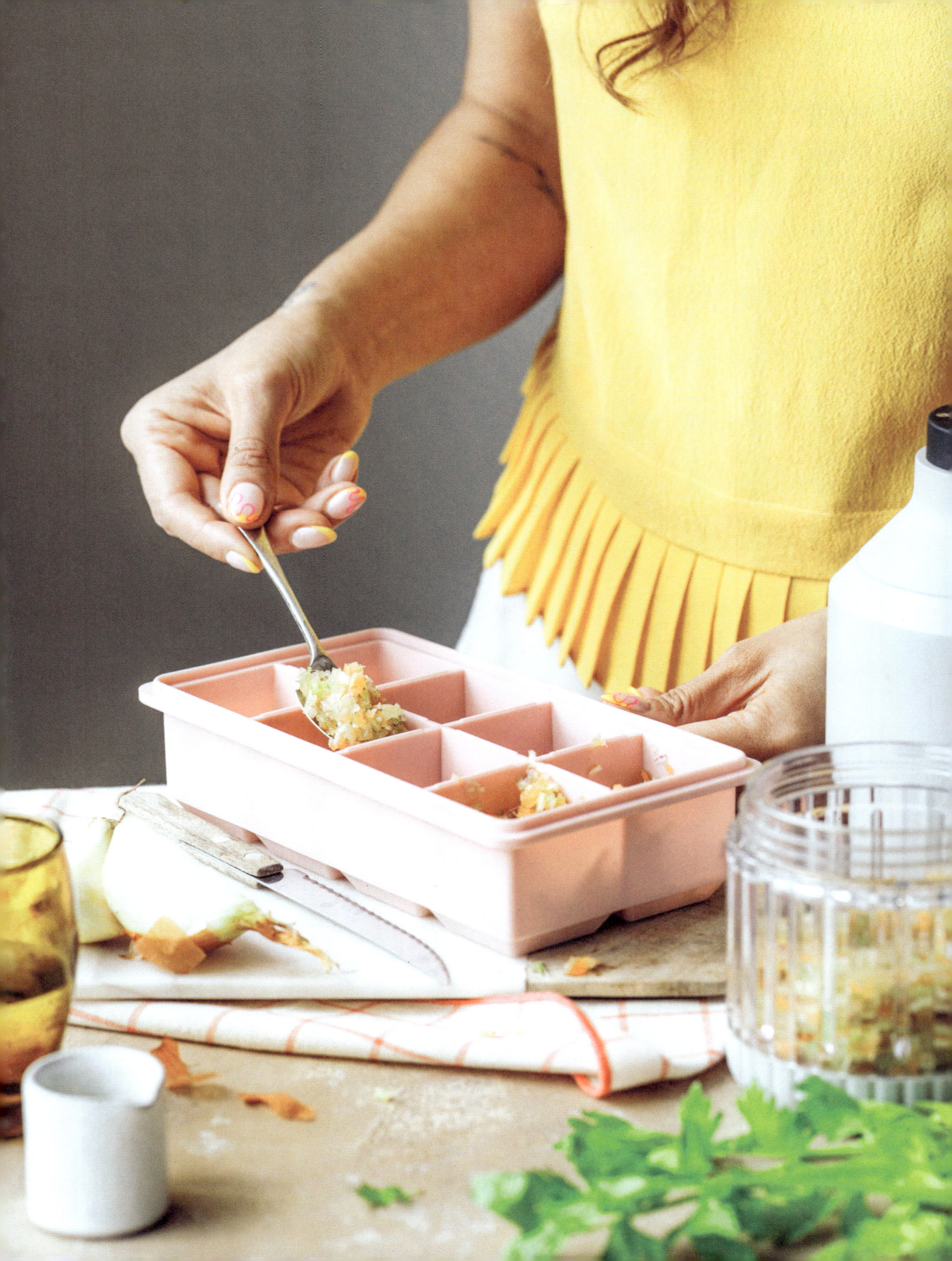

EASY PARMESAN-STYLE CHEESE

Let's face it, high-quality plant-based grated cheese can be pricey and is often a massive let down. So why not whip up your own blend at home? It's easy, economical and adds that cheesy flavour to your dishes without the dairy. And, what if I also told you that my recipe is high in protein? It's a win-win-win! Sprinkle this over pasta, salads or anything that needs a cheesy kick.

150g (5½oz/1 cup) raw cashews
5 tablespoons nutritional yeast
1 teaspoon onion granules
½ teaspoon sea salt

Combine all the ingredients in a food processor and blend until a crumbly texture is achieved. Be careful not to over-blend, or it will become a paste.

Store in an airtight container in the refrigerator for up to 2 weeks.

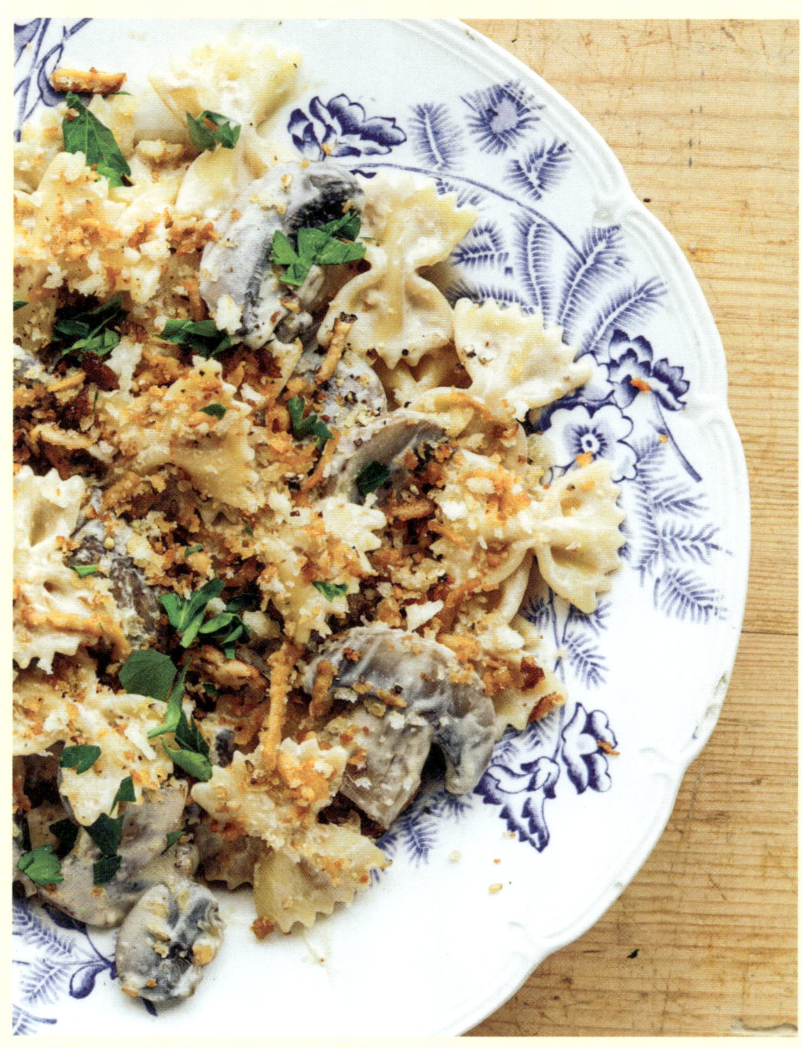

PREPARING TOFU

Tofu, our versatile vegan hero, can be a game-changer when prepared correctly. Tofu is like a sponge – the more moisture you remove, the more it will be able to soak up your marinades or sauces. Getting rid of the moisture also lets you achieve a crispy texture, which is great for stir-fries and similar recipes. Don't be scared – it's not rocket science. Here are three ways to turn your tofu from bland to grand.

PRESSING METHOD

CUT THE TOFU: slice the tofu into your desired size or shape.

WRAP IT UP: wrap the tofu pieces in a clean dish towel or paper towels.

APPLY PRESSURE: place the wrapped tofu on a flat surface (like a plate) and put a weight on top. This could be a heavy pan, tins, or any object that provides steady and even pressure.

PRESS AWAY: allow the tofu to press for at least 15–30 minutes, or longer for extra firmness. Change the towels if they become too wet during the process.

FREEZING AND THAWING METHOD

CUT THE TOFU: slice the tofu into your desired size or shape.

BAG IT: place the tofu in a sealable plastic bag and freeze it overnight.

THAW IT: thaw the tofu in the refrigerator or at room temperature.

PRESS AGAIN: when you press or squeeze the tofu after thawing, water will be released pretty much immediately, giving it a chewier texture perfect for stir-fries or grilling. Pressing after thawing is much quicker than pressing fresh tofu!

MICROWAVING METHOD

CUT THE TOFU: slice the tofu into your desired size or shape..

MICROWAVE IT: Place the tofu pieces on a microwave-safe plate and microwave on high for 2–3 minutes to evaporate some of the moisture.

PRESS AGAIN: Once microwaved, press the tofu further using the pressing method mentioned above.

Getting your tofu game on point can transform your meals, adding both texture and flavour that will turn even the hardest non-believers into tofu fans. Whether you press it, freeze it or microwave it, preparing your tofu the right way ensures it soaks up all the delicious flavours you add later.

BREAKFAST

MISO AND CHOCOLATE QUINOA POWER GRANOLA

Serves 8–10

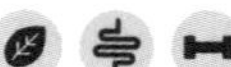

I know, mixing miso and chocolate might sound like a recipe for disaster, but bear with me on this and I promise that you won't be disappointed! The miso adds umami and depth of flavour to chocolate like nothing else. Once you try it, I guarantee you'll fall in love – and not only with the flavour, because adding quinoa to the mix packs in loads of great nutrients, too! Breakfast or snack, this granola will give you a great source of complete protein, healthy fats, fibre, vitamins and minerals.

2 tablespoons ground flaxseeds
50g (1¾oz/¼ cup) dark
    (bittersweet) chocolate chips,
    plus extra to taste
65g (2¼oz) coconut oil, melted
30g (1oz) miso paste
120g (4oz/1¼ cups) rolled oats
30g (1oz/3 tablespoons)
    tricolour quinoa
120g (4oz) unsalted mixed nuts (raw
    or toasted; I used hazelnuts,
    walnuts, pecans and cashews)
50g (1¾oz) mixed seeds (I used
    shelled hemp seeds, black
    and white sesame seeds and
    chia seeds)
20g (¾oz) raw cacao powder
100ml (3½fl oz/scant ½ cup)
    maple syrup
2 teaspoons vanilla extract
Pinch of salt

TO SERVE
Fresh seasonal fruits or berries
High-protein plant-based yoghurt

Preheat the oven to 180°C/160°C fan/350°F/Gas mark 4 and line a baking tray (pan) with baking parchment.

In a small bowl, combine the flaxseed powder with 5 tablespoons water, mix well and set aside for 10 minutes while you prepare the other ingredients. With time it will form a slurry.

Put the chocolate and 1 tablespoon of the coconut oil into a microwave-safe container and melt in the microwave on medium in 20-second intervals, stirring in between each one to prevent burning. Once the chocolate has melted, add the miso paste and stir until combined.

In a separate bowl, mix together the oats, quinoa, nuts, seeds and cacao powder.

Stir in the chocolate and miso mixture, then the flaxseed mixture, the remaining coconut oil, maple syrup, vanilla extract and salt. Mix until well combined.

Transfer the mixture to the prepared baking tray and press it down evenly across the tray. It should be a thin and even layer, no thicker than 5mm (¼ inch) otherwise it won't crisp up properly.

Bake the granola in the oven for 40 minutes, then switch the oven to fan grill (broiler) and grill for 5–8 minutes until crispy. Do not mix the granola when baking, and keep an eye on it to make sure it doesn't burn, especially towards the end of the cooking time.

Turn off the oven and let the granola cool completely, undisturbed, for at least 45 minutes.

Once completely cool, break the granola into uneven pieces with your hands, then mix in some more chocolate chips to taste and store in an airtight container.

Serve with plant-based yoghurt and fresh seasonal fruits or berries.

PROTEIN PER SERVING

10g

MAKE IT GLUTEN-FREE

Use certified gluten-free oats and miso paste.

STORAGE

Store up to 2 weeks in an airtight container and up to 3 months in the freezer.

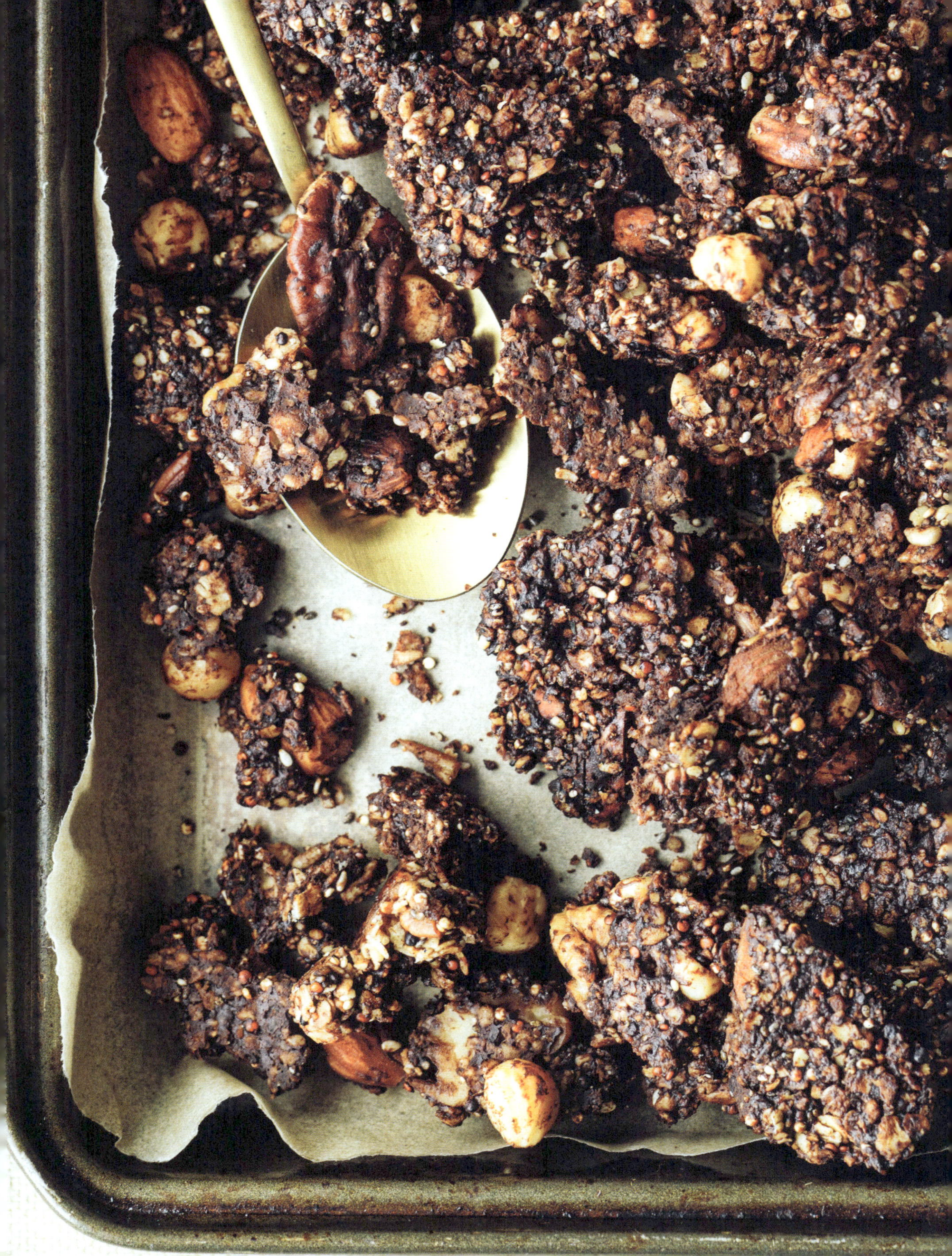

CHOCOLATE, CARAMEL AND PEANUT OVERNIGHT OATS

Serves 1

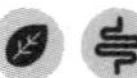 

There's nothing like waking up to find a jar of prepped Snickers-inspired overnight oats waiting in the refrigerator. They are the perfect blend of convenience and indulgence, with the irresistible flavours of the famous chocolate bar in a healthier, protein-packed form. These oats aren't just a tasty treat – they're a nutritional powerhouse, loaded with protein, healthy fats and fibre to fuel your day ahead. And the best part? They're ridiculously easy to prep – just mix, chill and enjoy the next morning.

CARAMEL LAYER

50ml (1¾fl oz/3½ tablespoons) soya milk (or any milk alternative)
2 medjool dates, pitted and finely chopped
1 tablespoon smooth peanut butter

OAT LAYER

50g (1¾oz/½ cup) quick oats
1 teaspoon chia seeds
50g (1¾oz/scant ¼ cup) high-protein plant-based yoghurt
15g (½oz) chocolate protein powder
200ml (7fl oz/scant 1 cup) soya milk (or any milk alternative)

CHOCOLATE LAYER

20g (¾oz) dark (bittersweet) chocolate
½ teaspoon coconut oil (optional, for a smoother finish)
2–3 salted peanuts, to decorate

First, make the caramel layer. Heat the soya milk in the microwave on high for 30 seconds, or in a small saucepan until steaming.

Put the dates and peanut butter into a small bowl and pour over the hot soya milk. Set aside to soak for 10–15 minutes until the dates have softened.

Meanwhile, put all the ingredients for the oat layer into a jar or bowl and mix thoroughly.

Next, make the chocolate layer. Put the chocolate and coconut oil (if using) into a microwave-safe container and melt in the microwave on medium in 20-second intervals, stirring in between each one to prevent burning.

Once the dates have softened, use a fork to mash them with the peanut butter and milk until you have a paste-like consistency.

Assemble the overnight oats by topping the oat mixture with the caramel layer, then generously drizzling the melted chocolate over the top. Garnish with the salted peanuts.

Cover and transfer to the refrigerator, then allow to sit overnight before eating.

NOTES

If you only have rolled oats, make sure to roughly blend them in a food processor first.

If you prefer to omit the protein powder, you can replace it with more oats or incorporate additional mashed banana for a fibre boost. Alternatively, add an extra tablespoon of high-protein plant-based yoghurt to focus on increasing the protein content.

PROTEIN PER SERVING	MAKE IT GLUTEN-FREE	STORAGE
31g	Use certified gluten-free oats.	Store for up to 4 days in the refrigerator. Not freezer friendly.

CHOCOLATE BROWNIE BAKED OATS

Serves 4–6

If your eyes (like mine) are shining at the idea of having dessert for breakfast, then you won't be disappointed by this brownie baked oats recipe. It has the best of both worlds – all the nice bits from brownies (rich, chocolatey and melt-in-your mouth delicious) while also being packed with nutrients to start your day off right. They're also great for meal prep – I always make a batch at the weekend so that we have breakfast ready for the week!

200g (7oz/2 cups) rolled oats
2 ripe bananas, mashed
40g (1½oz) chocolate
    protein powder
40g (1½oz) raw cacao powder
3 tablespoons maple syrup
150g (5½oz/scant ⅔ cup) high-
    protein plant-based yoghurt
400ml (14fl oz/generous 1½ cups)
    soya milk
1 teaspoon vanilla extract
1 teaspoon baking powder
Pinch of salt
Dark (bittersweet) chocolate chips,
    plus extra for sprinkling

TO SERVE

Peanut butter (crunchy or smooth)
High-protein plant-based yoghurt

Preheat the oven to 180°C/160°C fan/350°F/Gas mark 4.

Combine all the ingredients except the chocolate chips in a bowl and mix well until thoroughly combined.

Add the chocolate chips and stir through.

Pour the mixture into a 24 x 24cm (9½ x 9½ inch) baking dish, spreading it out evenly. Sprinkle more chocolate chips over the top.

Bake in the oven for about 30 minutes, or until the top is set and a skewer inserted into the centre comes out clean.

Remove from the oven and allow to cool slightly before serving.

NOTE

If you prefer to omit the protein powder, add an extra tablespoon of high-protein plant-based yoghurt, 1 additional tablespoon of maple syrup and 20g (¾oz) ground almonds (almond meal) to keep the protein quantity high.

PROTEIN PER SERVING	MAKE IT GLUTEN-FREE	STORAGE
25g	Use certified gluten-free oats.	Store for up to 4 days in the refrigerator and up to 3 months in the freezer.

BLENDED CHIA PUDDING

Serves 1–2

  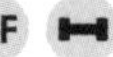

30g (1oz) chia seeds
2 tablespoons raw cacao powder
3 tablespoons maple syrup, plus
extra for drizzling
160ml (5½fl oz/⅔ cups) soya milk
200g (7oz/generous ¾ cup) high-
protein plant-based yoghurt
Fresh berries, to serve

Regular chia pudding is good, but have you tried blended chia pudding? You won't even have to wait for the chia seeds to set with this twist on the classic recipe. By blending chia seeds with plant-based milk, rich cacao powder and sweet maple syrup, you create a smooth and indulgent base that's high in fibre and bursting with flavour. Layered with high-protein plant-based yoghurt and topped with fresh berries, this blended chia pudding is not only delicious but also incredibly satisfying.

Put the chia seeds, cacao powder, maple syrup and soya milk into a food processor and blend until creamy. Allow to thicken for 5 minutes.

Serve by layering the yoghurt and fresh berries on top of your chia pudding base and finish with a drizzle of maple syrup.

PROTEIN PER SERVING	STORAGE
14g	Store for up to 3 days in the refrigerator. Not freezer friendly.

BREAKFAST

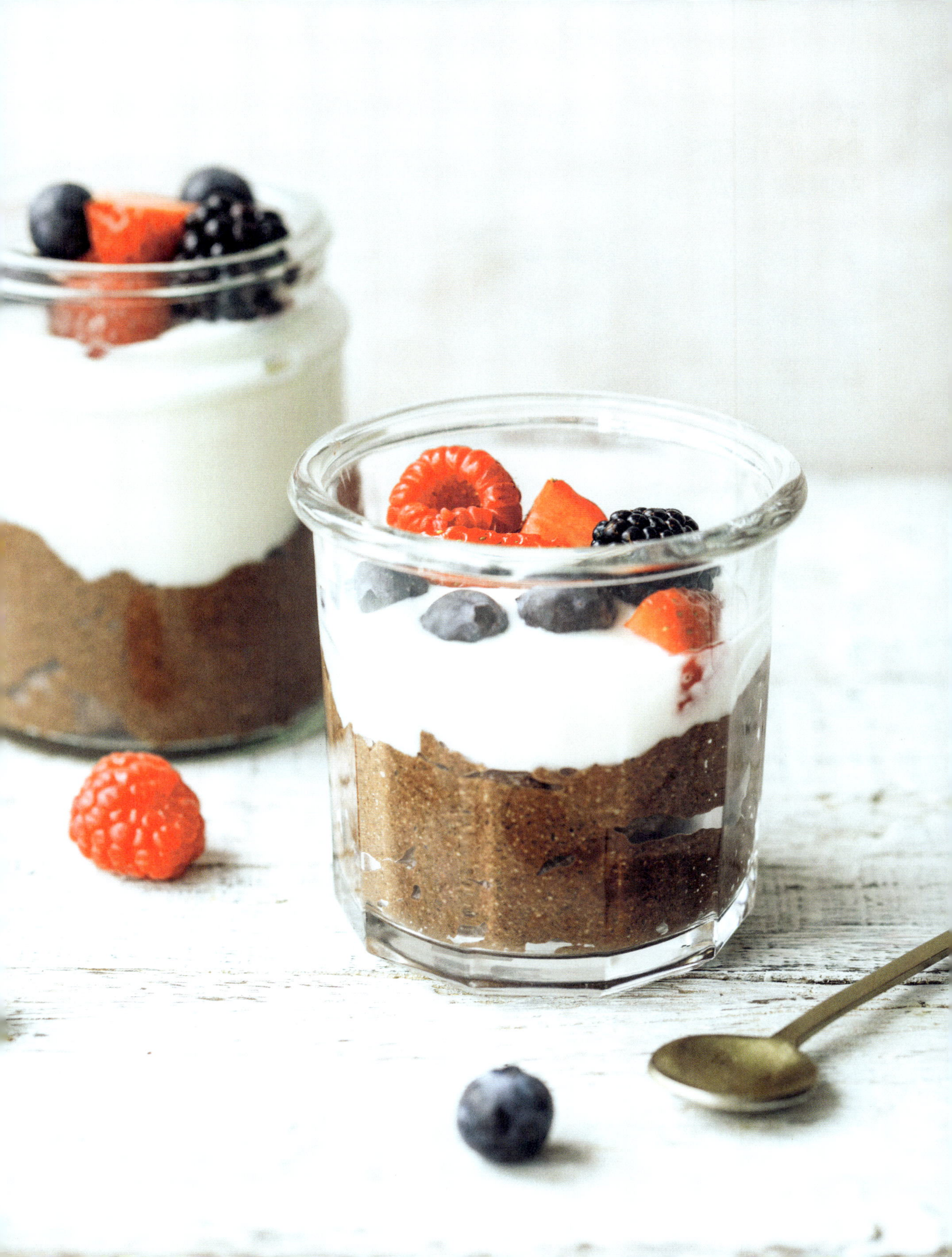

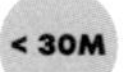

TOFU PANCAKES FOUR WAYS

Serves 1–2

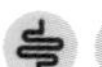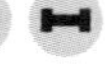

200g (7oz) silken tofu
130g (4½oz/1 cup) self-raising
    (self-rising) flour, sifted
2 tablespoons vegetable oil
130ml (4½fl oz/generous ½ cup)
    soya, oat or almond milk
½ teaspoon vanilla
    extract (optional)
Pinch of salt
Plant-based butter, for
    greasing (optional)

NOTE

Depending on the consistency of the silken tofu used (I used Satono Yuki), you may need to add more milk to get the right consistency, as some silken tofu brands tend to be firmer than others.

I had no idea how many types of tofu there were out there when I started my vegan journey, but I can happily say that the most lovely and revolutionary discovery of all was silken tofu. It is such an amazing, versatile and underrated high-protein ingredient. You'll see that it's used in many of my recipes in this book, even in some ways you might not expect – like these high-protein pancakes. You'd never guess that tofu was the star of the show, but it is what makes these pancakes so delicious and also so high in protein!

Combine all the ingredients in a blender and blend until smooth and bubbly. Transfer the batter to a bowl and allow to rest for 10 minutes. This step enhances the texture and flavour of the pancakes.

Meanwhile, preheat a non-stick frying pan (skillet) over a low-medium heat. If your pan is not non-stick, grease it with plant-based butter.

Pour 4 tablespoons of the batter into the pan and cook for 2–5 minutes until bubbles form on the surface and the edges appear set, then carefully flip and cook the other side until golden brown. Repeat with the remaining batter, then serve with your favourite toppings.

VARIATIONS

Love 'em with lemon

Add 1 tablespoon poppy seeds, 1 tablespoon lemon juice and 1 tablespoon lemon zest to the batter after blending and mix thoroughly. Top the pancakes with soya yoghurt, blueberries and maple syrup.

Go bananas

Add 1 mashed banana, ½ teaspoon ground nutmeg and ½ teaspoon ground cinnamon to the batter after blending and mix thoroughly. Top the pancakes with sliced bananas and maple syrup.

Go American

Serve the pancakes with crispy plant-based bacon, a drizzle of maple syrup and plant-based butter.

Everything's better with chocolate

Add 2 tablespoons dark (bittersweet) chocolate chips to the batter after blending and mix thoroughly. Top the pancakes with plant-based yoghurt and fresh berries.

PROTEIN PER SERVING
20g

MAKE IT GLUTEN-FREE
Use gluten-free flour.

STORAGE
Store for up to 4 days in the refrigerator and up to 3 months in the freezer with baking parchment.

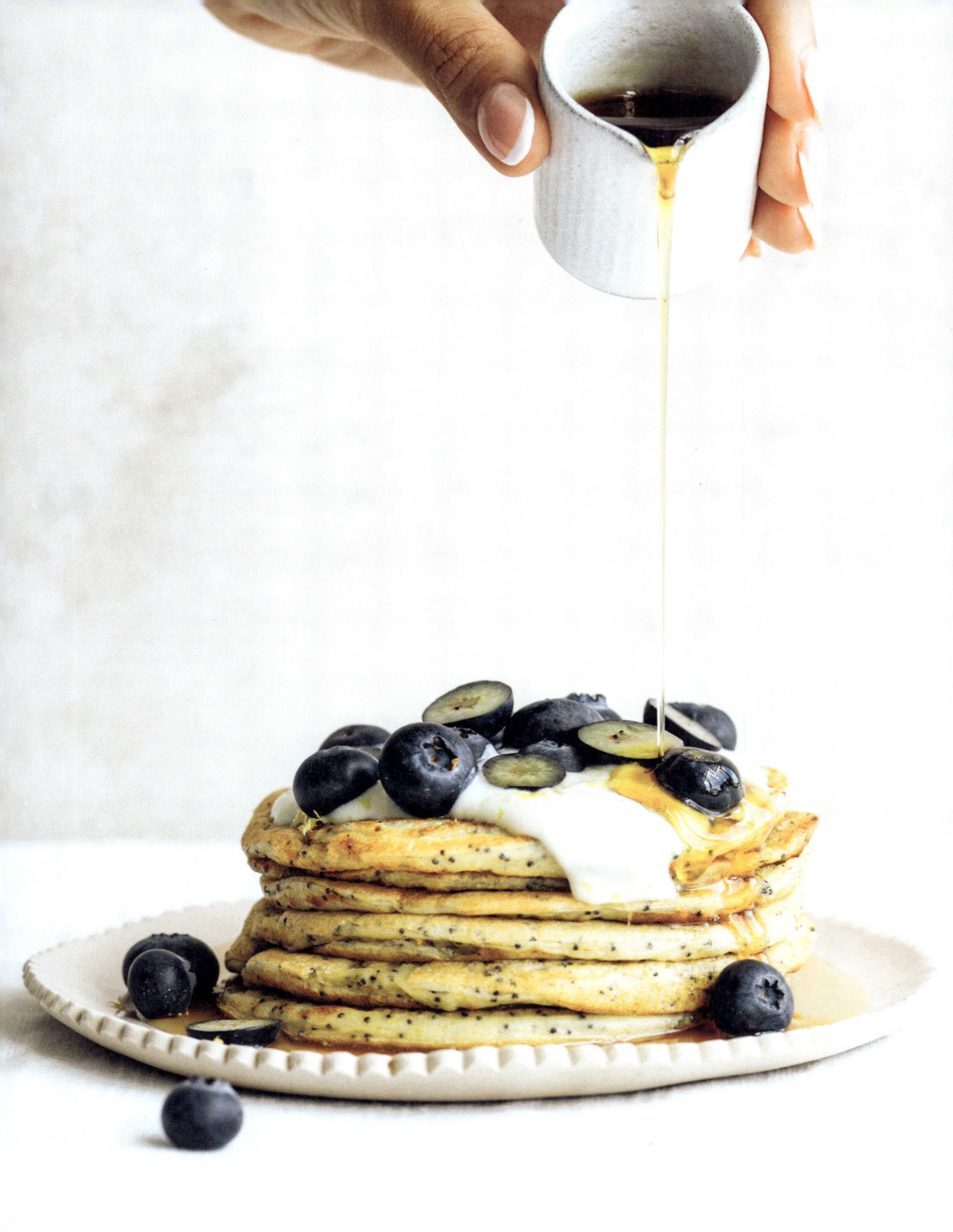

POWER SMOOTHIE FOUR WAYS

Serves 1

These smoothies are a deliciously creamy, filling and tasty way to end a workout or for breakfast on the go, especially during the warmer seasons. Depending on what my taste buds prefer that morning, I make sure I always have a source of protein paired with fresh fruit, super seeds and natural sweeteners to ensure I have enough vitamins, healthy fats and fibre to fuel my day. I've gone with four variations that should cover you whatever your mood!

NOTE

For a frothier texture, add ice cubes when blending. If you prefer to omit the protein powder, try adding the same amount of shelf-stable silken tofu, or swap for oats or nuts of your choice.

PROTEIÑACOLADA

- 100g (3½oz) frozen mango or pineapple
- 130–150ml (4½–5fl oz/generous ½–scant ⅔ cup) soya milk
- 50g (1¾oz/scant ¼ cup) high-protein plant-based yoghurt
- 20g (¾oz) vanilla protein powder
- 1 medjool date, pitted
- 1 teaspoon lemon or lime juice
- 1 tablespoon desiccated (dried shredded) coconut
- 1 teaspoon chia seeds

WHEN CASHEWS DATE VANILLA

- 1 small frozen banana
- 15g (½oz) raw cashews
- 100–130ml (3½–4½fl oz/scant ½–generous ½ cup) soya milk
- 50g (¾oz/scant ¼ cup) high-protein plant-based yoghurt
- 20g (¾oz) vanilla protein powder
- 1 medjool date, pitted
- 1 teaspoon chia seeds
- 1 teaspoon vanilla extract

GREEN GODDESS REINVENTED

- Handful of baby spinach
- 1 frozen banana or 100g (3½oz) frozen mango
- 130–150ml (4½–5fl oz/generous ½–scant ⅔ cup) soya milk
- 20g (¾oz) vanilla protein powder
- 50g (1¾oz/scant ¼ cup) high-protein plant-based yoghurt
- 1 medjool date, pitted
- 1 teaspoon spirulina powder (blue or green)
- 1 teaspoon shelled hemp seeds

NOTELLA

- 1 frozen banana
- 20g (¾oz) toasted hazelnuts
- 100–130ml (3½–4½fl oz/scant ½–generous ½ cup) soya milk
- 50g (1¾oz/scant ¼ cup) high-protein plant-based yoghurt
- 20g (¾oz) chocolate protein powder or 1 tablespoon raw cacao powder
- 20ml (1½ tablespoons) maple syrup
- 1 medjool date, pitted
- 1 tablespoon hazelnut or peanut butter (smooth or crunchy)
- 1 teaspoon chia seeds
- ½ teaspoon vanilla extract

Combine all the ingredients in a blender and blend until smooth, adjusting the quantity of soya milk to your taste.

PROTEIN PER SERVING

Proteiñacolada · 26g
When cashews date vanilla · 28g
Green goddess reinvented · 26g
Notella · 32g

STORAGE

Store for up to 2 days in the refrigerator and up to 3 months in the freezer.

CORN FRITTERS WITH SMOKY BAKED BEANS AND AVO SMASH

Serves 4

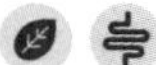

We don't do savoury breakfasts in Italy, but having now perfected this recipe I can't believe I was missing out for so long! The smoky beans combine beautifully with the sweetness of the corn fritters and a rich avocado smash to top it all off – what's not to love? It is rich in plant protein but also vitamin C, K, folate and antioxidants. Quite literally the perfect brunch recipe!

SMOKY BAKED BEANS

1 small-medium carrot, diced
½ celery stick, diced
1 small onion, diced
2–3 garlic cloves, very
    finely chopped
1 tablespoon tomato purée (paste)
½ teaspoon chilli (hot
    pepper) flakes
1 teaspoon smoked paprika
1 teaspoon ground cumin
5 sun-dried tomatoes, roughly
    chopped
1 x 400g (14oz) tin of
    chopped tomatoes
600g (1lb 5oz) drained tinned
    haricot (navy) beans
Small handful of flat-leaf
    parsley, chopped
Olive oil, for cooking
Salt and freshly ground
    black pepper

Preheat the oven to 220°C/200°C fan/425°F/Gas mark 7 and line a large baking tray (pan) with baking parchment.

To make the beans, heat a drizzle of olive oil in a saucepan and add the carrot, celery, onion and garlic. Cook for 5–8 minutes until soft, then add the tomato purée, chilli flakes, paprika, cumin and sun-dried tomatoes. Stir and allow the flavours to infuse for a minute, then add the tinned tomatoes and beans. Simmer for 10 minutes, or until the sauce has thickened to your liking. If it's too dry, add a splash of water. Season with salt and pepper, then stir in the chopped parsley and set aside.

RECIPE CONTINUES →

CORN FRITTERS

200g (7oz/1 cup) tinned or
    defrosted frozen sweetcorn
8 spring onions (scallions),
    chopped (green part included)
8 tablespoons chickpea
    (gram) flour
2 tablespoons ground flaxseed
2 teaspoons smoked paprika
2 teaspoons garlic granules
Handful of chopped
    coriander (cilantro)
Juice of 1 lemon
2 tablespoons olive oil

AVO SMASH

2 ripe avocados, peeled and
    stoned
1 tablespoon olive oil
1 teaspoon chilli (hot pepper) flakes
Juice of 1½ limes
5–6 sun-dried tomatoes,
    roughly chopped

Meanwhile, prepare the corn fritters. Put three quarters of the sweetcorn, the spring onions, chickpea flour, ground flaxseed, paprika, garlic, coriander, lemon juice, olive oil and a pinch of salt and pepper into a food processor and blend until a chunky mixture forms. Once the mixture has come together, mix through the remaining sweetcorn.

Scoop tablespoons of the batter onto the prepared baking tray, shaping them to form fritters. Bake the fritters in the oven for 15 minutes, then turn on the grill (broiler) and grill for 10 minutes to crisp up the fritters. Alternatively, if you have an air fryer, you can air-fry the fritters at 200°C (400°F) for 15 minutes.

Finally, make the avo smash by combining the avocado, oil, chilli and a pinch of salt and pepper in a bowl and mashing together with a fork. Squeeze over the lime juice and stir through the chopped sun-dried tomatoes.

To serve, divide the baked beans between plates, then top with the fritters and avocado.

NOTE
The soffritto base for the beans can be batch-cooked and used for many different recipes in this book. See page 34 for my pantry staple recipe.

PROTEIN PER SERVE

25g

STORAGE

Store for up to 3 days in the refrigerator. Freeze the fritters and baked beans separately for up to 3 months.

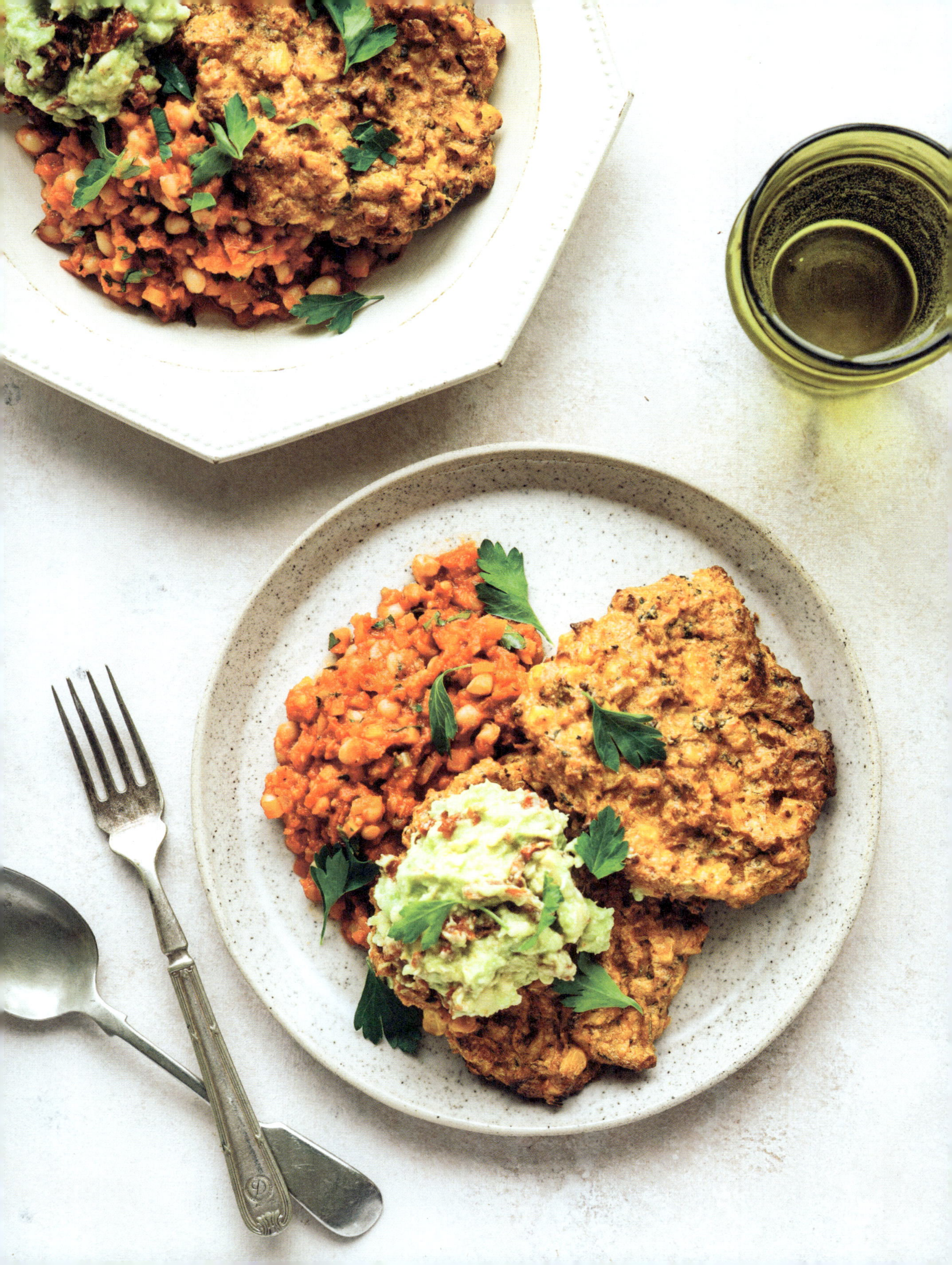

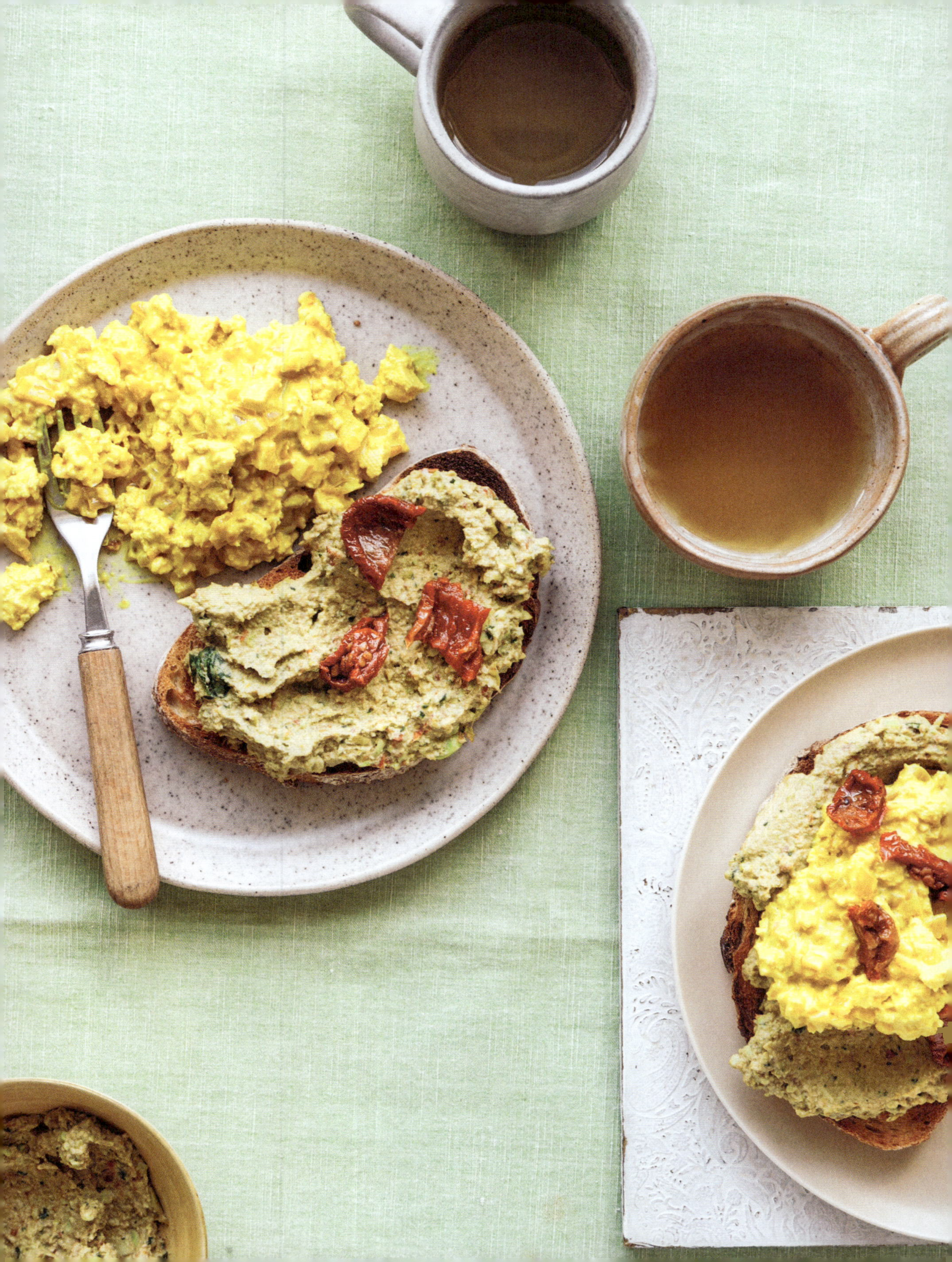

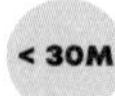

ENERGIZING EDAMAME TOAST WITH TOFU SCRAMBLE

Serves 2–3

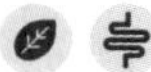

This is the perfect post-workout breakfast or brunch for the weekend. With creamy smashed edamame bursting with flavour from basil and sun-dried tomatoes, savoury scrambled tofu and crispy sourdough toast, it's a wholesome and satisfying meal that's sure to keep you energized throughout the morning. Try to make sure you use the kala namak (black salt), as this is what gives the tofu it's egg-like taste.

SMASHED EDAMAME

150g (5½oz/2½ cups) cooked edamame beans (defrosted if frozen)
75g (2½oz/generous ¼ cup) high-protein plant-based yoghurt
Small handful of basil, plus extra to serve
2 sun-dried tomatoes, chopped, plus extra to serve
1 garlic clove
2 tablespoons nutritional yeast
Juice of ½ lemon, plus 1 teaspoon zest
1 tablespoon olive oil
Salt and freshly ground black pepper

TOFU SCRAMBLE

100g (3½oz) silken tofu
4 tablespoons soya milk
1 teaspoon cornflour (cornstarch)
2 tablespoons nutritional yeast
1 tablespoon plant-based butter
1 small onion, finely chopped
½ teaspoon ground turmeric
100g (3½oz) firm smoked tofu, drained and pressed (see page 37), then roughly crumbled
½ teaspoon kala namak (black salt)

TOAST

2–3 slices of sourdough bread
Plant-based butter, for spreading

First, make the smashed edamame. Combine all the ingredients in a food processor and roughly blend until creamy but still with some visible chunks of edamame and tomato. Taste and check the seasoning, then transfer to a bowl and set aside.

Next, make the tofu scramble. In the clean bowl of the food processor, combine the silken tofu, soya milk, cornflour and nutritional yeast and blend until smooth, scraping down the sides as necessary. It should be liquid – it will thicken when it cooks.

Heat the plant-based butter in a frying pan (skillet) over a medium heat and fry the onion with the turmeric for 5 minutes until golden and soft. Add the crumbled firm tofu and stir gently to combine without breaking up the chunks.

Next, add the silken tofu mixture and black salt and season with regular salt and pepper to taste. Mix gently and warm through for an additional minute.

Toast the bread to golden perfection and generously spread each slice with plant-based butter, then spoon a generous portion of the creamy smashed edamame onto each slice and top with the tofu scramble. Finish with a few extra basil leaves or sun-dried tomatoes if desired.

PROTEIN PER SERVING	**MAKE IT GLUTEN-FREE**	**STORAGE**
39g	Use gluten-free bread.	Best eaten immediately, but the components can be stored separately in the refrigerator for up to 3 days.

TOFU OMELETTE

Serves 2

  GF

Is it possible to make an omelette without breaking eggs? Absolutely! This delicious omelette is a protein-packed breakfast made with firm tofu, nutritional yeast, balsamic mushrooms and a medley of savoury spices that's anything but bland. With its hassle-free preparation and wholesome ingredients, it's the perfect way to kickstart your day with a nutritious and satisfying meal. With the secret ingredient of kala namak (black salt), I promise you won't miss the eggs!

200g (7oz) firm tofu, drained
    and pressed (see page 37)
20g (¾oz) nutritional yeast
160ml (5½fl oz/⅔ cup) soya milk
10g (½oz) cornflour (cornstarch)
½ teaspoon kala namak (black salt)
¼ teaspoon ground black pepper
¼ teaspoon salt
½ teaspoon ground turmeric
Plant-based butter, for frying
Salad, to serve

FILLING

1 small onion, thinly sliced
150g (5½oz) chestnut (cremini) or
    oyster mushrooms, chopped
1 tablespoon balsamic vinegar
1 tomato, diced
Handful of spinach
Olive oil, for cooking
Salt and freshly ground
    black pepper

NOTES

The omelette batter can be made in advance and stored in the refrigerator for 2–3 days for a quicker breakfast!

If you use a high-quality non-stick pan, you won't need to grease it.

First, make the filling. Heat a good glug of olive oil in a frying pan (skillet) over a medium heat and fry the onion for about 5 minutes until soft and lightly browned.

Add the mushrooms, then deglaze with the balsamic vinegar. Cook for 5–8 minutes until the mushrooms are nicely browned and cooked, then add the spinach and tomato and stir for a minute until the spinach has wilted. Season with salt and pepper to taste, then set aside

To make the omelette batter, combine all the ingredients except the plant-based butter in a food processor and blend until smooth.

Lightly grease a non-stick frying pan over a medium heat, then pour in a ladle of the batter and immediately swirl the pan to coat the bottom. Alternatively, you can use the bottom of a ladle to help you spread the batter evenly on the surface.

Reduce the heat to low and cook for 5–8 minutes until the omelette starts to look brown and crispy on the bottom and the top changes from shiny to a matte finish, with lots of small holes on the surface. Add half of the filling mixture to one side of the omelette, then carefully fold the other side of the omelette over the filling using a spatula.

Transfer the omelette to a plate, then cover the plate with another plate or a lid and let the omelette steam for 5 minutes.

Repeat the process with the remaining batter, adding more butter if needed.

Serve with a side of salad.

PROTEIN PER SERVING	STORAGE
25g	Store for up to 3 days in the refrigerator. Not freezer friendly.

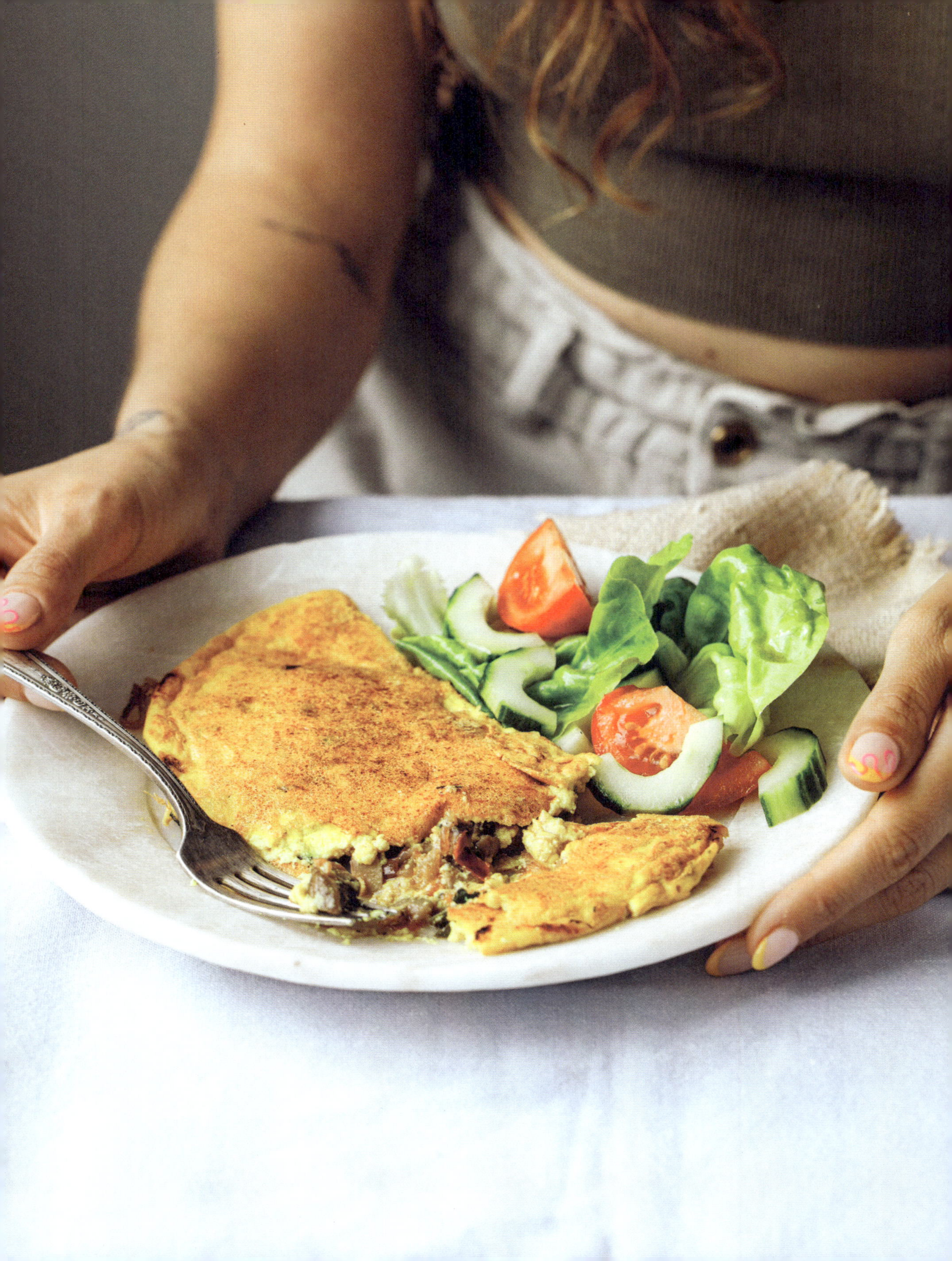

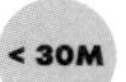

BREAKFAST BURRITO

Serves 2

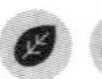 

This vegan breakfast burrito is the perfect high-protein post-workout meal, especially because it's ideal for prepping ahead. Packed with aromatic spiced scrambled tofu, creamy avocado, veggies and a touch of zesty hot sauce, this burrito is not just a meal, it's a celebration of savoury flavours and nutritious ingredients.

4 tablespoons tahini

½ teaspoon smoked paprika

½ teaspoon kala namak (black salt)

½ teaspoon ground turmeric

80ml (2¾fl oz/⅓ cup) soya milk

2 tablespoons nutritional yeast

1 heaped tablespoon plant-based butter

200g (7oz) firm smoked tofu, drained and pressed (see page 37), then crumbled into bite-sized pieces

Handful of fresh spinach

½ avocado, peeled, stoned and mashed

100g (3½oz) cherry tomatoes, halved

2 large wholemeal (whole-wheat) tortilla wraps

Juice of ½ lemon

Hot sauce (or your favourite sauce), to taste

Salt and freshly ground black pepper

Combine the tahini, paprika, kala namak, turmeric, soya milk and nutritional yeast in a bowl.

Heat the plant-based butter in a frying pan (skillet) over a medium heat, then add the tofu and cook for 8–10 minutes, or until it starts to brown. Do not over crumble the tofu because it will break down more when cooking.

Remove from the heat and pour over the tahini mixture, stirring gently until the tofu turns evenly golden. Season with salt and pepper to taste.

To assemble the burritos, divide the spinach, avocado, tofu scramble and tomatoes between the tortilla wraps. Drizzle with hot sauce and squeeze over the lemon juice. Fold in the sides and roll up, keeping the filling tucked in place. Cut in half and serve.

PROTEIN PER SERVE

28g

MAKE IT GLUTEN-FREE

Use gluten-free wraps.

STORAGE

Store for up to 3 days in the refrigerator and up to 3 months in the freezer.

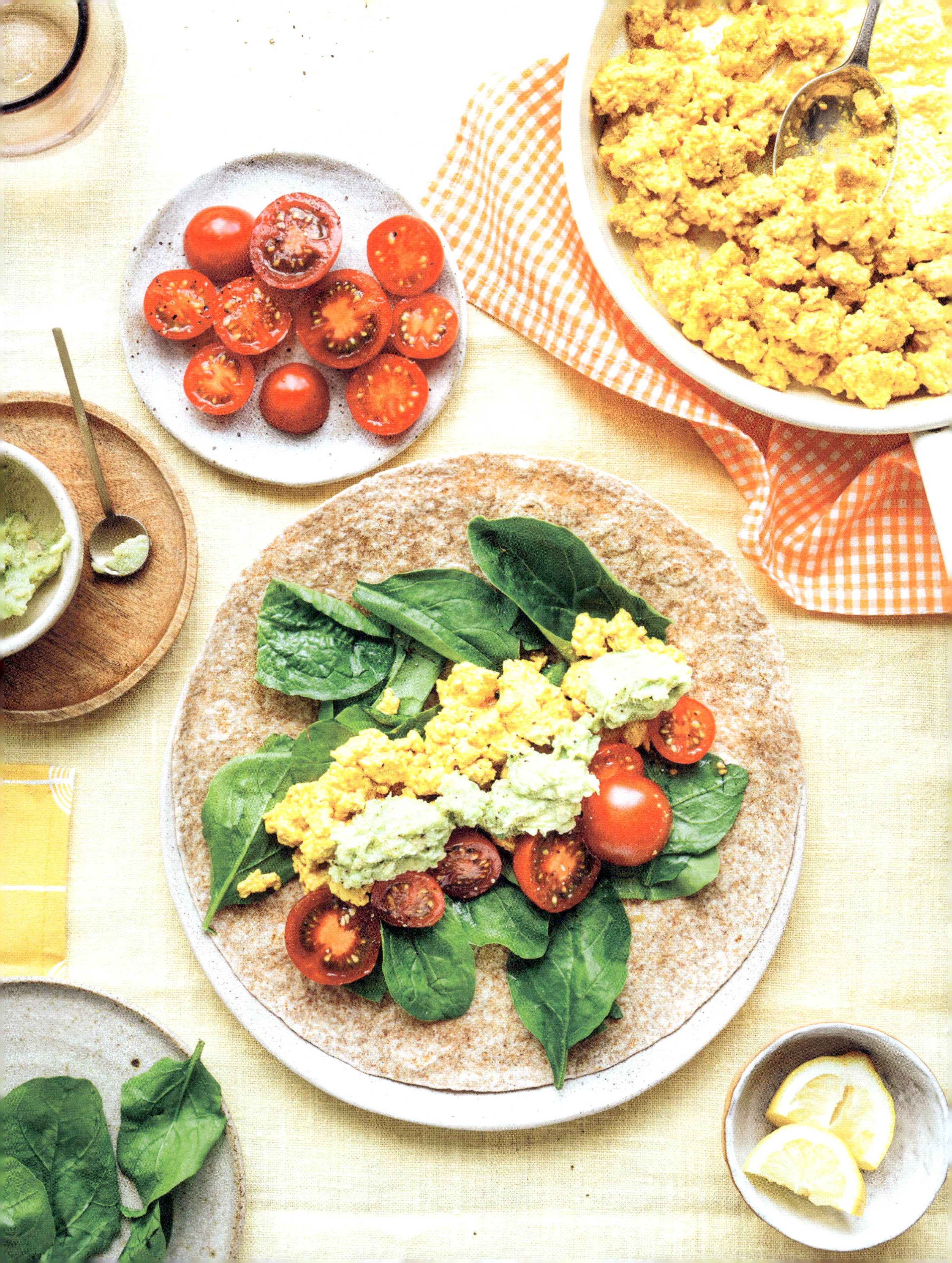

MUSHROOM, BUTTER BEAN AND CARAMELIZED ONION TOASTS

Serves 3

This loaded toast is the brunch you need to start your weekend right. Creamy butter bean purée, decadent caramelized onions and mushrooms set the perfect tone for a leisurely morning. Whether you're sharing it with loved ones or savouring it solo, this toast is sure to become a beloved weekend tradition.

CARAMELIZED ONIONS
1 red onion, thinly sliced
Pinch of salt
2 teaspoons balsamic vinegar
2 teaspoons light brown soft sugar
Olive oil, for cooking

MUSHROOMS
1 tablespoon plant-based butter
8–9 chestnut (cremini)
    mushrooms, sliced
Small handful of flat-leaf
    parsley, chopped

BUTTER BEAN PURÉE
1 x 400g (14oz) tin of butter
    (lima) beans
30ml (2 tablespoons) tahini
3 tablespoons nutritional yeast
Juice of ½ lemon
Salt and freshly ground
    black pepper

TO SERVE
3 slices of sourdough bread
1 garlic clove
Olive oil, for drizzling
Chilli (hot pepper) flakes (optional)

First, make the caramelized onions. Heat a glug of olive oil in a frying pan (skillet) over a low heat. Add the onion and salt and cook very slowly for 10 minutes, stirring occasionally to prevent the onion from burning. Once the onion is soft and lightly golden, add the balsamic vinegar and sugar. This will start the caramelization process. Cook for a further 2–3 minutes until sticky and caramelized, then set aside.

Melt the plant-based butter in a separate frying pan over a medium heat and add the mushrooms. Cook for 10–12 minutes until browned, stirring every 2 minutes to ensure the mushrooms cook evenly. Sprinkle with the parsley, season to taste, then set aside.

Meanwhile, pour the beans and half of their liquid (or a splash of water) into a food processor. Add the tahini, nutritional yeast, a pinch of salt and pepper and the lemon juice. Blend until thick and creamy. If it's too dry, add a splash of water.

Toast the bread, then rub the hot toast with the garlic on both sides. Drizzle with oil and season with a pinch of salt and pepper.

Generously spread the butter bean purée on the toast, then add the mushrooms and onions and top with chilli flakes (if using).

PROTEIN PER SERVING

22g

MAKE IT GLUTEN-FREE

Use gluten-free bread.

STORAGE

Best eaten immediately. Store ingredients separately in the refrigerator for up to 3 days.

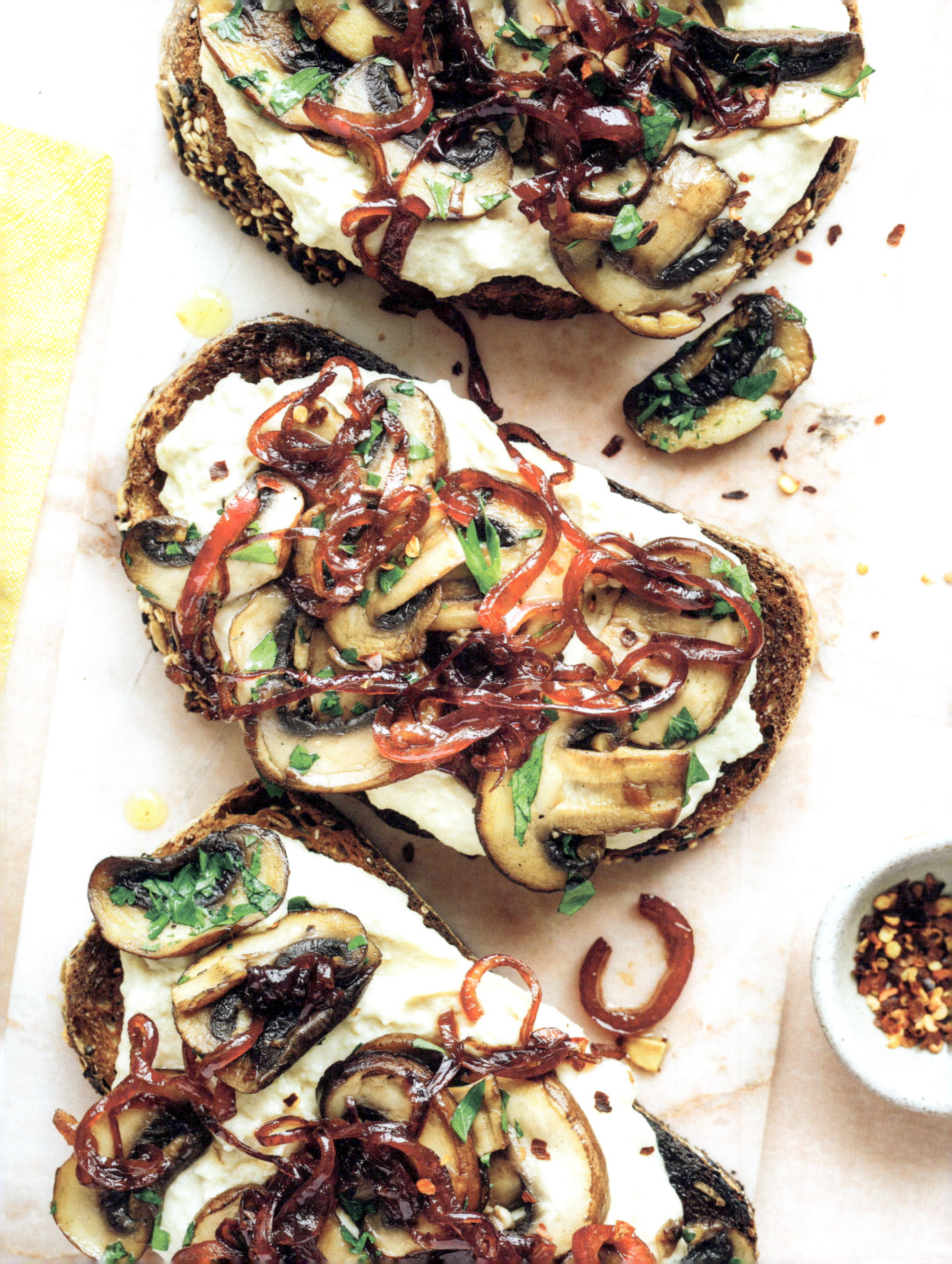

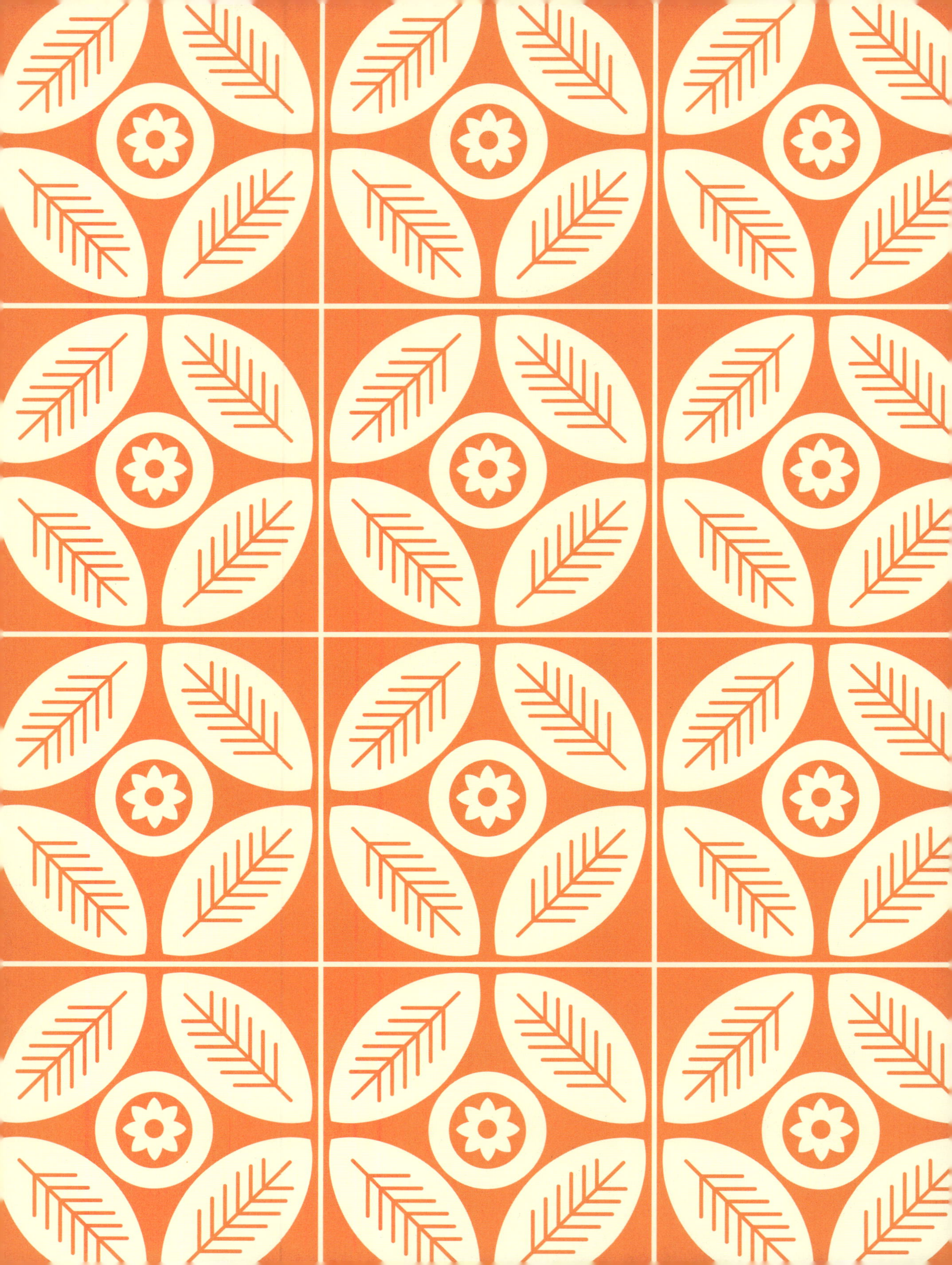

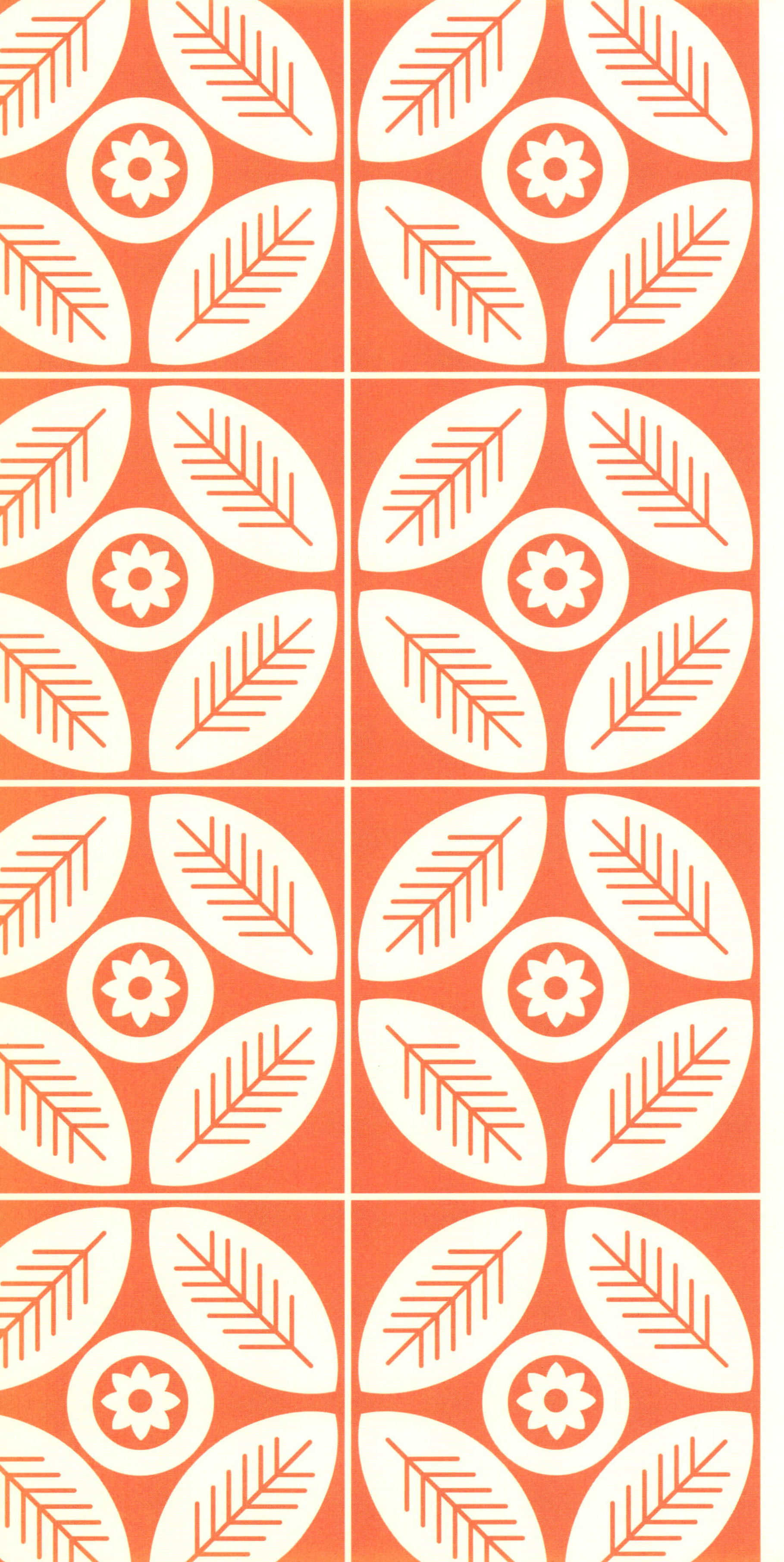

QUICK LUNCHES

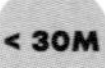

GREEK-INSPIRED SALAD WITH TOFU 'FETA'

Serves 2–3

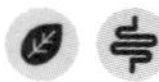

Salads often get a bad rap for being uninspiring, but once you discover the secret to crafting a truly satisfying blend that keeps you fuelled and nourished throughout your day, everything changes. Take this Greek-inspired salad – It's packed with tonnes of fresh veggies, tangy marinated tofu 'feta', and the most addictive crunchy seed blend. The perfect way to enjoy Mediterranean flavours.

TOFU 'FETA'
Juice of 1 lemon, plus
    2 tablespoons zest
1 teaspoon miso paste (or a pinch
    of salt)
2 tablespoons nutritional yeast
30ml (2 tablespoons) olive oil
250g (9oz) firm tofu, drained and
    pressed (see page 37), cut into
    1.5cm (½ inch) cubes

DRESSING
3 tablespoons apple cider vinegar
2 tablespoons olive oil
½ teaspoon Dijon mustard
1 teaspoon dried oregano
1 teaspoon flaky sea salt
1 teaspoon freshly ground
    black pepper

SALAD
20g (¾oz) mixed seeds (roughly
    equal amounts of chia
    seeds, sunflower seeds,
    pumpkin seeds)
½ cucumber, halved lengthwise,
    deseeded and sliced into 2cm
    (¾ inch) thick pieces
100g (3½oz) drained tinned
    chickpeas (garbanzos)
100g (3½oz) cherry
    tomatoes, halved
½ red onion, sliced
20g (¾oz) kalamata olives, pitted
    and chopped
Handful of mint leaves, chopped

First, marinate the tofu. Combine the lemon juice and zest, miso paste, nutritional yeast, olive oil and a splash of water in a lidded container and whisk until well combined. Add the cubed tofu, close the container and shake. Let the tofu marinade while you prepare the salad.

To make the dressing, combine all the ingredients in a bowl and whisk until combined.

Put the mixed seeds into a dry frying pan (skillet) and toast them over a low heat until they start to sizzle and pop. Remove from the heat and set aside to cool.

Meanwhile, combine the remaining ingredients for the salad in a large bowl. Add the marinated tofu 'feta' along with its marinade and the dressing and seeds. Toss to combine.

NOTE
The tofu 'feta' can be made the day before and kept in the refrigerator overnight to marinate.

PROTEIN PER SERVING	MAKE IT GLUTEN-FREE	STORAGE
38g	Use gluten-free miso paste.	Store in the refrigerator for up to 3 days. Not freezer friendly.

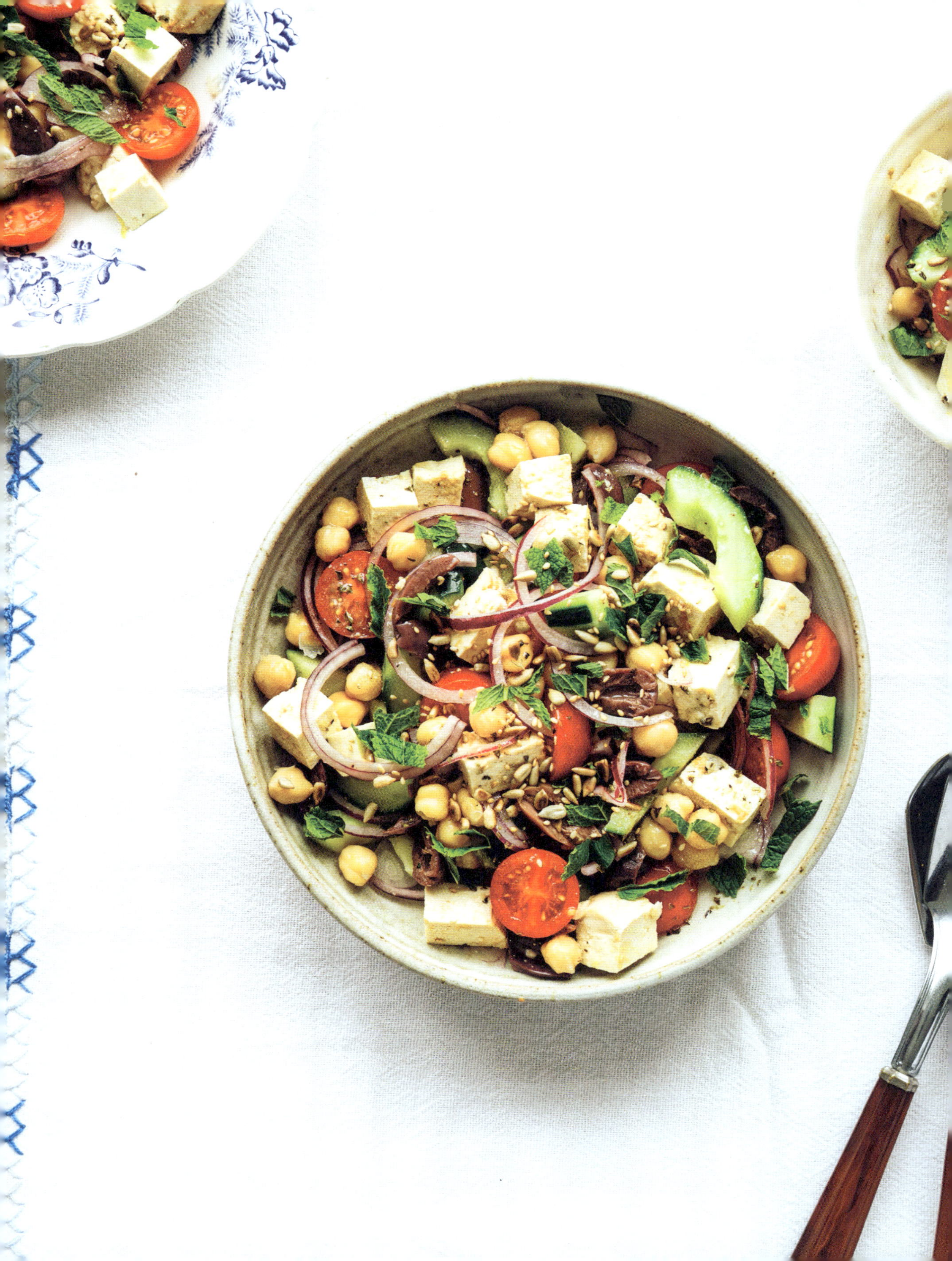

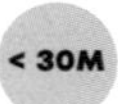

BUCKWHEAT TABBOULEH

Serves 2–3

100g (3½oz/⅔ cup) buckwheat
50g (1¾oz/scant ½ cup)
    sunflower seeds
1 x 400g (14oz) tin of brown
    lentils, drained
½ cucumber, diced
150g (5½oz) cherry tomatoes, diced
½ small red onion, diced
30g (1oz) curly or flat-leaf parsley
    leaves, chopped
15g (½oz) mint leaves, chopped
6 tablespoons shelled hemp seeds

DRESSING
40ml (1½fl oz/3 tablespoons)
    olive oil
Juice of 1 lemon
1 garlic clove, grated
Pinch of salt

As the warmer months approach, my appetite naturally gravitates towards the vibrant allure of raw, fresh foods, with salads taking centre stage in my culinary rotation. But fear not, for we're not settling for bland here. This wholesome dish marries nutty buckwheat, hearty brown lentils and a symphony of crisp, fresh vegetables, all harmonized by a zesty dressing. It's one of those recipes that invites you to truly savour each ingredient, leaving you feeling nourished and invigorated.

Bring a saucepan of salted water to the boil and cook the buckwheat according to the packet instructions, then drain.

Put the sunflower seeds into a dry frying pan (skillet) over a medium heat and toast for 8–10 minutes, tossing the pan frequently to prevent burning. Once brown, remove from the heat and set aside to cool slightly.

Meanwhile, combine all the ingredients for the dressing in a jar and shake to combine.

Put the cooked buckwheat, lentils, cucumber, tomatoes, red onion, parsley, mint and hemp seeds into a large bowl. Drizzle with the dressing and toss to combine, then serve.

PROTEIN PER SERVING

25g

STORAGE

Store for up to 3 days in the refrigerator.
Not freezer friendly.

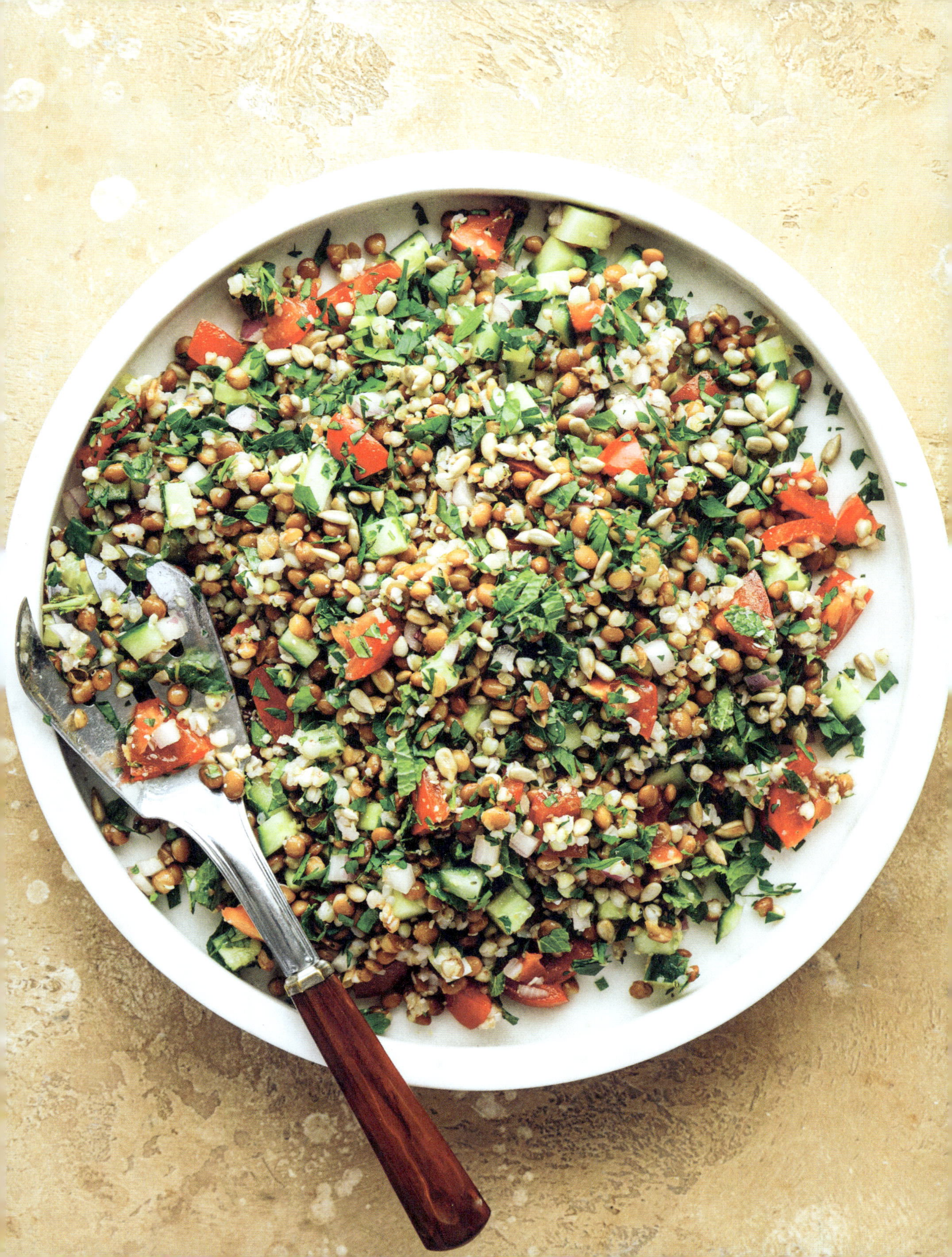

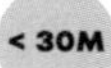

CHICKPEA AND MANGO SALAD

Serves 2–3

 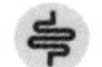 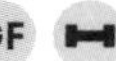

This salad takes inspiration from a popular starter at our favourite Indian restaurant in London, *chana chaat*. It's made with bright and nutritious ingredients like cooked chickpeas, fresh mango and pomegranate seeds. It's tangy, it's spicy and it's the perfect light yet filling lunch.

80g (2¾oz/generous ⅓ cup) tricolour quinoa
1 x 400g (14oz) tin of chickpeas (garbanzos), drained
1 small red onion, chopped
100g (3½oz) pomegranate seeds
60g (2oz/generous ⅓ cup) lightly salted peanuts
Small handful of coriander (cilantro), leaves chopped
200g (7oz) chopped mango

DRESSING

50ml (1¾fl oz/3½ tablespoons) olive oil
1 teaspoon garam masala
1 teaspoon chilli powder
1 teaspoon ground turmeric
½ teaspoon salt
1 tablespoon mango chutney (optional)

Bring a large saucepan of water to the boil and cook the quinoa according to the packet instructions, then drain and set aside to cool slightly.

Combine all the ingredients for the dressing in a small bowl and whisk to combine.

Put the chickpeas, onion, pomegranate seeds, peanuts, coriander and mango into a large bowl, then add the quinoa, drizzle with the dressing and mix to combine.

PROTEIN PER SERVING

25g

STORAGE

Store for up to 3 days in the refrigerator. Not freezer friendly.

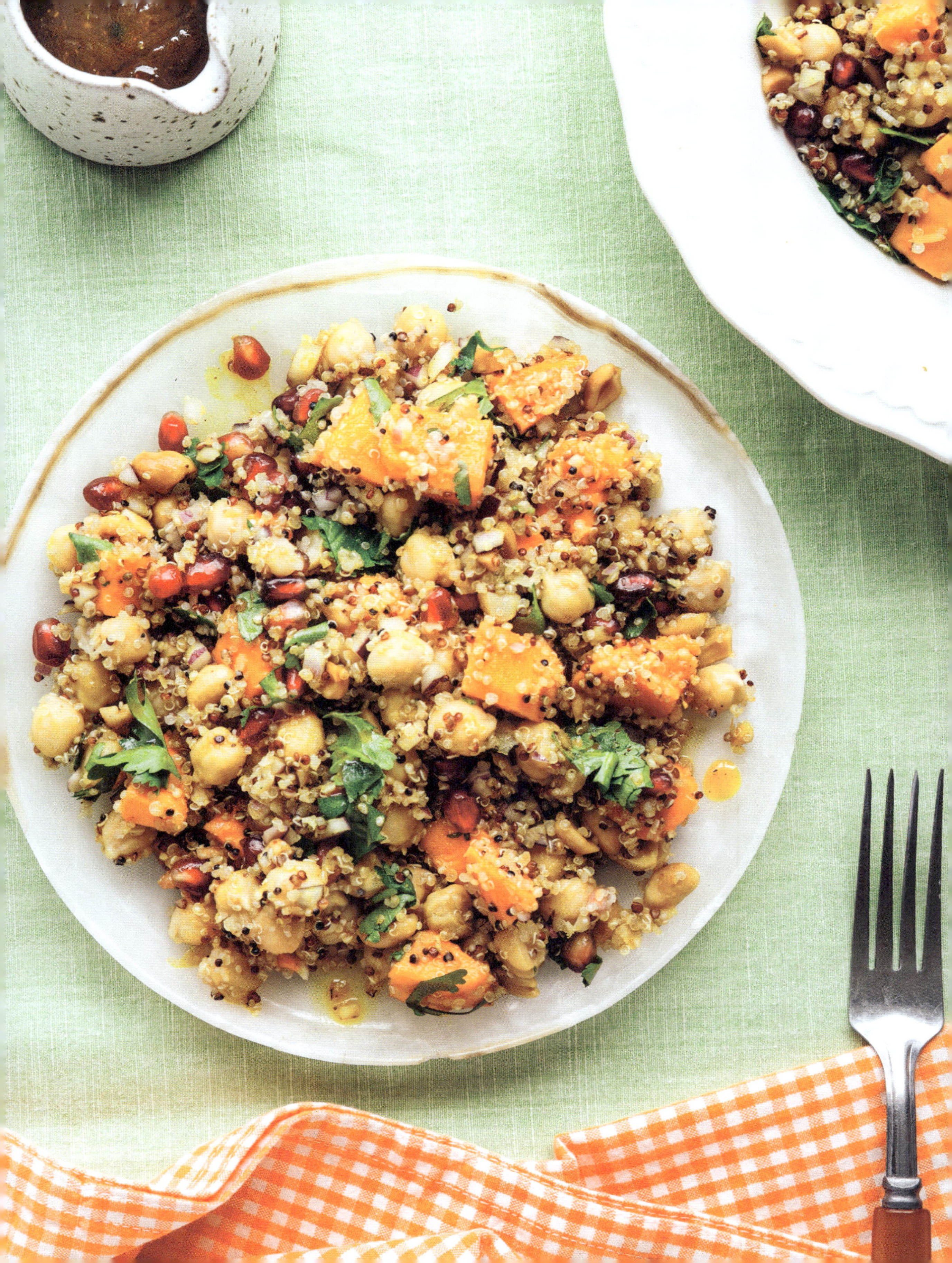

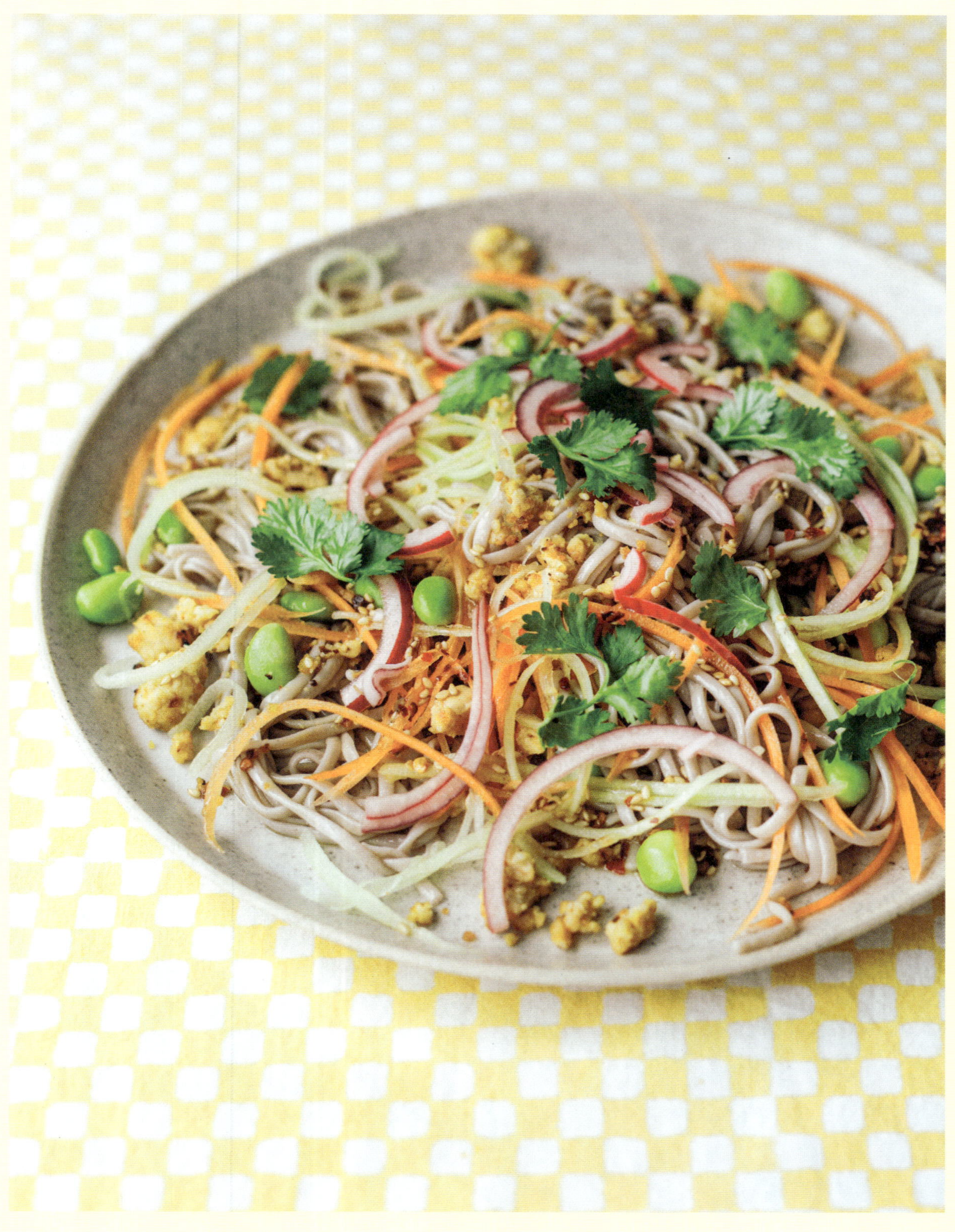

SPICY SOBA NOODLE SALAD WITH CRISPY TEMPEH

Serves 2–3

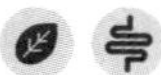

This vibrant salad is packed with fibre and protein. It requires minimal cooking yet delivers a substantial and satisfying meal that will keep you fuelled through your day. Tender buckwheat soba noodles, crunchy edamame and crumbled tempeh are tossed in a zesty, spicy sesame dressing. With vibrant veggies and a burst of flavour in every bite, it's a nutritious delight ready in no time!

180g (6¼oz) buckwheat
   soba noodles
100g (3½oz/1⅔ cups) frozen
   edamame beans
2 tablespoons sesame oil
200g (7oz) tempeh, finely crumbled
1 carrot, grated (shredded)
½ cucumber, thinly sliced
   or spiralized
Small handful of chopped
   coriander (cilantro),
   plus extra to serve
Pickled red onions

SPICY SESAME DRESSING
3 tablespoons apple cider vinegar
4 tablespoons toasted sesame oil
2 tablespoons maple syrup
2 tablespoons light soy sauce
1 teaspoon chilli (hot pepper) flakes
2 teaspoons sesame seeds

Bring a saucepan of water to the boil and cook the soba noodles according to the packet instructions, then drain and plunge the soba into cold water to stop the cooking process. This prevents the noodles from becoming gummy and sticking together.

Put the edamame into a bowl and cover with boiling water. Leave to soak for 10 minutes, then drain. This will defrost the edamame and cook them without them losing their crunch.

Heat the sesame oil in a frying pan (skillet) over a medium heat, then add the crumbled tempeh. Cook for 10 minutes, tossing occasionally, until crispy and brown.

Meanwhile, combine all the dressing ingredients in a jar and shake to combine.

Layer the carrot, cucumber, coriander, soba noodles, edamame and tempeh in a large bowl and drizzle the spicy sesame dressing on top.

Toss to combine, then serve topped with more coriander and some pickled red onions.

PROTEIN PER SERVING

39g

MAKE IT GLUTEN-FREE

Use gluten-free soba noodles and soy sauce.

STORAGE

Store for up to 3 days in the refrigerator. Not freezer friendly.

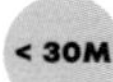

MEZZE BOWL WITH COURGETTE FALAFEL

Serves 2–3

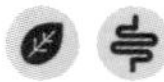

I'm absolutely sold on this dish – I could eat it every day for the rest of my life and never tire of it. This bowl features delicious courgette (zucchini) falafel and crisp parsley salad accompanied by the lively kick of zesty harissa red lentil hummus and the rich savouriness of kalamata olives. And the best part? It comes together in just 30 minutes. With its meal prep-friendly nature, it's poised to rescue your lunchtimes, ensuring a delicious meal every day without fail.

FALAFELS

2 medium courgettes (zucchini), grated (shredded)
1 carrot, peeled and grated (shredded)
100g (3½oz/scant 1 cup) chickpea (gram) flour
2 tablespoons cornflour (cornstarch)
Small handful of flat-leaf parsley, chopped
½ teaspoon salt
½ teaspoon freshly ground black pepper
½ teaspoon garlic granules
½ teaspoon ground cumin

PARSLEY SALAD

25g (1oz) curly or flat-leaf parsley, chopped
250g (9oz) tomatoes, diced
½ red onion, sliced
Juice of 1 lemon
20ml (1½ tablespoons) olive oil
Salt and freshly ground black pepper

TO SERVE

Harissa Red Lentil Hummus (see page 164)
Kalamata olives
Lemon wedges
Tofu Flatbread (see page 164)

Put the grated courgette and carrot into a clean dish towel and squeeze to remove the excess moisture, then place them in a bowl and add the remaining falafel ingredients. Mix well – I squeeze the mixture through my fingers to ensure it is properly combined.

Take spoonfuls of the mixture and form 2.5cm (1 inch) wide falafels. Once all falafels have been formed, air-fry them at 180°C (350°F) for 20 minutes, turning them halfway through, or else pan-fry them in a little olive oil over a medium heat for 5–10 minutes on each side.

Meanwhile, put the parsley, tomatoes and onion for the salad into a bowl. Whisk together the lemon juice, olive oil and a pinch of salt and pepper and pour over the salad. Mix to combine.

Divide the parsley salad and falafels between bowls and top with the harissa red lentil hummus, kalamata olives and lemon wedges for squeezing. Serve with the tofu flatbread.

PROTEIN PER SERVING	MAKE IT GLUTEN-FREE	STORAGE
40g	Use gluten-free flatbread.	Store for up to 3 days in the refrigerator. Not freezer friendly.

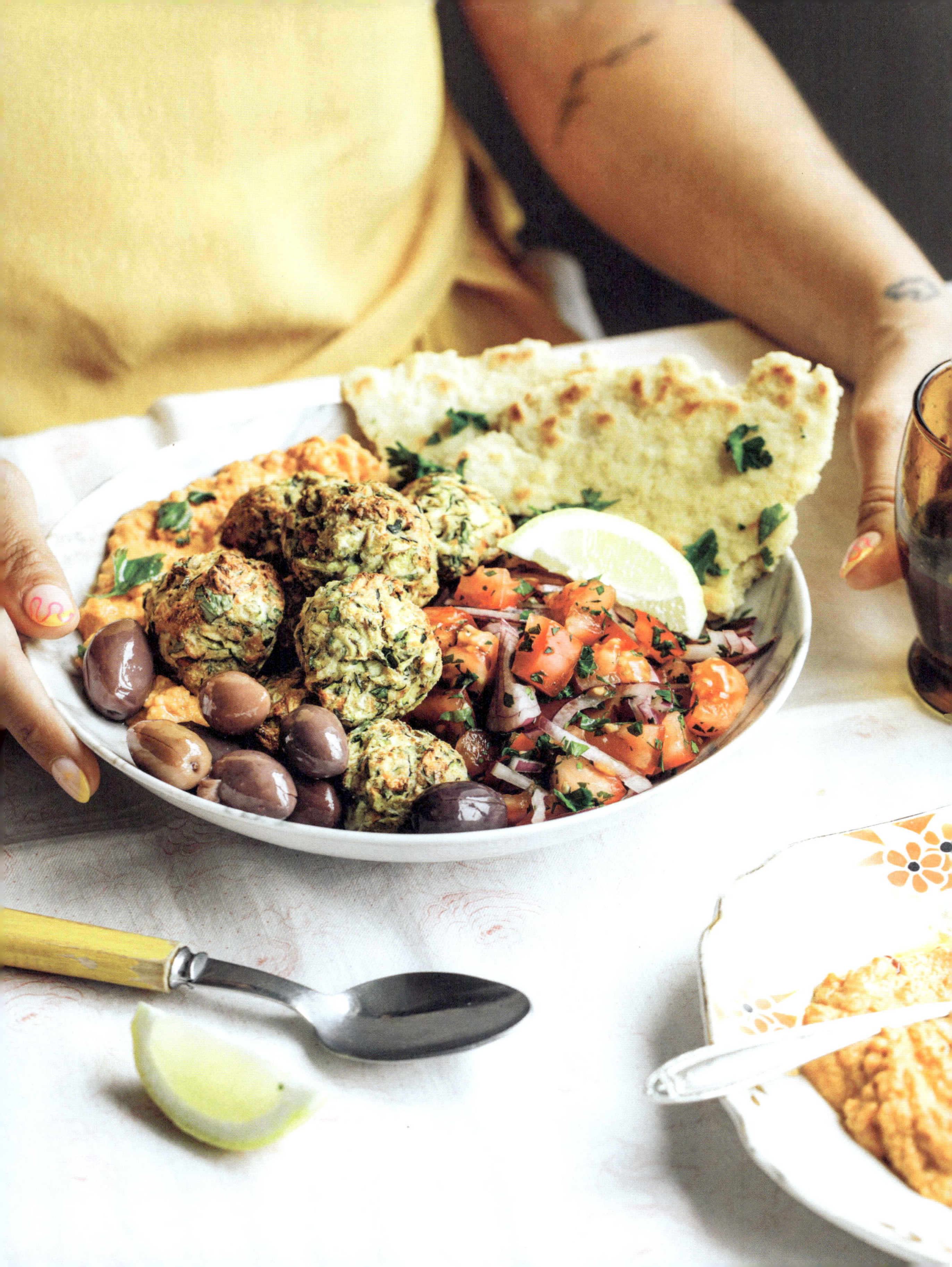

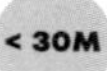

CRUNCHY THAI-STYLE QUINOA SALAD

Serves 2–3

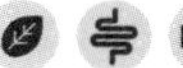

Packed with nutritious ingredients like quinoa, smoked tofu, crunchy vegetables and a luscious peanut dressing, this salad is a delightful fusion of Thai-inspired flavours and wholesome goodness. Bound to impress with its fresh, bold flavours and satisfying textures, it's the perfect vibrant lunch to pack for work or share with friends at a picnic.

80g (2¾oz/generous ⅓ cup) quinoa

100g (3½oz) smoked tofu, grated (shredded)

⅛ red cabbage, thinly sliced

5-6 spring onions (scallions), thinly sliced

1 carrot, peeled and julienned or grated (shredded)

150g (5½oz/ 2½ cups) cooked edamame beans (defrosted if frozen)

15g (½oz) coriander (cilantro), leaves, roughly chopped (optional), plus extra to serve

100g (3½oz) chopped mango (optional)

PEANUT DRESSING

30g (1oz/2 tablespoons) smooth peanut butter

2 tablespoons reduced-salt soy sauce

2 tablespoons maple syrup

Juice of 1 lime

4cm (1½ inch) piece of fresh ginger root, peeled and grated

1 garlic clove, very finely chopped or grated

TO SERVE

30g (1oz) lightly salted peanuts, roughly chopped

Black sesame seeds

Sliced red chillies (optional)

Bring a saucepan of water to the boil and cook the quinoa according to the packet instructions, then drain and set aside to cool.

Combine all the ingredients for the dressing in a jar with 2 tablespoons water and shake to combine.

Place the cooked quinoa in a bowl along with the remaining salad ingredients, then toss through the dressing.

Serve topped with chopped peanuts, coriander, black sesame seeds and sliced chilli (if using).

PROTEIN PER SERVING	MAKE IT GLUTEN-FREE	STORAGE
31g	Use gluten-free soy sauce.	Store for up to 3 days in the refrigerator. Not freezer friendly.

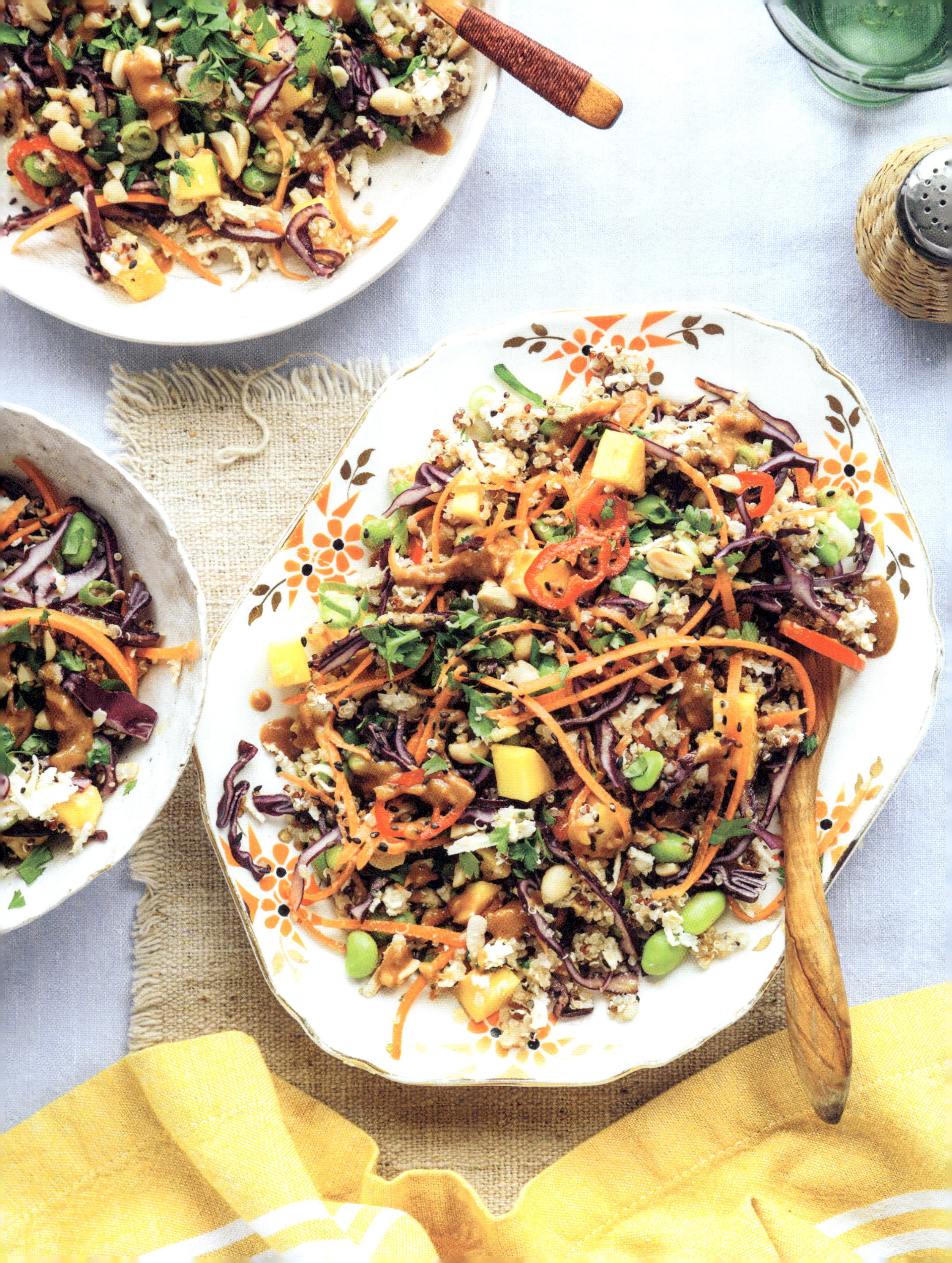

LEMONY SMASHED POTATO, COURGETTE AND BROAD BEAN SALAD

Serves 2–3

Fresh, zesty and bursting with texture, this dish is a celebration of seasonal produce and wholesome ingredients. With creamy smashed potatoes, crisp courgette (zucchini), tender broad (fava) beans and nutty pistachios, all tossed in a tangy lemon dressing, this salad is perfect for a light yet nutritious lunch.

1 courgette (zucchini), thinly sliced lengthwise (I use a vegetable peeler)
Juice and zest of ½ lemon
120g (4oz/1⅓ cups) kamut (Khorasan wheat), quick-cook spelt or giant couscous
250g (9oz) new (baby) potatoes
200g (7oz) fresh or frozen podded broad (fava) beans
40g (1½oz/¼ cup) shelled pistachios, roughly chopped
Small handful of mint, leaves chopped
Olive oil, for drizzling
Salt and freshly ground black pepper

LEMON DRESSING
Juice of 1 lemon
120g (4oz/½ cup) high-protein plant-based yoghurt
1 tablespoon olive oil
2 tablespoons nutritional yeast
1 teaspoon Dijon mustard
1 teaspoon maple syrup
½ teaspoon freshly ground black pepper
½ teaspoon salt

Preheat the oven to 220°C/200°C fan/425°F/Gas mark 7 and line a baking tray (pan) with baking parchment.

Place the sliced courgette in a bowl and add the lemon juice, a drizzle of oil and a pinch of salt and mix until combined. Set aside to marinate.

Bring a large saucepan of water to the boil and cook the kamut according to the packet instructions, then drain and set aside to cool slightly.

Bring another saucepan of salted water to the boil and cook the potatoes for 15 minutes until fork-tender. Add the broad beans for the last few minutes until tender. Drain and separate the potatoes from the beans.

Transfer the potatoes to the prepared baking tray and press down on them with a heavy cup or glass. Drizzle with oil and season with salt and pepper, then roast in the oven for 30 minutes, flipping them halfway through.

Meanwhile, combine all the ingredients for the dressing in a jar and shake until well combined.

In a bowl, combine the cooked kamut, marinated courgette, smashed potatoes, broad beans, most of the pistachios and the mint. Pour over the dressing, then toss to combine.

Garnish with the remaining pistachios and the lemon zest.

PROTEIN PER SERVING	MAKE IT GLUTEN-FREE	STORAGE
27.5g	Swap the kamut for brown rice.	Store for up to 4 days in the refrigerator. Not freezer friendly.

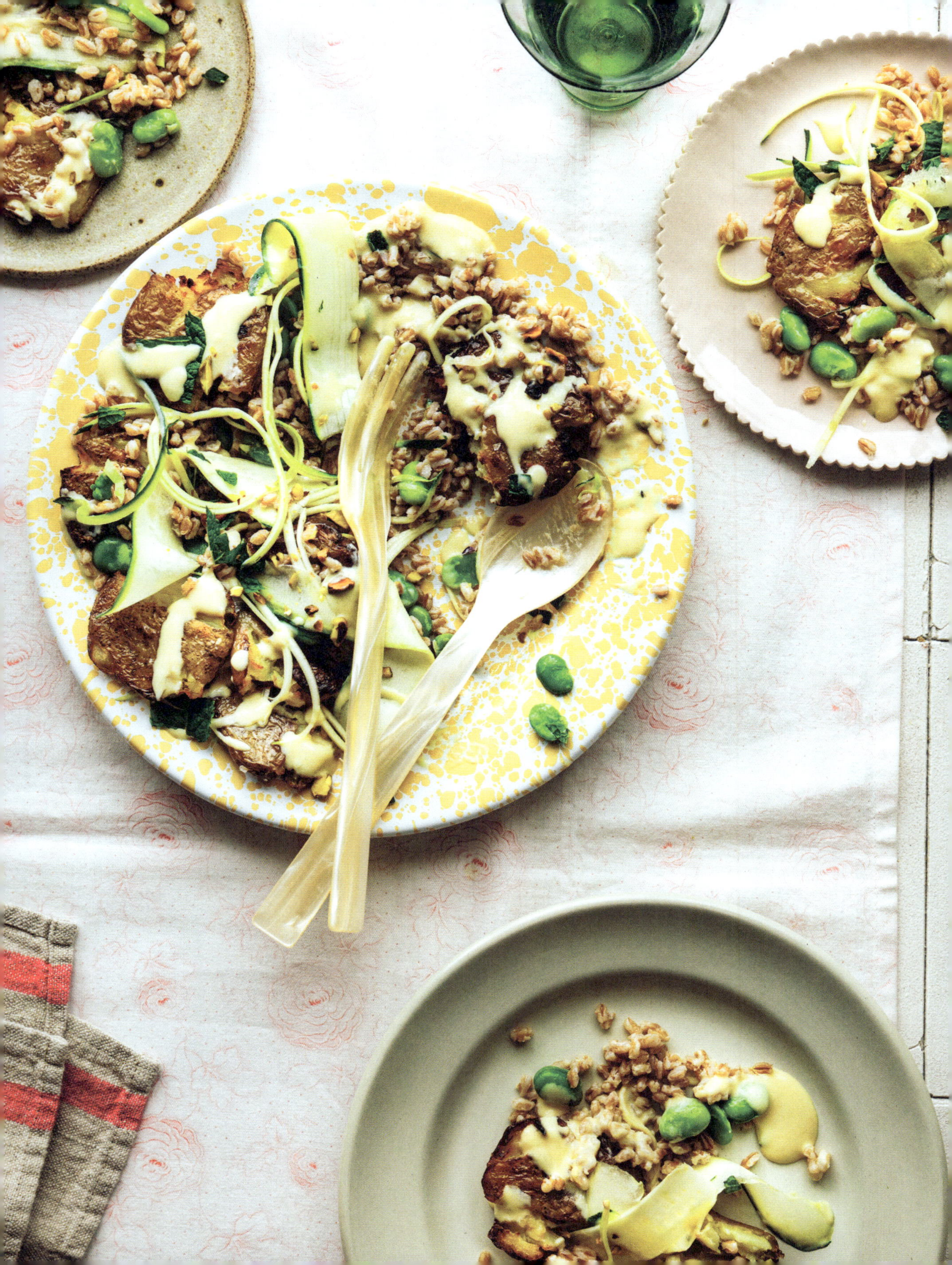

ROASTED SWEET POTATO **AND** CHICKPEA SALAD **WITH** HARISSA DRESSING

Serves 2–3

Bursting with aromatic spices and complemented by a zesty harissa dressing, this salad is a perfect balance of warmth and freshness. The sweet potatoes, rich in vitamins and fibre, mingle harmoniously with the protein-packed chickpeas and fluffy couscous, creating a wholesome and nourishing lunch.

1 teaspoon smoked paprika
½ teaspoon cayenne pepper
1 teaspoon ground cumin
½ teaspoon salt
1 tablespoon maple syrup
3 tablespoons olive oil
1 x 400g (14oz) tin of chickpeas (garbanzos), drained and patted dry
1 sweet potato (about 300g/10½oz), chopped into bite-sized pieces
80g (2¾oz/scant ½ cup) couscous
70g (2½oz) kale, stalks removed and leaves roughly chopped
Juice of ½ lemon, plus extra to serve
40g (1½oz) toasted almonds, chopped
20g (¾oz) toasted pumpkin seeds
Small handful of pomegranate seeds

CREAMY HARISSA DRESSING
1 tablespoon harissa paste
200g (7oz/generous ¾ cup) high-protein plant-based yoghurt
Juice of 1 lemon
Pinch of freshly ground black pepper

Preheat the oven to 220°C/200°C fan/425°F/Gas mark 7 and line a baking tray (pan) with baking parchment.

Whisk together the paprika, cayenne pepper, cumin, salt, maple syrup and 2 tablespoons of the olive oil in a small bowl.

Put the chickpeas and chopped sweet potato onto the prepared baking tray, then pour over the spice mixture and toss to coat. Roast in the oven for 30–40 minutes until the sweet potato is tender and the chickpeas are crunchy.

Meanwhile, put the couscous into a bowl and pour in just enough boiling water (or hot vegetable stock) to cover. Cover and steam for 5–10 minutes until the couscous is soft, then fluff it with a fork.

Put the kale into a large bowl, drizzle with the remaining 1 tablespoon of oil and the lemon juice and gently massage the kale with your hands. Set aside.

Whisk together all the ingredients for the dressing in a bowl.

Add the sweet potatoes and crispy chickpeas to the kale, then add the almonds, pumpkin seeds and pomegranate seeds. Drizzle with the harissa dressing and toss to combine. Serve with one last squeeze of lemon juice.

PROTEIN PER SERVING	MAKE IT GLUTEN-FREE	STORAGE
32.5g	Swap the couscous for brown rice.	Store for up to 3 days in the refrigerator. Not freezer friendly.

RED LENTIL SOUP WITH SMOKY, CRUNCHY CHICKPEAS AND A TOASTIE

Serves 3–4

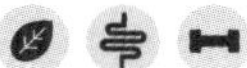

This is one of my favourite soups of all time. I love eating it in winter after a cold day out (or a run). I call it a hug in a bowl! The hearty mixture of lentils and chickpeas (garbanzos) – with balanced herbs and spices to give it a robust flavour – is an excellent source of plant-based protein. It's also rich in dietary fibre and antioxidants, which means it is great for recovery, supports digestive health and the immune system and fights inflammation. The best part is that this soup freezes well, so I love to double the portions so I have something ready in the freezer for when I can't be bothered to cook! I hope you'll love it as much as I do.

SMOKY CRUNCHY CHICKPEAS

- 150g (5½oz) tinned drained chickpeas (garbanzos)
- 1 heaped teaspoon ground cumin
- 1 heaped teaspoon smoked paprika
- Pinch of salt
- Olive oil, for drizzling

RED LENTIL SOUP

- 1 carrot, diced
- 1 celery stick, diced
- 1 small onion, diced
- 2–3 garlic cloves, very finely chopped
- 1 heaped teaspoon smoked paprika
- 1 heaped teaspoon ground cumin
- 200g (7oz/generous 1 cup) split red lentils, washed
- 750ml (25fl oz/3 cups) vegetable stock (or more or less as preferred)
- 1 x 400g (14oz) tin of chopped tomatoes
- Small handful of thyme, leaves stripped, plus extra to serve
- Small handful of basil, leaves roughly chopped, plus extra to serve
- 350g (12oz) tinned drained chickpeas (garbanzos)
- 4 tablespoons nutritional yeast
- Handful of spinach
- Olive oil, for cooking
- Salt and freshly ground black pepper
- Plant-based cream or high-protein plant-based yoghurt, to serve

Preheat the oven to 220°C/200°C fan/425°F/Gas mark 7 and a line a baking tray (pan) with baking parchment.

First, make the crunchy chickpeas. Put the chickpeas onto a clean dish towel and pat them dry to remove any excess moisture. This step is very important to ensure the chickpeas crisp up, so don't skip it.

Spread the chickpeas out on the prepared baking tray. Roast them in the oven for 35–40 minutes, then turn on the grill (broiler) and grill for 5–10 minutes to ensure they're crunchy. Alternatively, if you have an air fryer, you can air-fry the chickpeas at 200°C (400°F) for 15–20 minutes.

Meanwhile, start the soup. Heat a good glug of oil in a large saucepan over a medium heat and fry the carrot, celery, onion and garlic for 5–8 minutes until soft and golden. Add the smoked paprika and cumin and stir for a couple of minutes to allow the flavours to infuse, then add the red lentils and toast for 2 minutes. This will ensure the lentils don't break up too much when cooking. Pour in the stock, then add the tomatoes and herbs. Stir and bring to the boil, then reduce the heat and simmer for 10 minutes. Finally, add the chickpeas and cook for a further 5 minutes, stirring occasionally.

RECIPE CONTINUES →

3 slices of sourdough bread
Plant-based mozzarella-style
cheese or plant-based cheese
of your choice

NOTE

The soffritto base can be batch-cooked and used for many different recipes in this book. See page 34 for my pantry staple recipe.

Remove about a third of the soup and blend with the nutritional yeast in a food processor or with a hand-held blender until smooth. Return the blended soup to the pan, then add spinach and stir until completely wilted. Taste and adjust the seasoning as needed.

Make the toasties by toasting the bread until golden and crispy, then halve them and layer one side with the plant-based cheese. Top with the remaining toast.

Ladle the soup into bowls, topping each with a drizzle of plant-based cream or high-protein plant-based yoghurt.

Garnish with the crispy chickpeas, thyme and basil, and serve with the toasties.

PROTEIN PER SERVING	MAKE IT GLUTEN-FREE	STORAGE
25g	Use gluten-free bread.	Store for up to 3 days in the refrigerator and up to 3 months in the freezer.

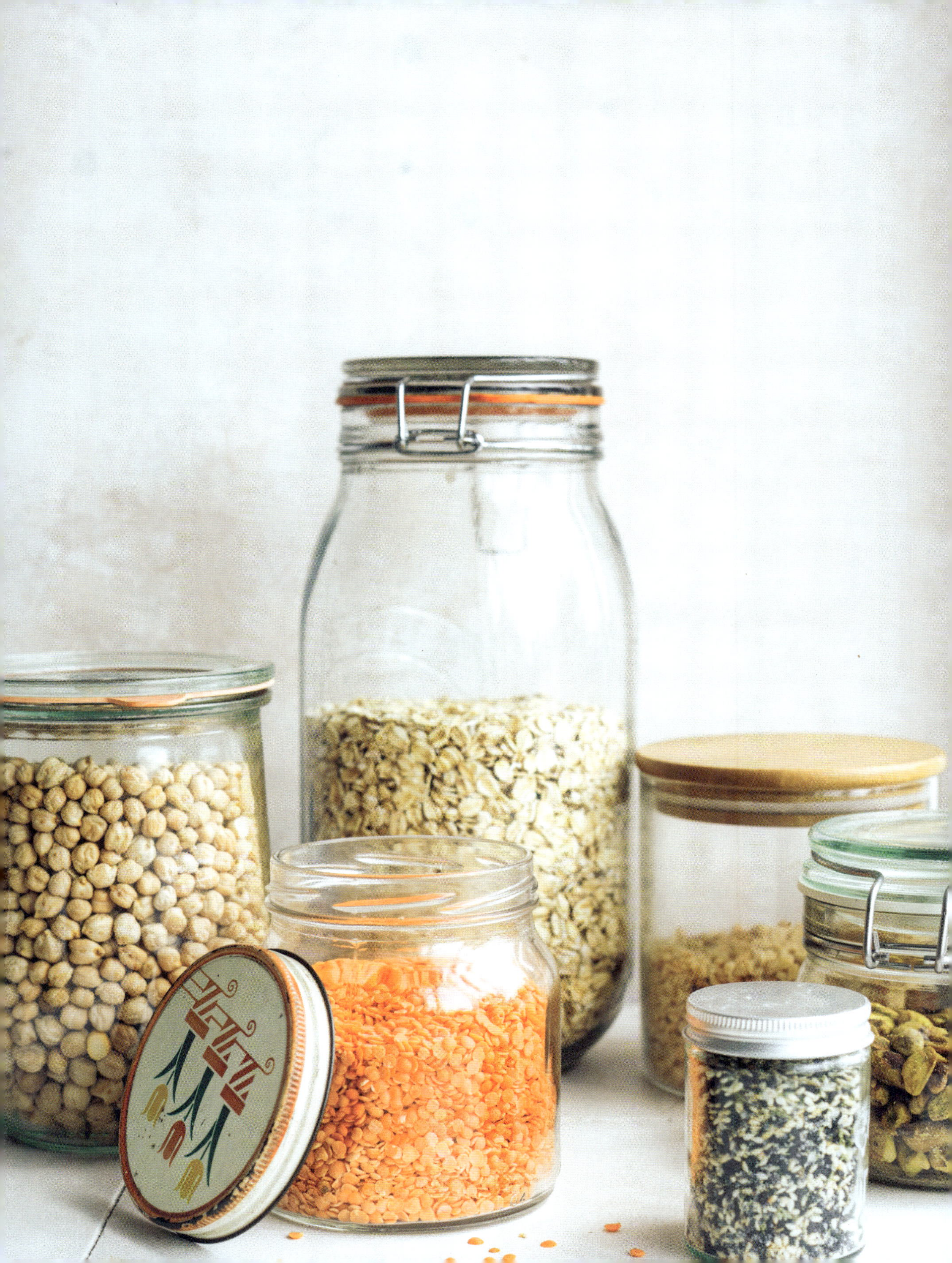

GOLDEN SPLIT PEA AND LEMON SOUP

Serves 2–4

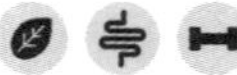

This soup is a golden elixir, perfect for those times of the year when you feel like you're constantly on the brink of getting sick. It's a delicious, very low effort and filling way to incorporate ingredients with anti-inflammatory and immune-boosting properties into your diet. It is of course also high in protein and, most importantly, absolutely delicious!

1 small-medium carrot, diced
½ celery stick, diced
1 small onion, diced
2–3 garlic cloves, very
    finely chopped
1 thumb-sized piece of fresh ginger
    root, peeled and grated
1 heaped teaspoon
    ground turmeric
1 teaspoon ground cumin
1 small sweet potato, peeled
    and diced
100g (3½oz/scant ½ cup) yellow
    split peas (see Notes)
500ml (17fl oz/generous 2 cups)
    vegetable stock (or more or
    less as preferred)
100g (3½oz) orzo
400ml (14fl oz/generous 1½ cups)
    coconut milk
Handful of spinach or cavolo nero
    (lacinato kale), stalks removed
4 tablespoons nutritional yeast
Juice of 1 lemon
Olive oil, for cooking and drizzling
Salt and freshly ground
    black pepper

TO SERVE
Plant-based Parmesan-style
    cheese (see page 36, or use
    shop-bought; optional)
Small handful of flat-leaf parsley

Heat a good glug of oil in a large saucepan over a medium heat and fry the carrot, celery, onion, garlic and ginger for 5–8 minutes until soft and golden. Add the turmeric and cumin and fry for a further 4–5 minutes, then add the sweet potato, split peas and stock. Cover and simmer for about 30 minutes until the split peas are cooked, adding more stock if needed.

Once the split peas have softened, add the orzo and coconut milk and simmer for a further 10 minutes. Remove from the heat, add the spinach or cavolo nero, nutritional yeast and lemon juice and stir until the spinach has completely wilted. Add more stock if you like a creamier consistency. Season with salt and pepper.

Serve topped with plant-based Parmesan-style cheese (if using), a drizzle of oil and a sprinkle of parsley.

NOTES
The soffritto base can be batch-cooked and used for many different recipes in this book. See page 34 for my pantry staple recipe.

Swap the split peas for split red lentils if you are in a hurry as they cook faster – they will only need about 10 minutes.

PROTEIN PER SERVE	MAKE IT GLUTEN-FREE	STORAGE
20g	Use gluten-free orzo.	Store for up to 3 days in the refrigerator and up to 3 months in the freezer.

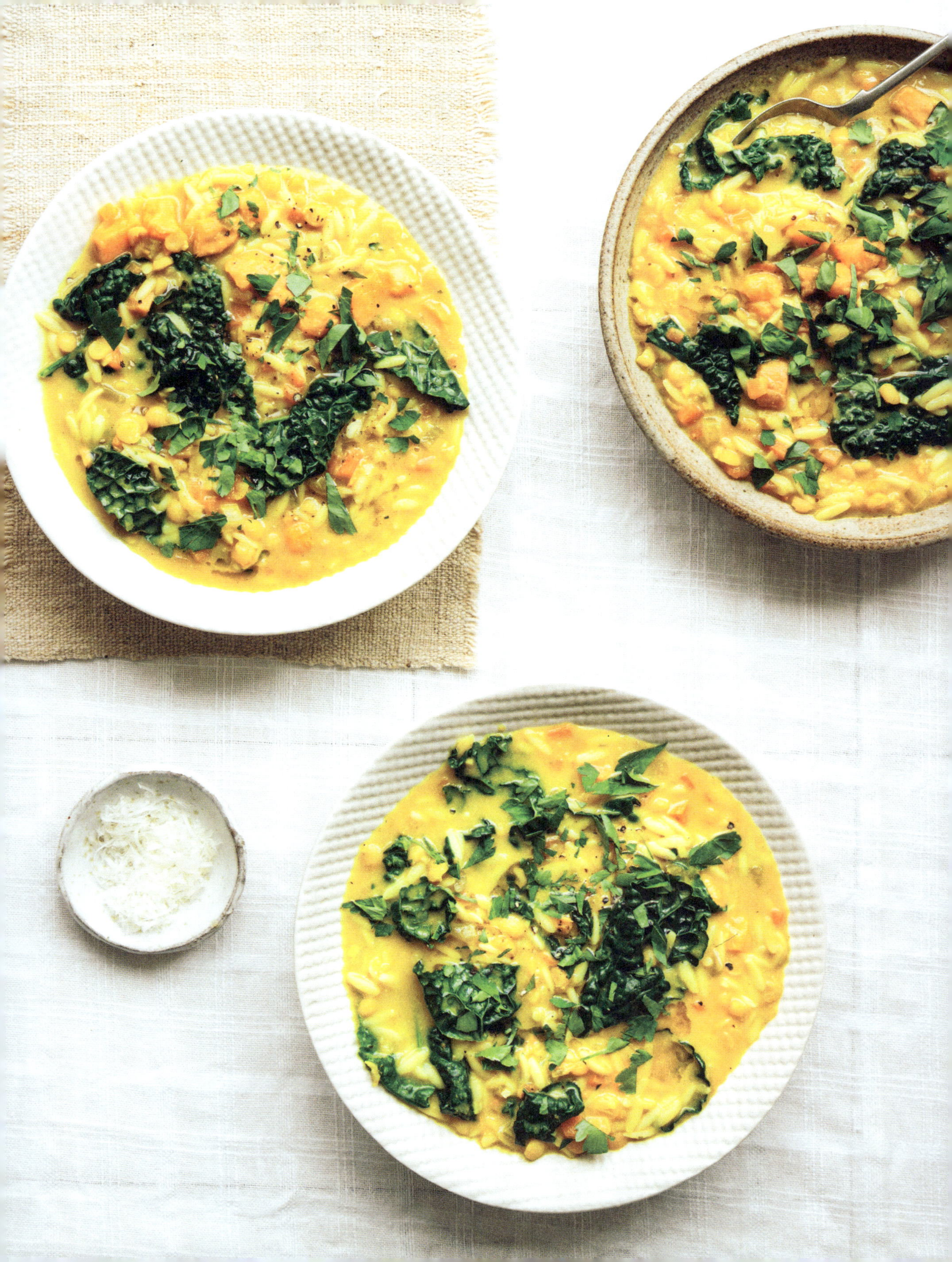

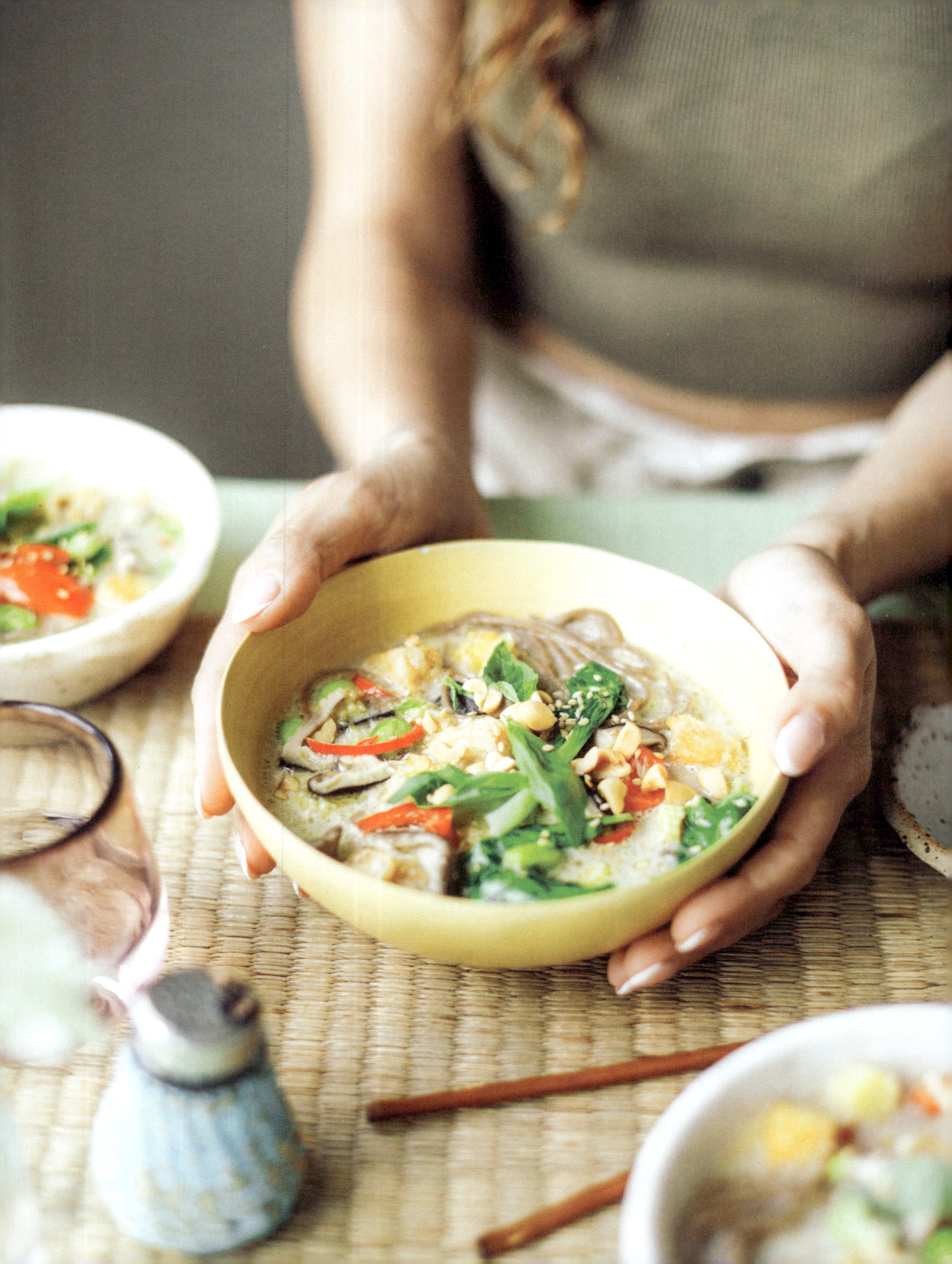

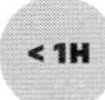

COCONUT AND LIME NOODLE SOUP

Serves 3–4

This recipe reminds me of the nearly two years I spent living (and eating!) in Asia. When we were living in Hong Kong, I used to travel often to countries like Japan, Vietnam and Thailand. My favourite place to visit? The food markets, of course! I used to spend hours looking at the different stalls filled with veggies and spices, so different from Europe! This recipe packs in all the flavours I love most, from the fresh lemongrass and ginger to the sweet coconut and the unique flavour of lime leaves. It is of course tailored so that it is high in protein, too!

300g (10½oz) firm tofu, drained and pressed (see page 37), then cut into 1cm (½ inch) cubes
1 tablespoon cornflour (cornstarch)
Pinch of salt
1 green chilli (deseed if you prefer)
2 lemongrass stalks, hard outer layer removed
1 thumb-sized piece of fresh ginger root, peeled
3 garlic cloves
6 spring onions (scallions)
1 tablespoon miso paste
100g (3½oz) shiitake mushrooms, roughly chopped
800ml (27fl oz/3⅓ cups) coconut milk
2 lime leaves
1 pak choi (bok choy), quartered lengthwise
Half red (bell) pepper, diced
3 baby corn, chopped (optional)
1 red chilli, deseeded and sliced (optional)
200g (7oz) buckwheat soba noodles
100g (3½oz/1⅓ cups) frozen edamame beans
1 lime
Sesame oil, for frying and drizzling

TO SERVE
Coriander (cilantro) or Thai basil
Lime wedges
Lightly salted roasted peanuts, chopped
Sesame seeds

Preheat the oven to 200°C/180°C fan/400°F/Gas mark 6 and line a baking tray (pan) with baking parchment.

Put the cubed tofu into a bowl and add the cornflour and salt, then toss to coat.

Transfer the tofu to the prepared baking tray, making sure to leave a gap between each cube, then drizzle with sesame oil and bake on the middle shelf of the oven for 30 minutes, or until golden and crispy, flipping the tofu halfway through to ensure even baking.

While the tofu is baking, move onto the soup. Put the green chilli, lemongrass, ginger, garlic and spring onions into a food processor along with 2 tablespoons water and blend to form a curry paste.

Heat a good glug of sesame oil in a saucepan over a medium heat, then add the miso paste, curry paste and mushrooms. Fry for 10 minutes, or until the mushrooms are soft and the flavours from the paste have infused.

Pour in the coconut milk and 300ml (10fl oz/1¼ cups) water, then add the lime leaves, pak choi, red pepper, baby corn and red chilli (if using). Simmer for 10 minutes.

Meanwhile, bring a saucepan of water to the boil and cook the soba noodles according to the packet instructions, then drain.

Add the noodles, edamame beans and lime juice to the soup and stir.

Serve in bowls, topped with coriander or Thai basil, lime wedges, roasted peanuts and sesame seeds.

PROTEIN PER SERVING	MAKE IT GLUTEN-FREE	STORAGE
31g	Use gluten-free soba noodles.	Store for up to 3 days in the refrigerator and up to 3 months in the freezer without the noodles.

SWEET POTATO GOCHUJANG SOUP WITH CRISPY CHICKPEAS

Serves 3–4

This is the *perfect* soup to slurp in colder months. Where to begin? It combines the earthy sweetness of sweet potatoes with the bold flavour of gochujang paste, creating a rich and aromatic broth. Silken tofu adds creaminess while nutritional yeast contributes an umami depth of flavour. It takes roughly 45 minutes to make and you'll honestly never guess that it is packed with so much protein!

1 small-medium onion,
   finely chopped
2–3 garlic cloves, very
   finely chopped
1 tablespoon gochujang paste
350g (12oz) sweet potatoes,
   chopped into 1cm (½ inch) cubes
450–600ml (15¼–20fl oz/scant 2–2½
   cups) vegetable stock
1 x 400g tin of chickpeas
   (garbanzos), drained
   and patted dry
1 heaped teaspoon smoked paprika
½ teaspoon ground cumin
1 teaspoon onion granules
300g (10½oz) silken tofu
2–3 tablespoons nutritional yeast
200g (7oz) vermicelli rice noodles
Olive oil, for cooking and drizzling
Salt and freshly ground
   black pepper

TO SERVE
Sesame seeds
Spring onions (scallions),
   finely chopped

Preheat the oven to 220°C/200°C fan/425°F/Gas mark 7 and a line a baking tray (pan) with baking parchment.

Heat a glug of olive oil in a saucepan over a medium heat and fry the onion, garlic and gochujang paste for 5–8 minutes until the onions are soft and golden.

Add the sweet potatoes and a splash of stock to prevent sticking, then stir and cover. Cook for 20–30 minutes, or until fork tender, adding a little more stock to prevent sticking.

Meanwhile, toss the chickpeas in a bowl with a drizzle of olive oil, the paprika, cumin, onion granules and salt. Spread the chickpeas out on the prepared baking tray. Roast them in the oven for 35–40 minutes, then turn on the grill (broiler) and grill for 5–10 minutes to ensure they're crunchy. Alternatively, if you have an air fryer, you can air-fry the chickpeas at 200°C (400°F) for 15–20 minutes.

In a food processor, combine the cooked sweet potato mixture, silken tofu, nutritional yeast, vegetable stock and a pinch of salt and pepper. Blend until creamy. You might have to do this in batches.

Cook the rice noodles according to the packet instructions.

Assemble the bowls by ladling in the creamy soup, followed by the noodles. Garnish with the crispy chickpeas, sesame seeds and finely chopped spring onions.

PROTEIN PER SERVE	MAKE IT GLUTEN-FREE	STORAGE
25g	Use gluten-free gochugang paste.	Store for up to 3 days in the refrigerator and up to 3 months in the freezer without the noodles.

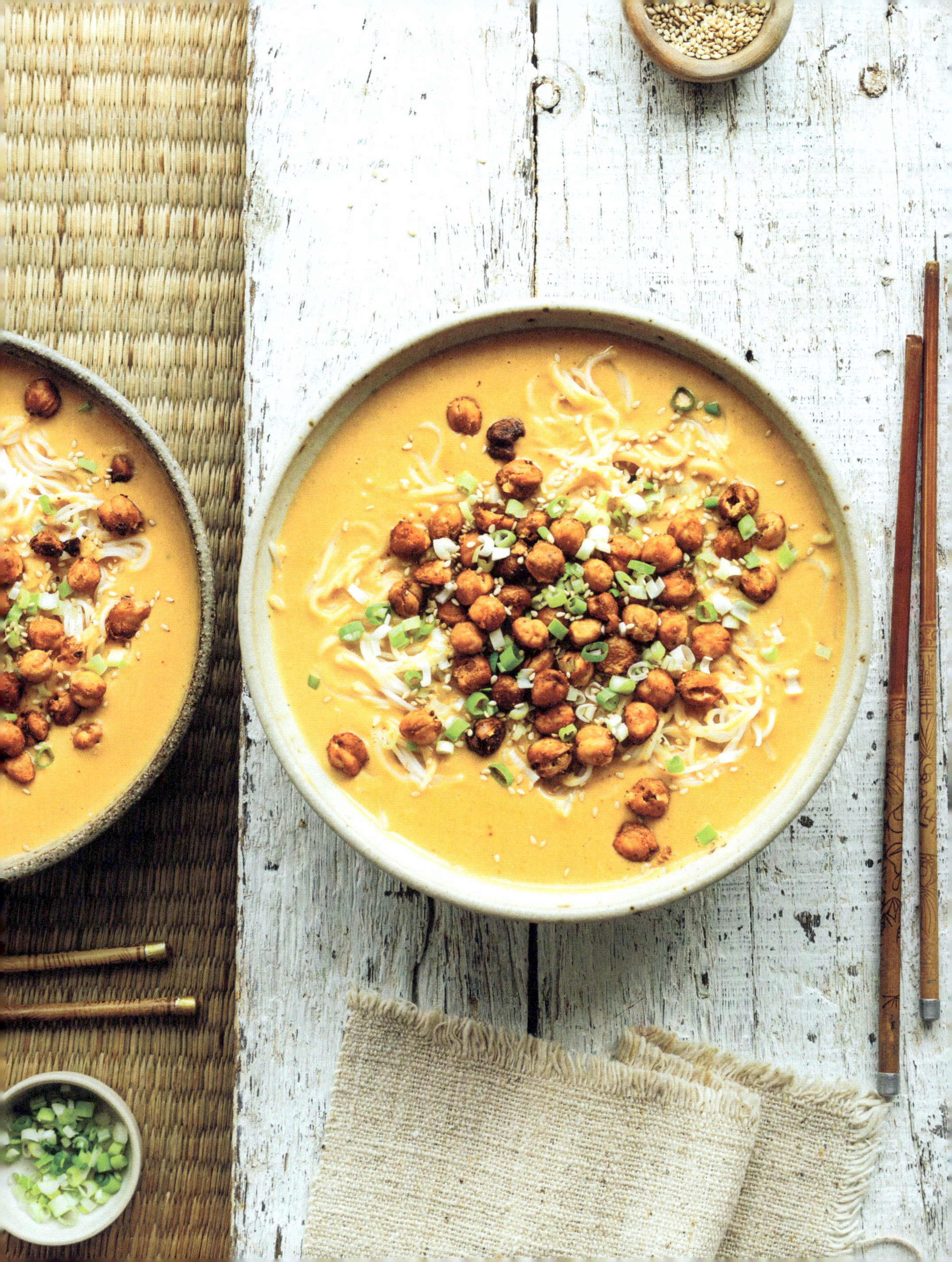

HEARTY PASTA E FAGIOLI

Serves 2–3

  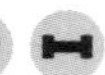

This recipe is dedicated to my nonna. When I was a kid, I remember growing up with the smell of this soup. It was my nonno's favourite, especially during the winter months, and Nonna used to welcome him home with a bowl of steaming *pasta e fagioli*. I remember he used to enjoy it with a drizzle of chilli oil (which I recommend you do too). I've tweaked the recipe slightly, but all the important bits are there! And don't forget Nonna's most important ingredient: love. *Buon appetito!*

2–3 tablespoons olive oil
1 small-medium carrot, diced
½ celery stick, diced
1 small onion, diced
2–3 garlic cloves, very finely
    chopped
½ teaspoon chilli (hot
    pepper) flakes
1 sprig of rosemary
4 tablespoons tomato purée (paste)
300g (10½oz) tinned drained
    borlotti (cranberry) beans
800ml (27fl oz/3⅓ cups)
    vegetable stock
1 bay leaf
150g (5½oz) short pasta,
    such as ditalini rigati,
    cavatelli or conchiglie
3 tablespoons nutritional yeast
Small handful of spinach
Salt and freshly ground
    black pepper

TO SERVE

Plant-based Parmesan-style
    cheese (see page 36, or use
    shop-bought; optional)
Chilli oil (optional)
Croutons (shop-bought
    or homemade)
Chilli (hot pepper) flakes

Heat the oil in a large saucepan over a medium heat and fry the carrot, celery, onion, garlic and chilli flakes for 5–8 minutes until soft and golden.

Add the sprig of rosemary, cook gently for a further 3–4 minutes to infuse the flavours, then reduce the heat to low, remove the rosemary and add the tomato purée. Stir to combine. Add the borlotti beans, stirring well to allow them to absorb the flavours, then gradually pour in the stock. Add the bay leaf and season with salt. Bring to the boil, then add the pasta, stir, cover and cook until the pasta is al dente.

Remove the pan from the heat and, if you like, mash some of the beans with a fork to create an even creamier, soup-like consistency.

Remove the bay leaf, add the nutritional yeast and spinach, season with salt and pepper and stir until the spinach has completely wilted. Add a splash of hot water or vegetable stock if it's too dry.

Serve in bowls with the plant-based Parmesan-style cheese and chilli oil (if using), croutons and chilli flakes.

NOTE

The soffritto base can be batch-cooked and used for many different recipes in this book. See page 34 for my pantry staple recipe.

PROTEIN PER SERVING	MAKE IT GLUTEN-FREE	STORAGE
29g	Use gluten-free pasta.	Store for up to 3 days in the refrigerator and up to 3 months in the freezer.

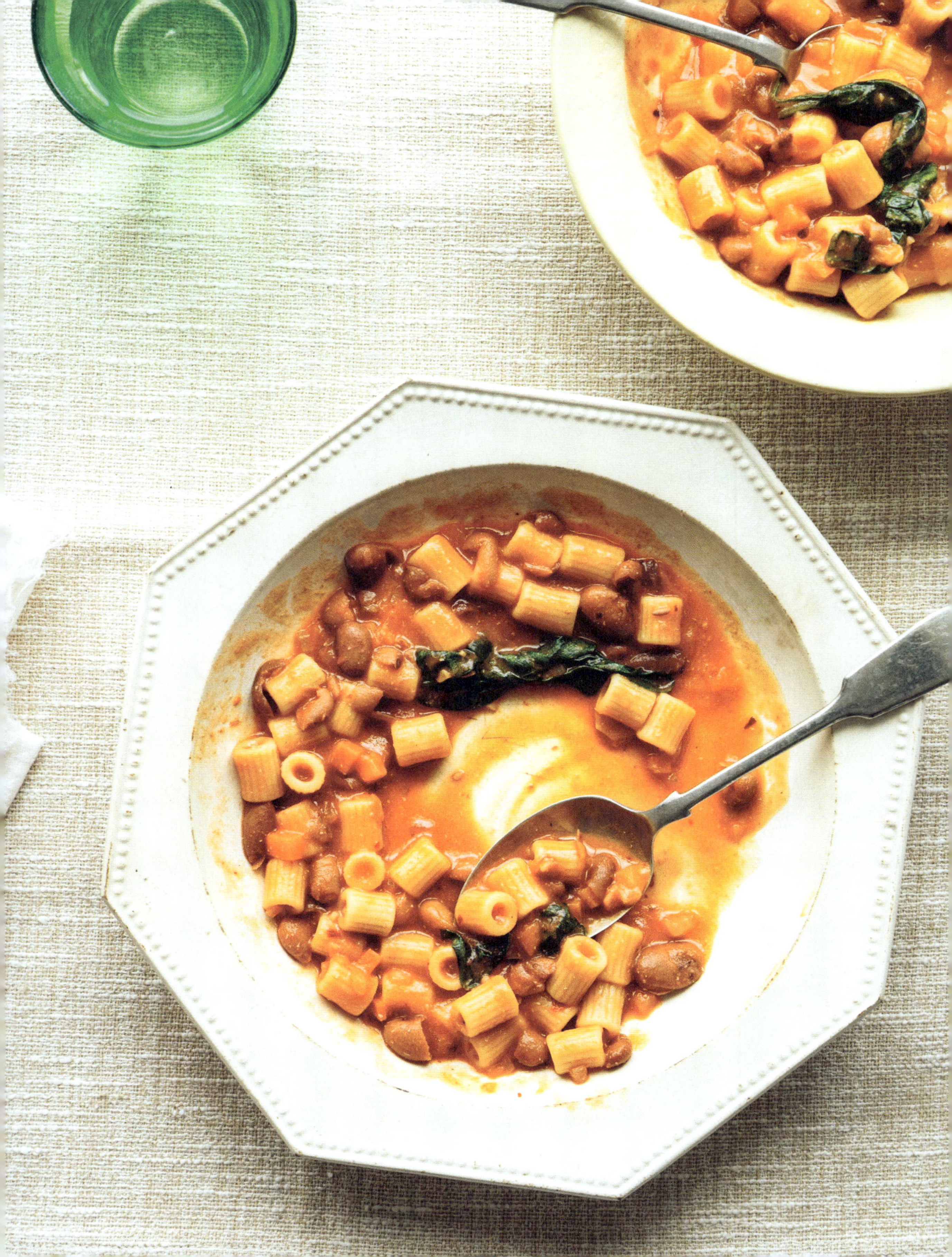

LIVE TO 100 MINESTRONE SOUP

Serves 3–4

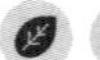  

1 small-medium carrot, diced
½ celery stick, diced
1 small onion, diced
2–3 garlic cloves, very
    finely chopped
100g (3½oz) fennel, finely chopped
1 sprig of rosemary
1 tablespoon tomato purée (paste)
100g (3½oz) fregola or conchigliette
1 small waxy potato (about
    150g/5½oz), peeled and cubed
800ml (27fl oz/3⅓ cups)
    vegetable stock
1 bay leaf
1 x 400g (14oz) tin of borlotti
    (cranberry) beans, drained
1 x 400g (14oz) tin of black
    beans, drained
Handful of cavolo nero (lacinato
    kale), stalks removed (or chard,
    cabbage or spinach)
30g (1oz) nutritional yeast
Olive oil, for cooking and drizzling
Salt and freshly ground
    black pepper
Plant-based Parmesan-style
    cheese (see page 36, or use
    shop-bought), to serve

According to the world's longest-living family, if you're aiming for a century of life, there's one dish you should prioritize: minestrone soup. A cornerstone of Italian cuisine, this hearty recipe combines vegetables, whole grains and legumes, delivering a comforting and nutritious meal that nourishes both body and soul. I can't guarantee it will mean you live to 100, but I can guarantee you'll love the taste!

Heat a good glug of oil in a large saucepan over a medium heat and fry the carrot, celery, onion, garlic, fennel, rosemary and tomato purée for 5–8 minutes until the vegetables are soft and golden.

Remove the rosemary, then add the pasta, potato, stock, bay leaf and borlotti and black beans. Stir to combine. Simmer for 15 minutes, or until the pasta is cooked and the potato is soft. Add the cavalo nero to the soup a couple of minutes before the end.

Remove the bay leaf and add the nutritional yeast, stir and season with salt and pepper to taste.

Serve with a drizzle of olive oil and a sprinkle of plant-based Parmesan-style cheese.

NOTES

The soffritto base can be batch-cooked and used for many different recipes in this book. See page 34 for my pantry staple recipe.

PROTEIN PER SERVING	MAKE IT GLUTEN-FREE	STORAGE
24g	Use gluten-free pasta.	Store for up to 3 days in the refrigerator and up to 3 months in the freezer.

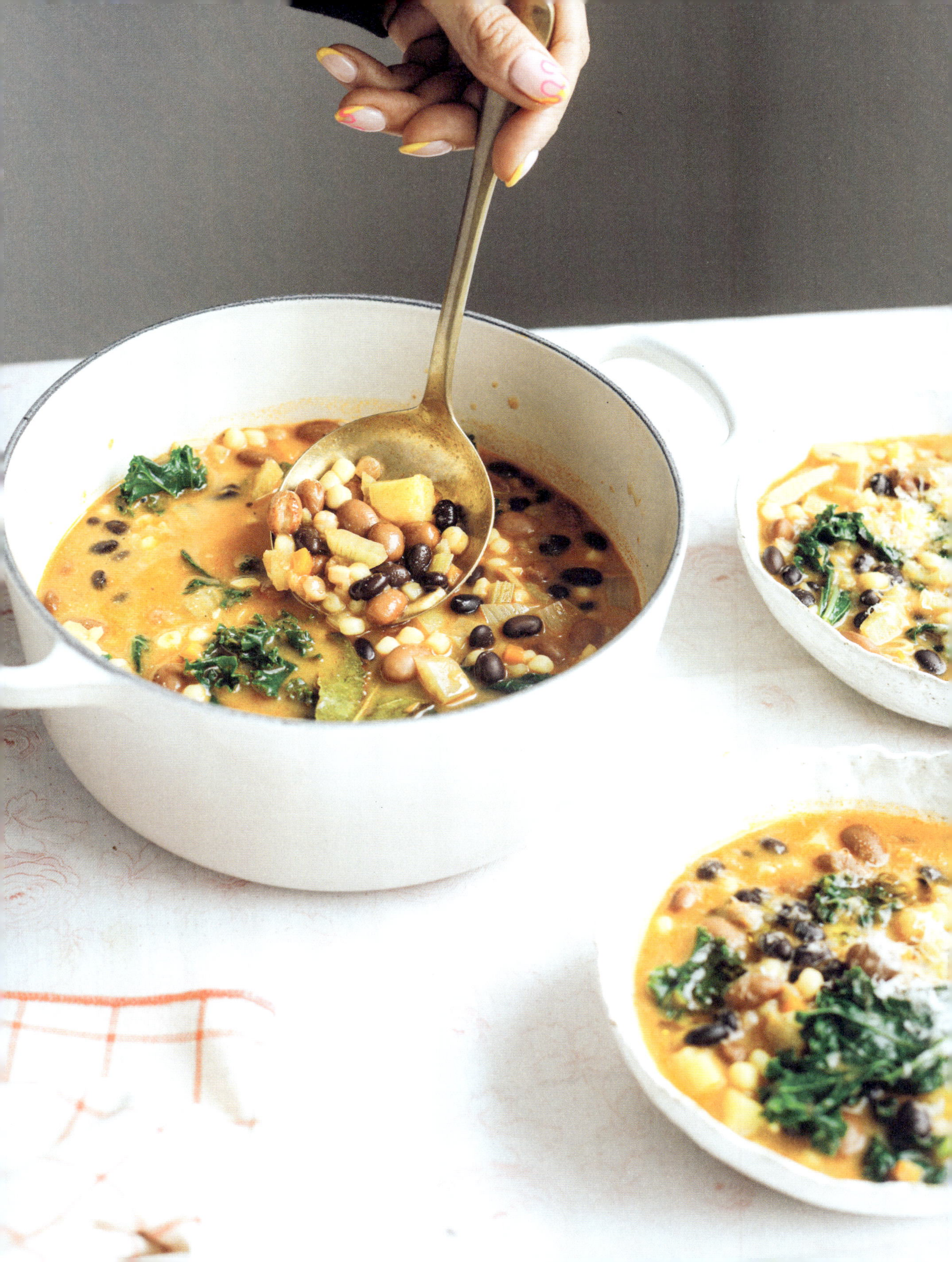

HARISSA-ROASTED TOMATO AND PEPPER SOUP WITH CRUNCHY BUTTER BEANS

Serves 2–3

  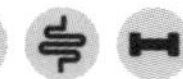

This is the perfect recipe for you when the day calls for soup but your schedule doesn't. In just a few simple steps you will be rewarded with a bowl of warmth and vitality. It's the perfect remedy for colder seasons, offering a soul-warming solution to your cravings.

1 x 400g (14oz) tin of butter (lima) beans, drained and patted dry
1 teaspoon smoked paprika
4–5 tomatoes, halved
2 red or orange (bell) peppers, sliced (or use jarred roasted peppers and skip the roasting)
1 red onion, halved
1 bulb of garlic
Few sprigs of thyme, leaves picked
1 tablespoon harissa paste
2 tablespoons olive oil, plus extra for drizzling
150g (5½oz) firm tofu, crumbled
300–350ml (10–11¾fl oz/1¼–1½ cups) vegetable stock
4 tablespoons nutritional yeast
Salt and freshly ground black pepper

TO SERVE
Plant-based sour cream or crème fraîche
Small handful of thyme
Small handful of basil
Sourdough or gluten-free bread, toasted

Preheat the oven to 200°C/180°C fan/400°F/Gas mark 6 and line two baking trays (pan) with baking parchment.

Put half the butter beans into a bowl and drizzle with olive oil, then sprinkle with the smoked paprika and a pinch of salt and pepper. Spread out on one of the prepared trays and cook in the oven for 30 minutes until crunchy. Alternatively, if you have an air fryer, you can air-fry the chickpeas at 200°C (400°F) for 15–20 minutes.

Arrange the tomatoes, peppers, onion and whole bulb of garlic on the second prepared tray and sprinkle with the thyme.

In a small bowl, combine the harissa paste and oil with a pinch of salt, and pepper. Mix thoroughly, then brush over the vegetables. Roast in the oven for 40–45 minutes until the vegetables are soft and juicy.

Once roasted, transfer the vegetables and their juices to a food processor. Squeeze the garlic cloves into the mixture and discard the skins. Add the remaining butter beans, the tofu, stock and nutritional yeast, and season with salt and pepper. Blend until creamy.

Ladle the soup into bowls, topping each with some of the crunchy butter beans. Drizzle with a touch of plant-based sour cream or crème fraiche and a final flourish of olive oil. Finish with a sprinkle of thyme and basil, and serve with toast.

PROTEIN PER SERVING	MAKE IT GLUTEN-FREE	STORAGE
30g	Use gluten-free bread.	Store for up to 3 days in the refrigerator and up to 3 months in the freezer without the butter beans.

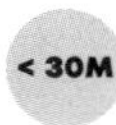

CHOPPED SANDWICH

Serves 1–2

One of the problems with sandwiches is that you don't often get all the flavours in a single bite. The solution? A chopped sandwich! You get a bit of everything in each mouthful, from the smoky richness of tofu and the intense sweetness of sun-dried tomatoes to the crisp freshness of lettuce and umami pesto. Perfect if you have only 10 minutes, it's a quick and satisfying meal option that doesn't compromise on taste or nutrition.

3 leaves of Little Gem lettuce
1 small tomato
¼ red onion, thinly sliced (optional)
150g (5½oz) smoked tofu
3 sun-dried tomatoes
2 tablespoons hummus
1 tablespoon vegan pesto
   (homemade or shop-bought)
Balsamic vinegar, for drizzling
1 small baguette

Put the lettuce, tomato, onion, tofu and sun-dried tomatoes onto a clean cutting board, then chop and mix everything together until finely diced and well combined.

Add the hummus, pesto and a drizzle of balsamic glaze and chop one more time to incorporate.

Halve and then slice open the baguette, then scoop a pile of the chopped ingredients into the baguette halves and serve.

PROTEIN PER SERVING

25g

MAKE IT GLUTEN-FREE

Use gluten-free bread.

STORAGE

Store for up to 3 days in the refrigerator. Not freezer friendly.

HARISSA TOFU CIABATTA

Serves 1

Harissa's unique flavour and hint of spice adds a special touch to any dish. In this recipe, we use its distinctive taste to turn simple tofu into something mouth-watering. Paired with a light lemon sauce in a soft ciabatta, this sandwich is a perfect balance of flavours and textures.

HARISSA TOFU

150g (5½oz) extra-firm tofu, drained and pressed (see page 37)
2 tablespoons harissa paste
1 tablespoon maple syrup
1 tablespoon olive oil

CREAMY LEMON SAUCE

50g (1¾oz/scant ¼ cup) high-protein plant-based yoghurt
Juice of ½ lemon
Pinch of salt

TO SERVE

1 small ciabatta
Small handful of spinach
Sliced cucumber

Preheat the oven to 220°C/200°C fan/425°F/Gas mark 7 and line a baking tray (pan) with baking parchment.

Slice the tofu into roughly 1cm (½ inch) thick slices, then score each piece in a criss-cross pattern on one side and transfer them to the prepared baking tray.

Combine the harissa paste, maple syrup and oil in a bowl and pour it over the tofu pieces, then use a spoon to push the sauce into the criss-cross incisions.

Bake the tofu in the oven for 15 minutes, then flip the slices and spoon the sauce on the tray over the unbaked side. Bake for a further 20 minutes

Slice open the ciabatta and add it to the oven for the last 6–9 minutes to toast.

Meanwhile, prepare the lemon sauce by whisking together all the ingredients in a bowl.

Spoon the lemon sauce on one side of the ciabatta, then top with the spinach, tofu and cucumber. Close and serve.

PROTEIN PER SERVING

30g

MAKE IT GLUTEN-FREE

Use gluten-free bread.

STORAGE

Store for up to 3 days in the refrigerator. Not freezer friendly.

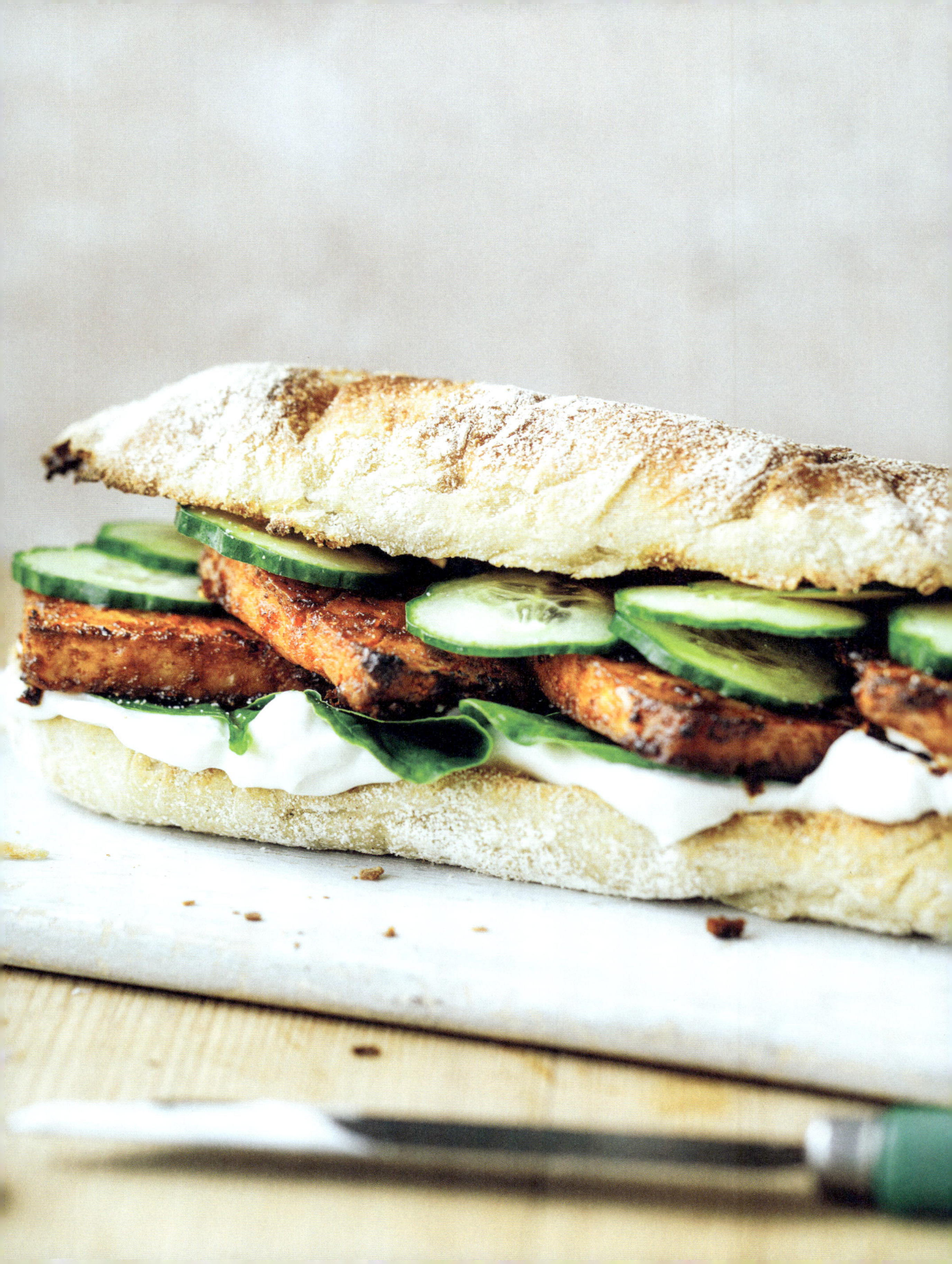

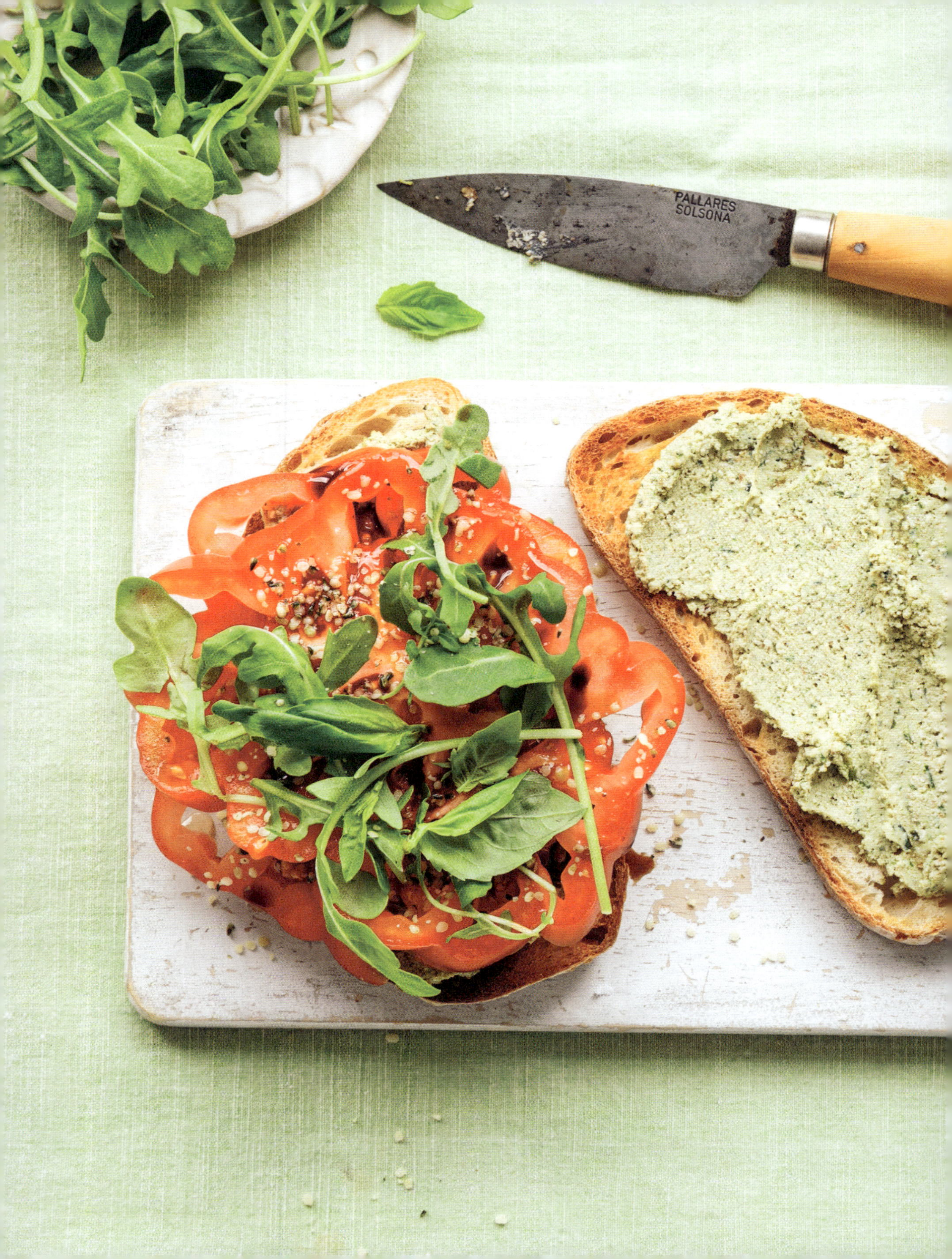
PALLARES
SOLSONA

 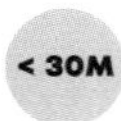

HEIRLOOM TOMATO SANDWICH WITH PESTO CREAM CHEESE

Serves 1

It may be the Italian in me, but there's nothing better than the taste of juicy, sweet tomatoes. In this recipe, I celebrate their unparalleled flavour. It's a delightful fusion of flavours and textures, where ripe, fresh tomatoes meet creamy tofu-based pesto cream cheese, nestled between slices of toasted sourdough. Italian summer in a bite!

2 slices of sourdough bread
Pinch of salt
Small handful of rocket (arugula)
2–3 thick slices of heirloom tomato
1 teaspoon shelled hemp seeds
Few basil leaves (optional)
Balsamic glaze, for drizzling
Olive oil, for drizzling

PESTO CREAM CHEESE
100g (3½oz) firm tofu, drained
10g (½oz) nutritional yeast
15g (½oz) walnuts
Small handful of basil leaves

First, make the pesto cream cheese. Combine all the ingredients in a food processor and blend until a thick paste forms.

Toast the bread, then drizzle the slices with olive oil and sprinkle with salt.

Spoon the cream cheese over both slices, then layer the rocket, sliced tomato and a drizzle of balsamic glaze on one. Sprinkle over the hemp seeds and basil leaves (if using), then top with the remaining slice of bread.

PROTEIN PER SERVING	MAKE IT GLUTEN-FREE	STORAGE
32g	Use gluten-free bread.	Store for up to 3 days in the refrigerator. Not freezer friendly.

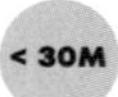

HOISIN TEMPEH AND ROASTED PEPPER SANDWICH

Serves 1

Tangy, sweet, salty and smoky, this sandwich has it all. It features tender hoisin-glazed tempeh, paired perfectly with the crisp crunch of cucumber and the richness of roasted peppers in seeded bread. Sure to hit the spot!

1 tablespoon hoisin sauce
½ tablespoon tomato purée (paste)
1 tablespoon maple syrup
1 tablespoon light soy sauce
100g (3½oz) tempeh, sliced
2 slices of seeded sourdough bread
2 tablespoons hummus
1–2 roasted (bell) peppers, sliced
    (from a jar or homemade)
¼ cucumber, sliced
Sesame oil, for frying
Sesame seeds (optional),
    for sprinkling

First, make the hoisin tempeh. Whisk together the hoisin sauce, tomato purée, maple syrup and soy sauce in a small bowl.

Heat a glug of sesame oil in a frying pan (skillet) over a medium heat, then fry the tempeh for 10–12 minutes until brown all over. Pour the sauce over the tempeh and wait for it to thicken, then remove the pan from the heat and set aside.

Toast the bread, then layer the hummus, roasted peppers, hoisin tempeh and cucumber on one slice. Top with sesame seeds (if using) and the remaining slice of bread.

PROTEIN PER SERVING	MAKE IT GLUTEN-FREE	STORAGE
27g	Use gluten-free bread, hoisin sauce and tamari.	Store for up to 3 days in the refrigerator. Not freezer friendly.

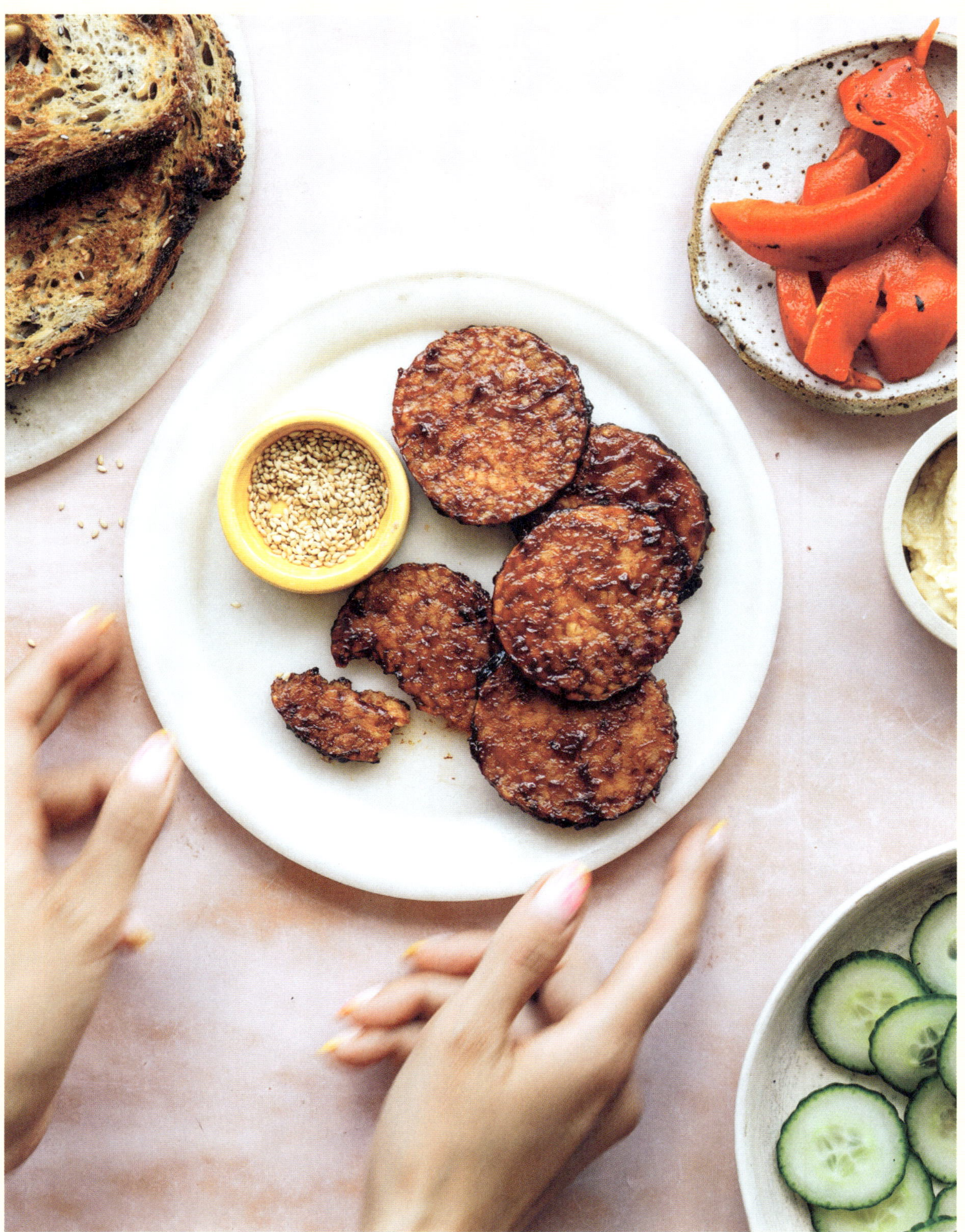

'MEATBALL' SUB

Serves 1–2

If I had to choose one sandwich for the rest of my life, it'd be this meatball sub. Bursting with flavour and texture, it combines hearty lentil 'meatballs' with a rich tomato sauce, all nestled within a warm baguette. It's a humble yet immensely satisfying dish that's sure to hit the spot.

LENTIL 'MEATBALLS'

150g (5½oz) drained tinned lentils
3 tablespoons dried breadcrumbs
5 sun-dried tomatoes, chopped
1 teaspoon Dijon mustard
½ teaspoon dried oregano
½ teaspoon dried basil
½ teaspoon dried parsley
3 tablespoons nutritional yeast
Polenta (cornmeal) or panko
   breadcrumbs, to coat
Olive oil, for cooking
Salt and freshly ground
   black pepper

TOMATO SAUCE

½ small-medium carrot, diced
½ celery stick, diced
¼ onion, diced
2–3 garlic cloves, very finely
   chopped
250g (9oz/1 cup) passata
   (sieved tomatoes)
Small handful of basil, plus
   extra to serve

TO SERVE

1 x 30cm (1ft) baguette or 2 bread
   rolls of your choice
Handful of chopped spinach
Plant-based Parmesan-style
   cheese (see page 36, or use
   shop-bought), to serve

First, make the meatballs. Combine all the ingredients except the breadcrumbs in a food processor along with a pinch of salt and pepper and blend until well combined.

Shape the mixture into three or four balls, then roll each one in the polenta or panko breadcrumbs.

Heat a good glug of oil in a deep frying pan (skillet) and pan-fry the meatballs for 10–15 minutes until golden all over, then remove from the pan and set aside.

Heat another glug of oil in the pan used for the meatballs and start the sauce. Add the carrot, celery, onion and garlic to the pan and fry for 5–8 minutes until soft and golden.

Add the passata and basil and season with salt and pepper. Simmer for 7–10 minutes until the flavours meld together.

Finally, add the meatballs to the sauce, gently coating them in the sauce (be careful, otherwise they might break) and simmer for a further 2–3 minutes.

Meanwhile, toast the baguette or bread rolls and slice open.

Place the chopped spinach on the bread, then generously ladle over the meatballs and tomato sauce. Sprinkle with plant-based Parmesan-style cheese and chopped basil and close.

PROTEIN PER SERVING	MAKE IT GLUTEN-FREE	STORAGE
30g	Use gluten-free bread and certified gluten-free polenta (cornmeal).	Store for up to 3 days in the refrigerator. The cooked meatballs can be frozen for up to 3 months.

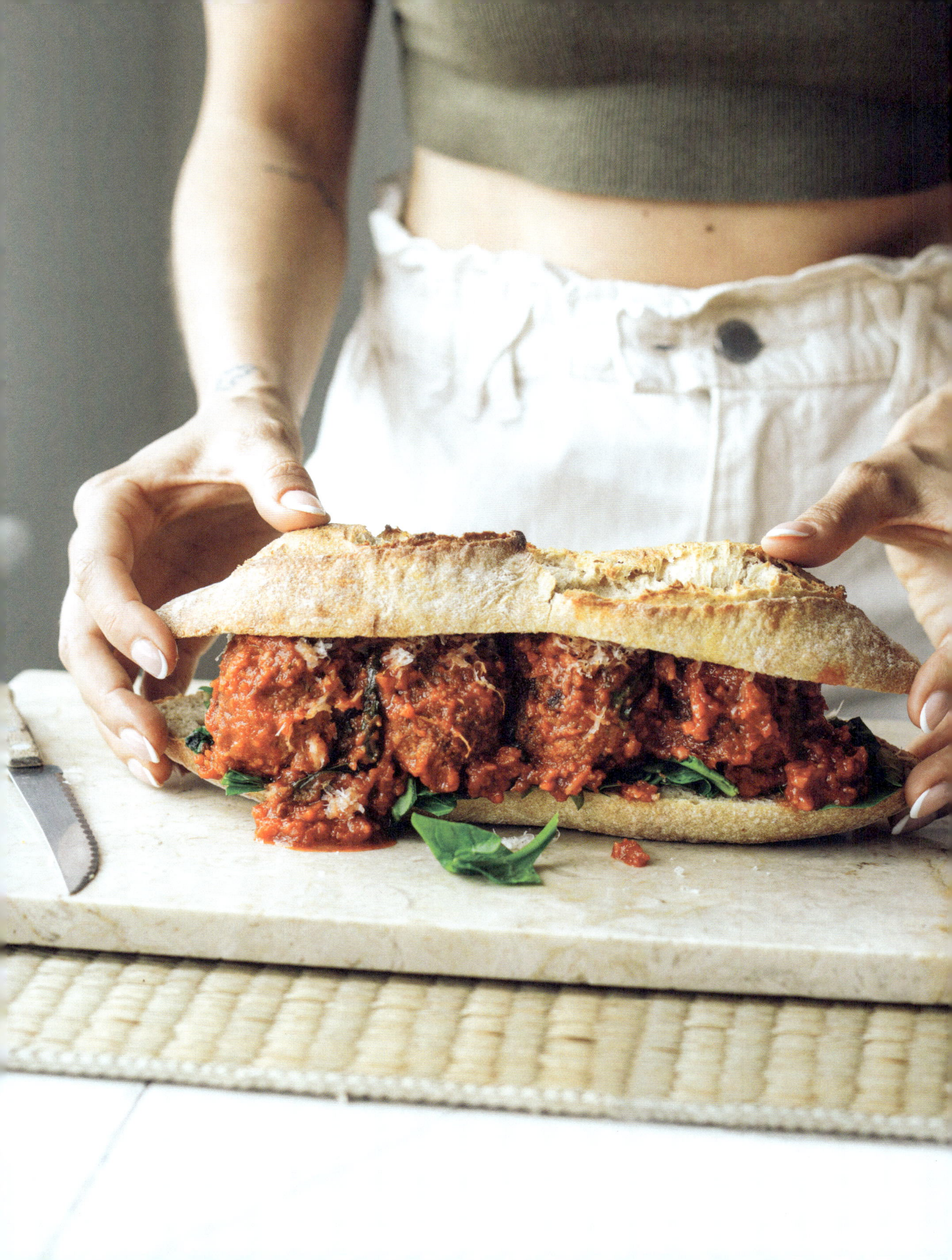

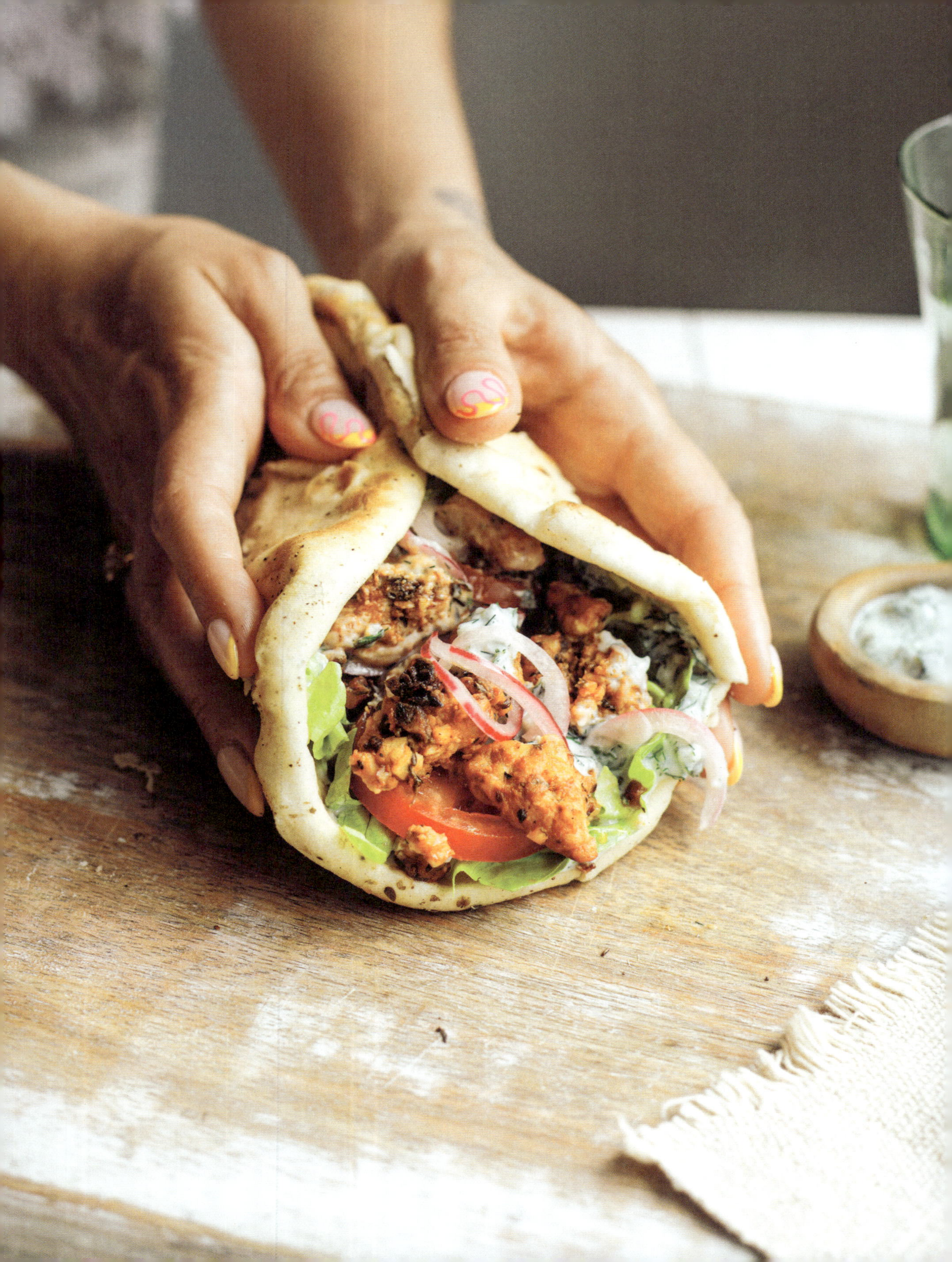

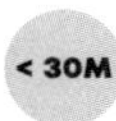

TEMPEH GYROS WITH TZATZIKI AND PROTEIN FLATBREAD

Serves 1

Finding time to prepare a satisfying and nutritious meal can feel like a daunting task, especially in the whirlwind of a hectic week! But fear not, this Greek-inspired tempeh gyros is the perfect solution! The zesty tzatziki combines with the juicy marinated tempeh to create a quick and easy lunch that is straight from the islands of Greece.

TEMPEH GYROS

80g (2¾oz/scant ⅓ cup) high-protein plant-based yoghurt
50ml (1¾fl oz/3½ tablespoons) warm vegetable stock
1 tablespoon tomato purée (paste)
1 tablespoon thyme leaves
1 tablespoon dried oregano
2 tablespoon light soy sauce
Juice of ½ lemon
100g (3½oz) tempeh, crumbled
Olive oil, for frying

TZATZIKI

1 thumb-sized piece of cucumber, grated (shredded) and squeezed
80g (2¾oz/scant ⅓ cup) high-protein Greek-style plant-based yoghurt
Small handful of dill, finely chopped
Small handful of mint, finely chopped
2 tablespoons lemon juice
1 garlic clove, very finely chopped or grated (optional)
½ teaspoon salt

TO SERVE

1 Tofu Flatbread (see page 164) or Middle Eastern flatbread, or 2 small pitas
Lettuce
Sliced tomato
Sliced red onions (fresh or pickled)

First, make the tempeh gyros. Mix together the yoghurt, warm stock, tomato purée, thyme, oregano, soy sauce and lemon juice in a bowl, then stir through the crumbled tempeh. Set aside to marinate while you make the tzatziki.

Meanwhile, combine all the ingredients for the tzatziki in a bowl.

Heat a small glug of oil in a frying pan (skillet) over a low heat and add the tempeh, discarding the excess marinade. Fry for 10–12 minutes until all the moisture has evaporated and the tempeh starts to brown. Don't flip it too often otherwise it may crumble too much.

Warm the flatbread or pita, then spread over generous layer of tzatziki. Top with lettuce, the tempeh gyros, tomatoes and onion, then serve.

PROTEIN PER SERVING	MAKE IT GLUTEN-FREE	STORAGE
35g	Use gluten-free bread and tamari.	Store for up to 3 days in the refrigerator. The tempeh gyros can be frozen for up to 3 months.

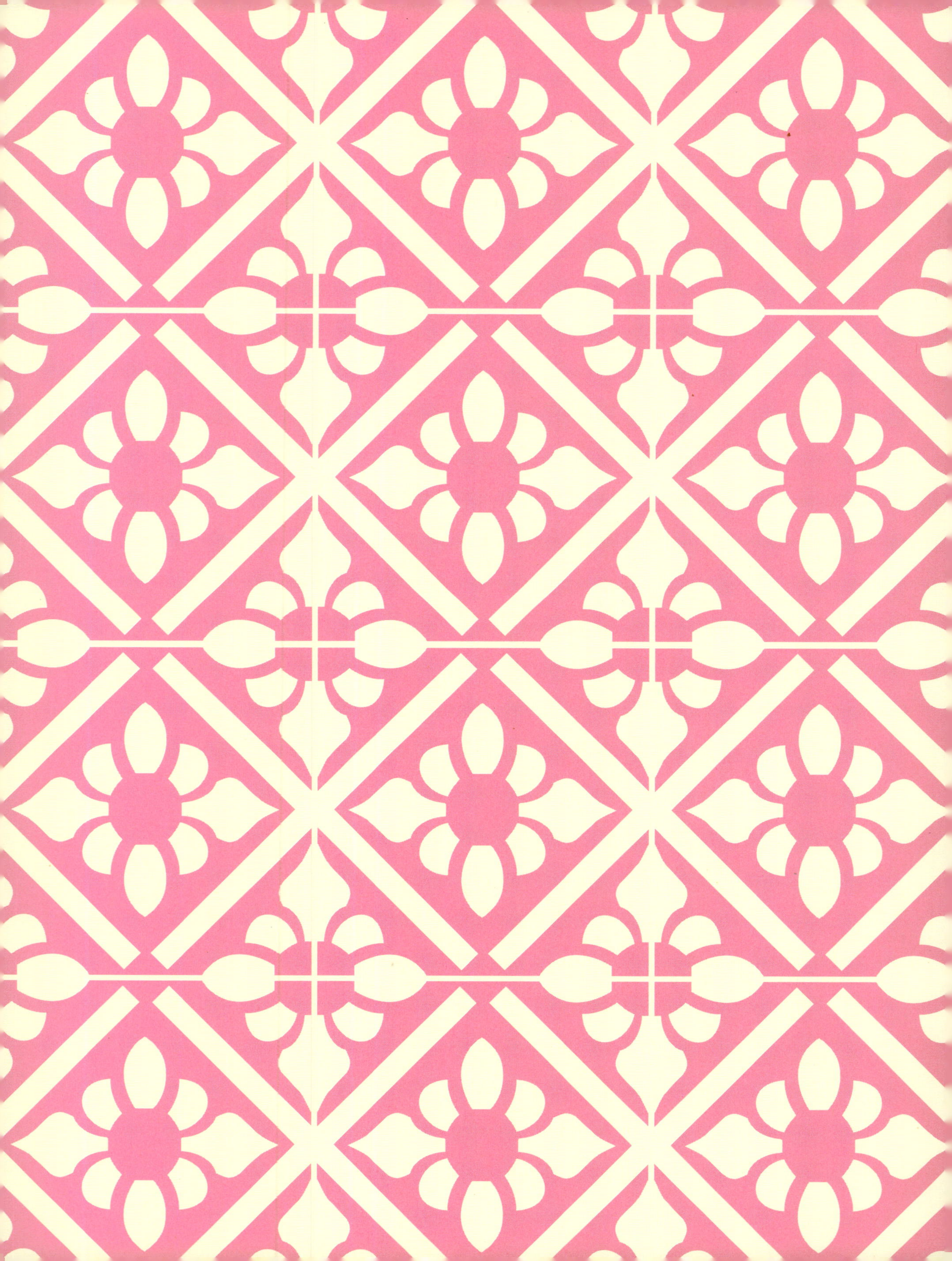

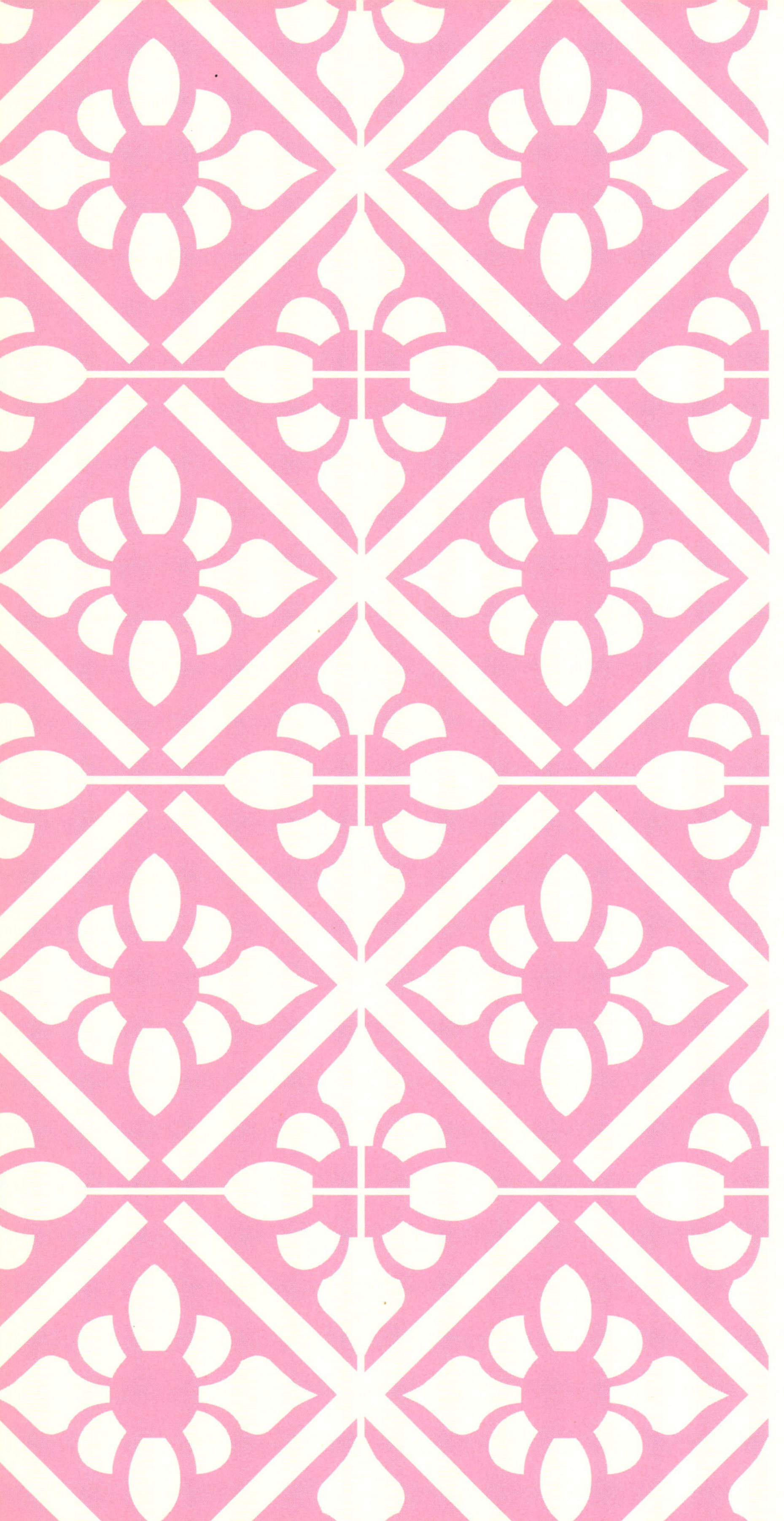

DINNERS

TOFU GNOCCHI WITH ITALIAN-STYLE TOMATO SAUCE

Serves 2–3

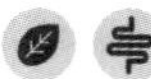

I have a deep love for gnocchi (comes with being Italian, I guess!) but I often wondered how to make an alternative that is high in protein. That is how these gnocchi were born! Don't worry, even if you have never made fresh pasta before, these gnocchi are very easy to make and don't require any specific tools (just willingness to knead!). And did someone mention the sauce? It's a ticket straight to Italy. *Buon appetito!*

GNOCCHI
300g (10½oz) firm tofu, drained
3 tablespoons nutritional yeast
200g (7oz/1⅔ cups) plain (all-purpose) flour, plus extra for dusting
1 tablespoon oil
Pinch of salt
Pinch of onion granules (optional)

TOMATO SAUCE
1 small-medium carrot, diced
½ celery stick, diced
1 small onion, diced
2–3 garlic cloves, very finely chopped
1 sprig of rosemary
1 sprig of sage (optional)
1 x 400g (14oz) tin of chopped tomatoes
Splash of vegetable stock
Small handful of basil, plus extra to serve
3–4 tablespoons nutritional yeast
Olive oil, for cooking
Salt and freshly ground black pepper
Plant-based Parmesan-style cheese (see page 36, or use shop-bought), to serve

NOTE
The soffritto base can be batch-cooked and used for many different recipes in this book. See page 34 for my pantry staple recipe.

To make the gnocchi, put the tofu and nutritional yeast into a food processor and blend to a paste.

Transfer the blended tofu to a bowl, then gradually incorporate the flour, followed by all the remaining ingredients. Mix thoroughly with a fork, then use your hands to gently form into a dough.

Transfer the dough to a well-floured work surface. It is important that you keep your surface floured as it will prevent the dough from sticking to it. While you knead, sprinkle the dough with more flour as needed (this will stop your hands getting too sticky). Knead the dough until it is uniform and has come together fully but is not dense or dry.

Divide the dough into two or three portions and then roll each portion into a long, rope-like shape, about 1cm (½ inch) in diameter. Cut the ropes into bite-sized gnocchi, about 2cm (1 inch) long. Set the gnocchi aside on a lightly floured surface, separated from each other and away from direct heat.

Next, make the sauce. Heat a good glug of oil in a large saucepan over a medium heat and fry the carrot, celery, onion, garlic, rosemary and sage (if using) for 5–8 minutes until soft and golden. Remove the rosemary and sage and add the chopped tomatoes and a splash of stock. Season with salt and pepper, then add the basil and cook for 10 minutes, stirring regularly. Finally, stir in the nutritional yeast.

Bring a large saucepan of salted water to the boil, then drop the gnocchi into the boiling water and cook until they float to the surface. This usually takes about 1 minute. To avoid the gnocchi sticking to each other while cooking, you can boil them in batches. Drain the gnocchi using a slotted spoon and add to the sauce, then allow to warm through for a couple of minutes. Serve hot with plant-based Parmesan-style cheese and more basil.

PROTEIN PER SERVING	MAKE IT GLUTEN-FREE	STORAGE
38g	Swap the plain (all-purpose) flour for 170g (6oz/1½ cups) chickpea (gram) flour.	Store for up to 3 days in the refrigerator. Freeze the uncooked gnocchi (not touching each other) and sauce separately for up to 3 months.

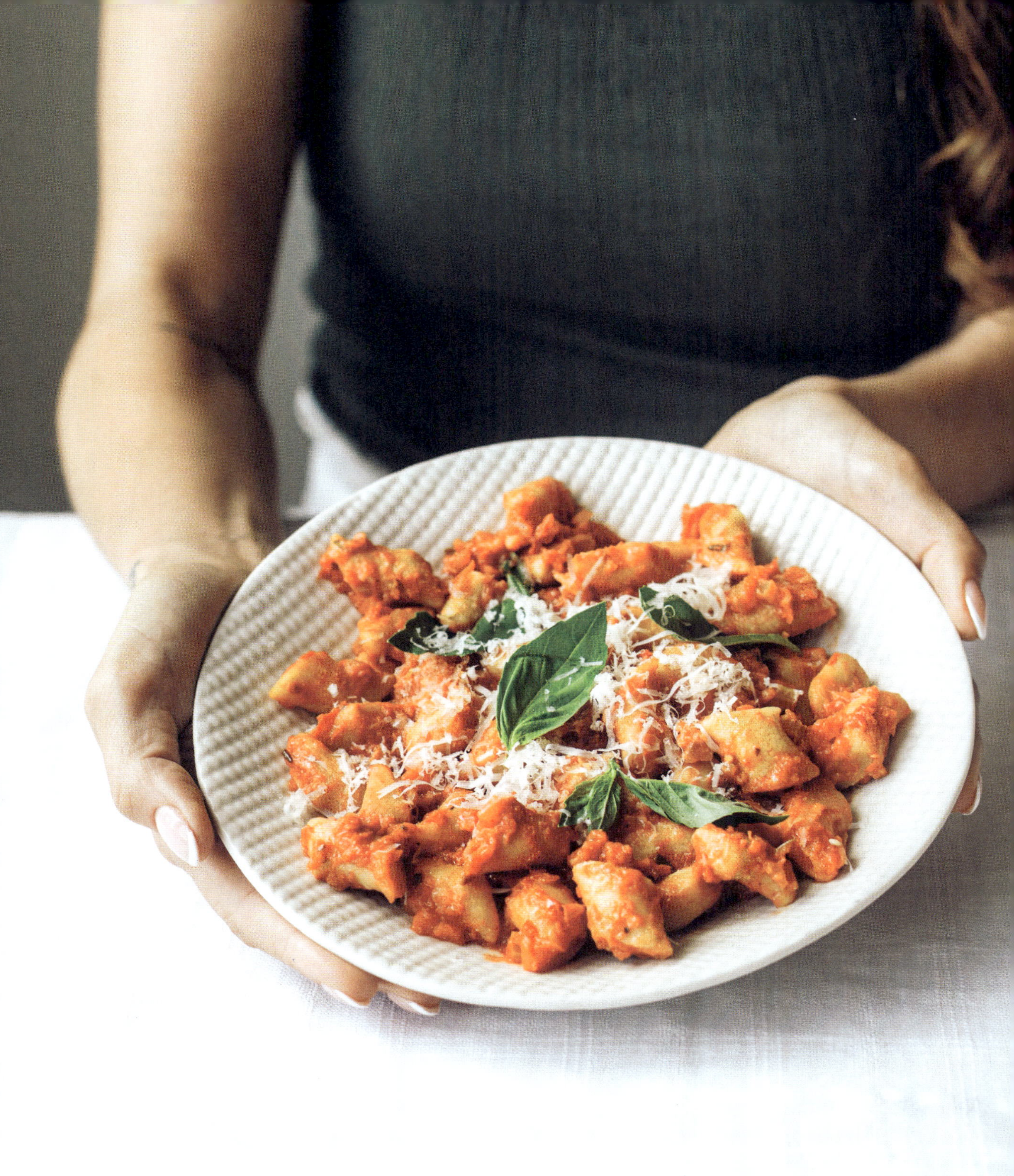

CHICKPEA GNOCCHI WITH BROCCOLI AND MINT PESTO

Serves 2–3

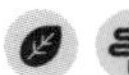

Making your own gnocchi sounds daunting, but fear not – these chickpea (garbanzo) gnocchi are a breeze to whip up! They offer a delightful change from the traditional potato gnocchi, providing a boost of fibre and protein from the chickpeas. While they come together harmoniously with all your favourite pasta sauces, I have gone with a springy broccoli pesto sauce featuring pistachios and a bit of zing from fresh mint.

GNOCCHI

1 x 400g (14oz) tin of chickpeas (garbanzos), drained
2 tablespoons olive oil
50g (1¾oz/scant ½ cup) plain (all-purpose) flour, plus extra as needed
1 tablespoon nutritional yeast
½ teaspoon onion granules (optional)
Salt and freshly ground black pepper

BROCCOLI AND MINT PESTO

½ broccoli (about 150g/5½oz), roughly chopped
Small handful of mint leaves
40g (1½oz) nutritional yeast
30ml (2 tablespoons) olive oil, plus extra for frying
2 tablespoons pine nuts
Pinch of salt
3 garlic cloves, very finely chopped
1 teaspoon chilli (hot pepper) flakes (optional)

TOPPINGS

Toasted pistachios, crushed

First, make the gnocchi. Combine the chickpeas, oil and a pinch of salt and pepper in a food processor and blend until smooth.

Transfer the mixture to a bowl, then gradually add the flour and nutritional yeast, gently kneading until a dough forms. Add more flour if needed, and avoiding overworking the dough.

Divide the dough into two portions and then roll each one into a long, rope-like shape, about 1cm (½ inch) in diameter. Cut the ropes into bite-sized gnocchi, about 2cm (1 inch) long. Set the gnocchi aside on a lightly floured surface, separated from each other and away from direct heat.

Next, make the sauce. Bring a saucepan of water to the boil and cook the broccoli for about 8 minutes until soft.

Transfer the cooked broccoli to a food processor and add the mint leaves, nutritional yeast, oil, pine nuts, 50ml (1¾fl oz/3½ tablespoons) water and pinch of salt and blend until smooth.

Heat a glug of olive oil in a deep frying pan (skillet) over a medium heat and fry the garlic and chilli flakes (if using) for a couple of minutes. Add the broccoli mixture, stir and keep warm while you cook the gnocchi.

Bring a large saucepan of salted water to the boil, then drop the gnocchi into the boiling water and cook for 2–3 minutes until they float to the surface. Drain the gnocchi using a slotted spoon and add to the sauce along with a ladle of the gnocchi water, then stir and allow to warm through for a couple of minutes.

Serve hot, topped with pistachios.

PROTEIN PER SERVING

20g

MAKE IT GLUTEN-FREE

Use gluten-free flour.

STORAGE

Store for up to 3 days in the refrigerator. Freeze the uncooked gnocchi (not touching each other) and sauce separately for up to 3 months.

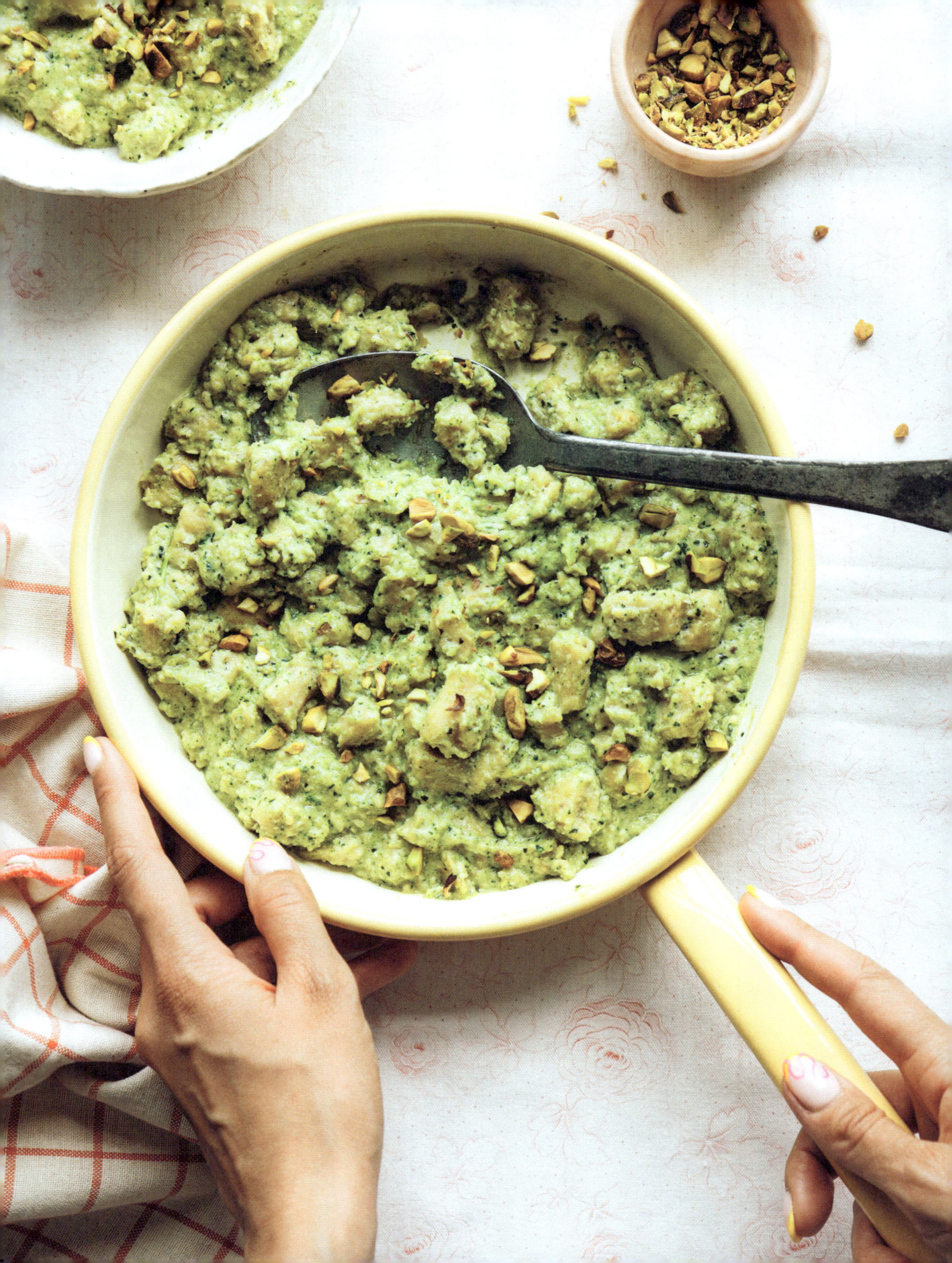

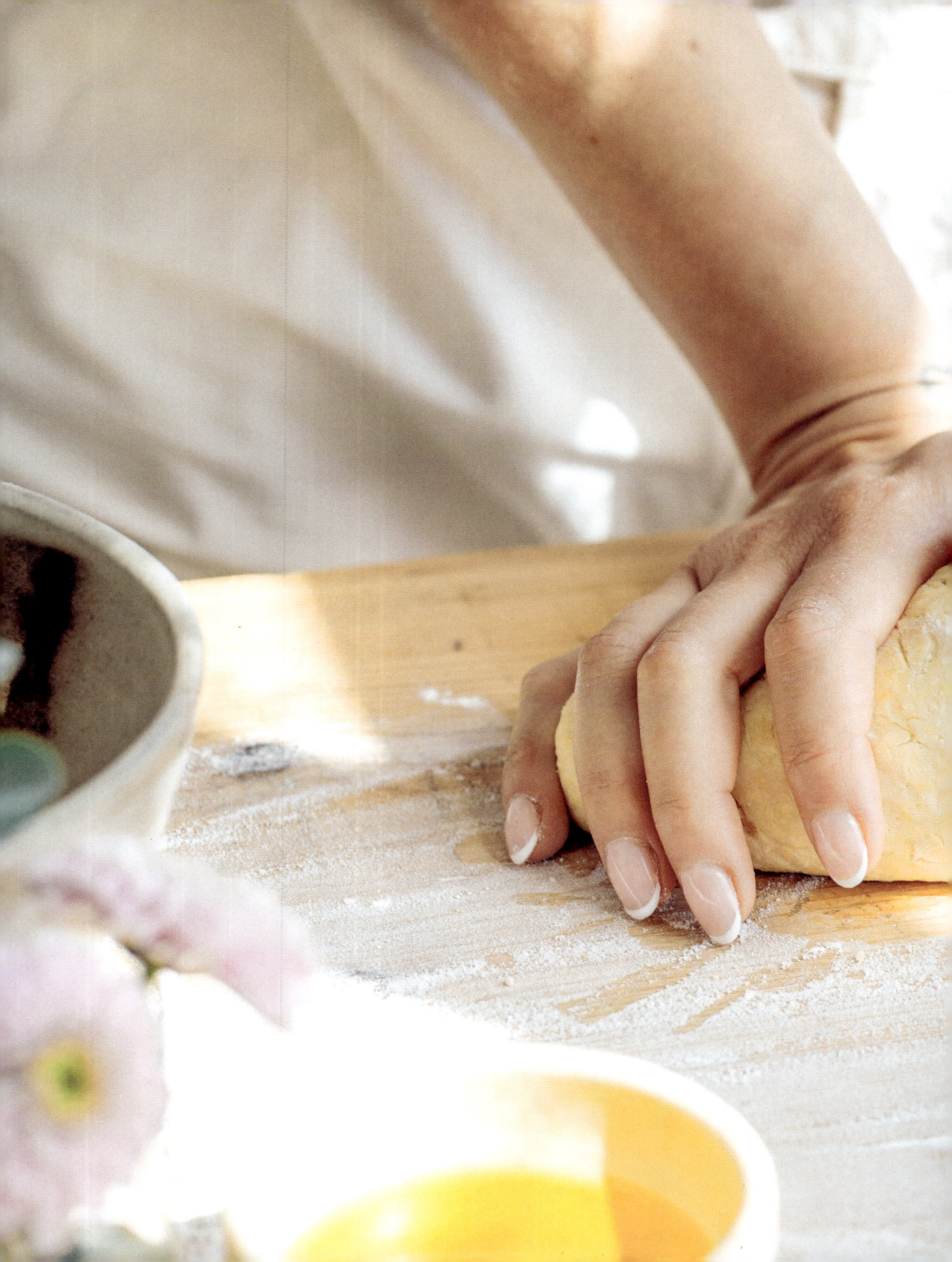

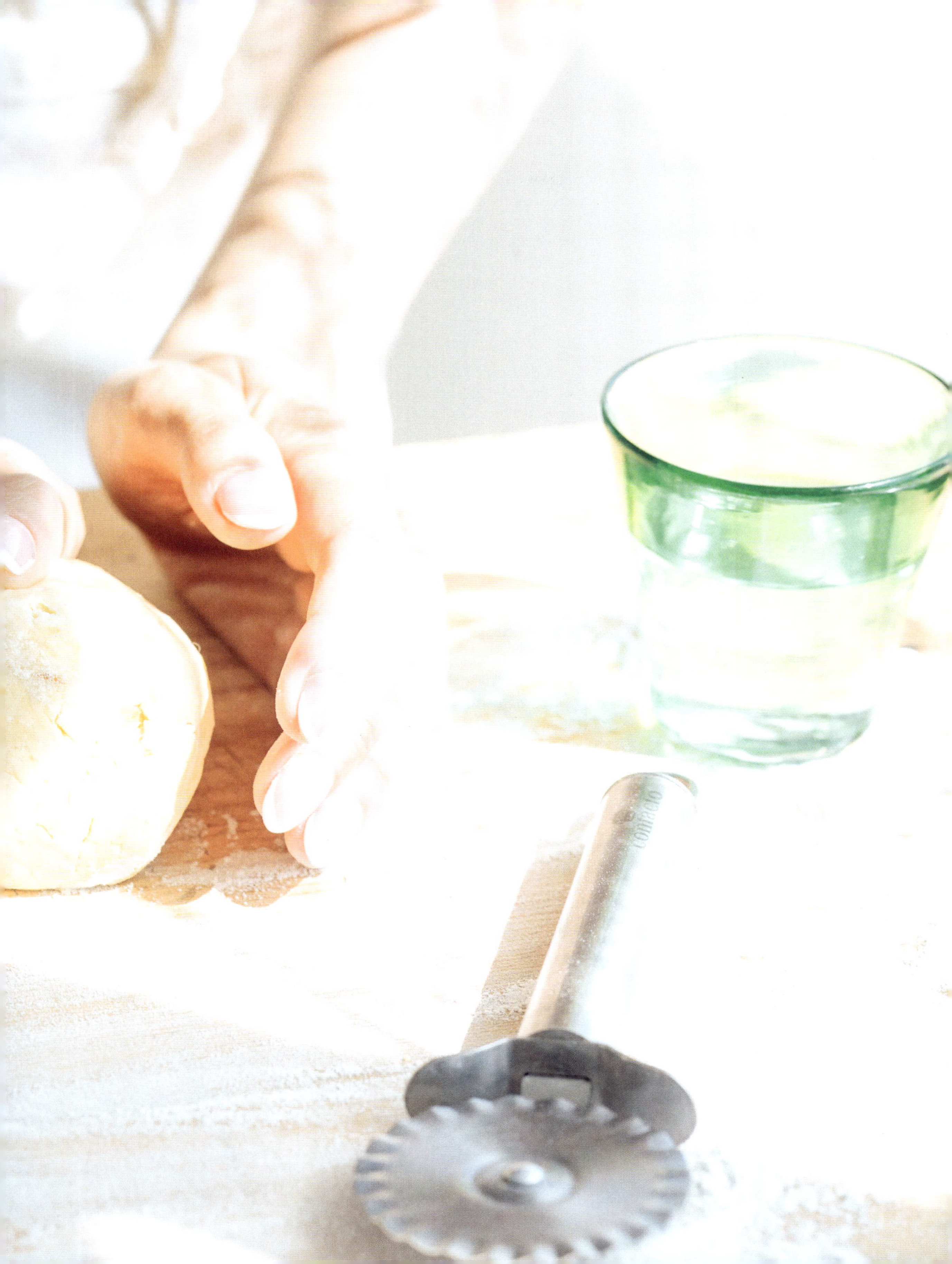

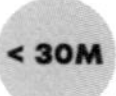

SMOKED TOFU CARBONARA

Serves 2

Pasta alla carbonara has a special place in my heart. When I was a kid, my dad used to take me on his work trips to Rome and we would stay in a hotel in the Vatican City and dine in a little family run *taverna* nearby, which used to make a special carbonara. It was our tradition and a happy memory I'll always treasure in my heart. When I became vegan I gave up guanciale, eggs and pecorino cheese, but I perfected this recipe to capture the same lip-smacking experience. It uses smoked tofu and kala namak (black salt) to recreate that iconic smoky, rich and eggy flavour I remember from my trips with my dad.

200g (7oz) smoked tofu, drained and pressed (see page 37)
3 tablespoons light soy sauce
1 tablespoon maple syrup
1 tablespoon tomato purée (paste)
½ teaspoon smoked paprika
250g (9oz) mezze maniche pasta
200g (7oz) silken tofu
150ml (5fl oz/scant ⅔ cup) soya milk
2 tablespoons nutritional yeast
1 teaspoon cornflour (cornstarch)
½ teaspoon kala namak (black salt)
½ teaspoon ground turmeric
Olive oil, for cooking

TO SERVE
Freshly ground black pepper
Plant-based Parmesan-style cheese (see page 36, or use shop-bought)

Cut half of the smoked tofu into 1cm (½ inch) cubes.

In a container, combine the soy sauce, maple syrup, tomato purée and paprika. Mix to combine, then add the cubed tofu, mixing well ensuring even coating. Cover and set aside to marinade.

Bring a large saucepan of generously salted water to the boil and cooking the pasta according to the packet instructions.

While the pasta is cooking, prepare the creamy sauce. Combine the silken tofu, the remaining smoked tofu, soya milk, nutritional yeast, cornflour, kala namak and turmeric in a food processor and blend until smooth and creamy.

Heat a good glug of oil in a frying pan (skillet) and add the cubed tofu and the marinade. Fry for 5–6 minutes, or until the tofu starts to brown.

When the pasta is cooked, drain it, reserving half a ladle of pasta water.

Add the pasta and reserved pasta water back to the pan along with the creamy sauce and stir over a low heat for about 30 seconds until the sauce has thickened a little and is evenly coating the pasta. Don't heat it too long or it might thicken too much and become clumpy.

Serve topped with the smoky tofu, a generous pinch of black pepper and plant-based Parmesan-style cheese.

PROTEIN PER SERVING
43g

MAKE IT GLUTEN-FREE
Use gluten-free pasta and tamari.

STORAGE
Store for up to 3 days in the refrigerator and up to 3 months in the freezer.

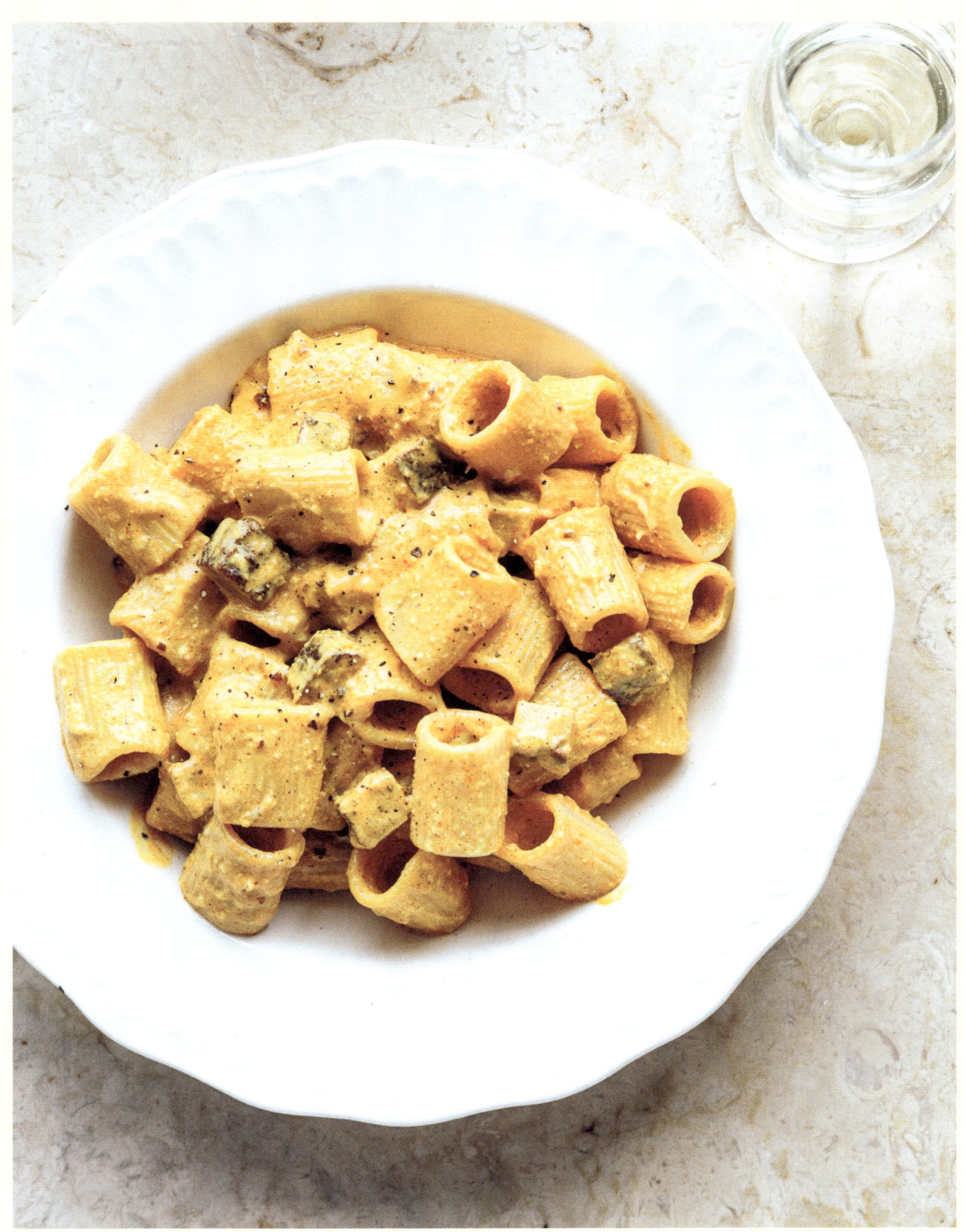

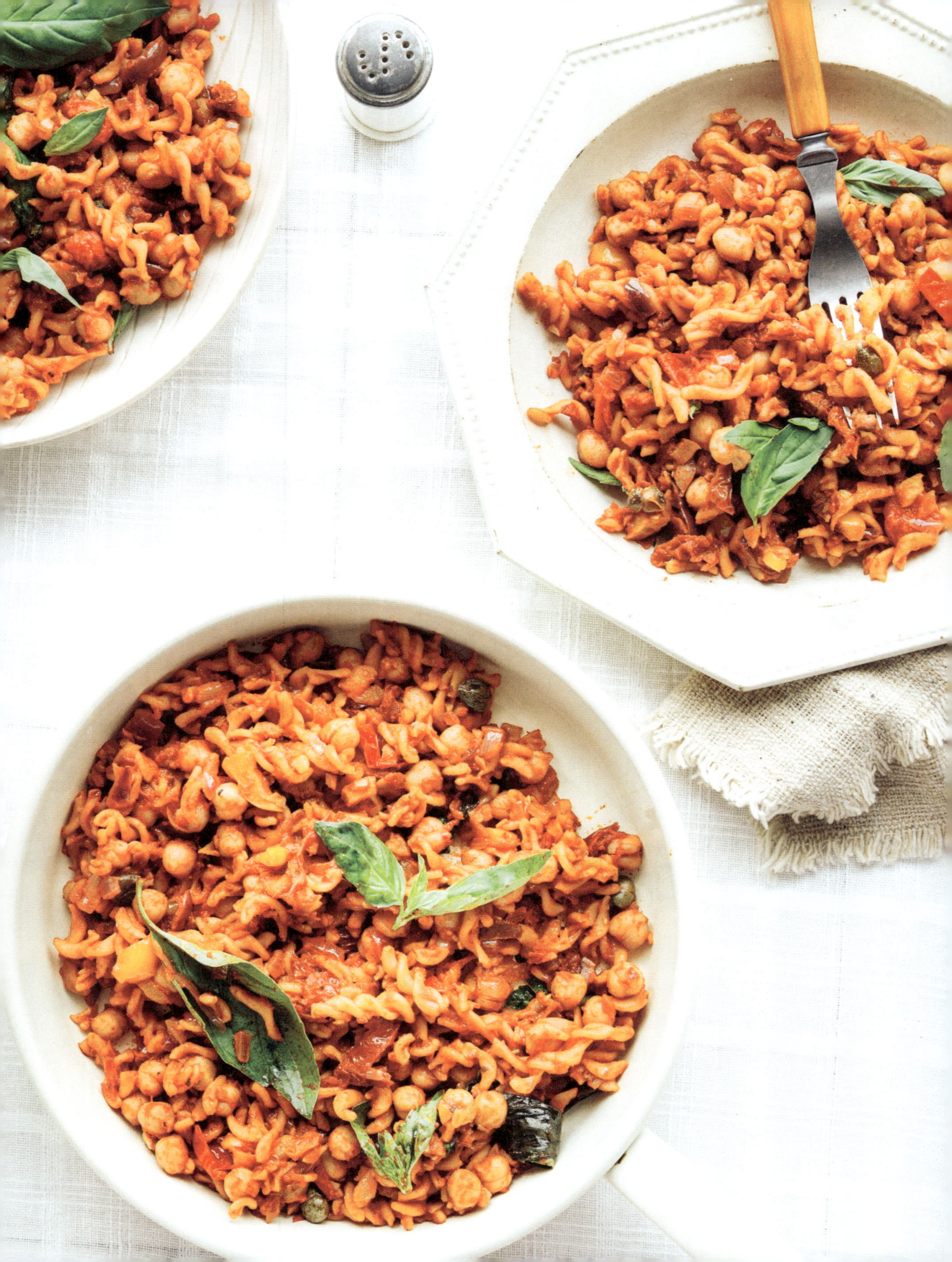

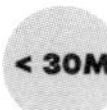

SALTY DELICIOUS RED LENTIL PASTA

Serves 2–3

  GF

This recipe is dedicated to Bryn, as it's actually a tweaked version of his own recipe. Legend has it that he used to make this recipe for his roommates when he was studying in New Zealand and got such positive reviews that when we started dating, he made the famous 'salty delicious' for me too. It was the first time he cooked for me, but it was a huge success! It is a take on spaghetti puttanesca and combines sun-dried tomatoes, black olives, capers and tomatoes with chickpeas for body and protein. It's such an easy win and it comes together in less than 30 minutes!

1 red onion, finely chopped
2–3 garlic cloves, very
    finely chopped
1 teaspoon chilli (hot pepper) flakes
150g (5½oz) cherry tomatoes
300g (10½oz/generous ¾ cup)
    passata (sieved tomatoes)
1 yellow (bell) pepper, chopped
360g (12½oz) drained tinned
    chickpeas (garbanzos)
10 sun-dried tomatoes, chopped
Handful of kalamata olives, pitted
    and chopped
1 teaspoon salted capers
200g (7oz) red lentil fusilli
Small handful of basil
Olive oil, for frying
Salt and freshly ground
    black pepper

TO SERVE
Small handful of rocket (arugula)
    or basil
Plant-based Parmesan-style
    cheese (see page 36, or use
    shop-bought)

Heat a good glug of oil in a saucepan over a medium heat and fry the onion, garlic and chilli flakes for 5–8 minutes until softened.

Add the cherry tomatoes, passata, yellow pepper, chickpeas, sun-dried tomatoes, olives and capers and simmer for 10 minutes until the tomatoes start to break down.

Meanwhile, bring a large saucepan of salted water to the boil and cook the pasta according to the packet instructions, then drain.

Add the pasta to the sauce along with the basil and stir to combine. Season with salt and pepper to taste.

Serve topped with rocket or basil and a generous sprinkle of plant-based Parmesan-style cheese.

PROTEIN PER SERVING

30g

STORAGE

Store for up to 3 days in the refrigerator and up to 3 months in the freezer.

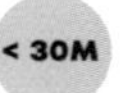

CREAMY HIGH-PROTEIN SPINACH MAFALDINE

Serves 2–3

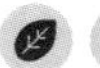 

This recipe ticks so many boxes. It's quick, it's high in protein, it's rich in iron and vitamins, it's a great source of fibre and it will stand out thanks to its bright colour. Perfect for those quick weeknight dinners when you need to fight off the blues of the week.

200g (7oz) mafaldine pasta
1 small onion, diced
2 garlic cloves, very finely chopped
½ teaspoon chilli (hot pepper) flakes
260g (9¼oz) baby spinach
150g (5½oz) silken tofu
2 tablespoons shelled hemp seeds, plus extra to serve
3–4 tablespoons nutritional yeast
Olive oil, for cooking
Salt and freshly ground black pepper
Plant-based Parmesan-style cheese (see page 36, or use shop-bought), to serve

Bring a large saucepan of salted water to the boil and cook the pasta according to the packet instructions.

While the pasta cooks, make the sauce. Heat a generous glug of oil in a deep frying pan (skillet) and fry the onion, garlic and chilli flakes for 5–8 minutes until the onion is soft. Add the spinach and stir until fully wilted.

Transfer the cooked spinach mixture to a food processor and add the silken tofu, hemp seeds, nutritional yeast, a pinch of salt and pepper and a ladle of the pasta water. Blend until smooth.

Pour the blended sauce back into the pan that you cooked the spinach in. Drain the pasta, reserving a little pasta water, and add it to the pan and stir until well combined. If the pasta sauce is too thick for your taste, just add a splash more pasta water until you get to the desired texture.

Serve the pasta with a sprinkling of hemp seeds and plant-based Parmesan-style cheese.

PROTEIN PER SERVING

32g

MAKE IT GLUTEN-FREE

Use gluten-free pasta

STORAGE

Store for up to 3 days in the refrigerator and up to 3 months in the freezer.

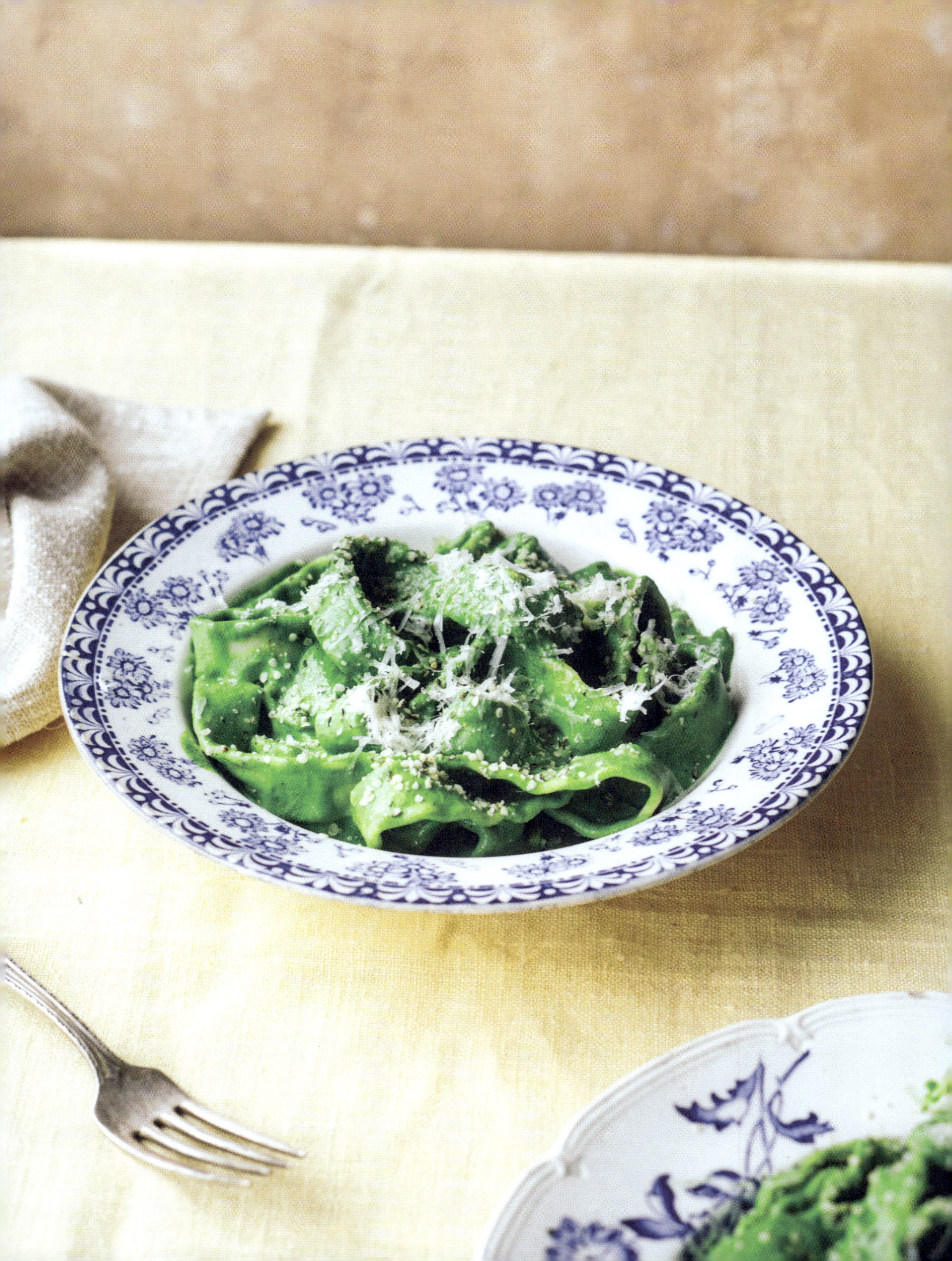

CREAMY MISO MUSHROOM FARFALLE WITH CRISPY TOFU

Serves 2–3

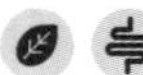

Did you know that a simple kitchen hack can significantly increase the protein content of your pasta dishes? This simple and yummy pasta recipe gets a sneaky protein boost from the crispy tofu – it adds nutrients but also flavour and texture. What's more, it's ready in under 30 minutes, so it's great for midweek dinners (and any leftovers are perfect for lunch, too!).

70g (2½oz) smoked tofu, drained and pressed (see page 37), then grated (shredded)

2 tablespoons dried breadcrumbs

½ teaspoon each of any spice you like (I added onion granules and Italian herbs)

1 tablespoon plant-based butter

2 garlic cloves, very finely chopped

200g (7oz) mushrooms of your choice (chestnut/cremini or button mushrooms work well), sliced

230g (8¼oz) farfalle

200g (7oz) silken tofu

2 tablespoons white miso paste

100ml (3½fl oz/scant ½ cup) unsweetened soya milk (or any unsweetened milk alternative)

3 tablespoons nutritional yeast

1 teaspoon light soy sauce

Olive oil, for cooking

Salt and freshly ground black pepper

Small handful of flat-leaf parsley, chopped, to serve

Heat a good glug of olive oil in a deep frying pan (skillet) over a medium heat, then add the grated smoked tofu, breadcrumbs and spices. Cook for 8–10 minutes, stirring frequently, until the tofu has reduced, most of the moisture has evaporated and it is golden. Remove from the pan and set aside.

In the same pan, heat the plant-based butter. Once melted, add the garlic and mushrooms. Sauté for about 10 minutes until the mushrooms are golden brown and the garlic is fragrant.

Meanwhile, bring a large saucepan of salted water to the boil and cook the pasta according to the packet instructions until al dente, then drain.

Combine the silken tofu, white miso paste and soya milk in a food processor and blend until smooth and creamy.

Pour the creamy tofu mixture into the pan with the mushrooms and stir to combine. Let it simmer gently for a few minutes to allow the flavours to meld together, then stir in the nutritional yeast and soy sauce. Season with salt and pepper to taste.

Add the cooked farfalle to the pan and toss until the pasta is evenly coated with the sauce and everything is warmed through. If the sauce is too thick, you can add a splash of soya milk to thin it out.

Serve the pasta topped with the crispy tofu, black pepper and parsley.

PROTEIN PER SERVING

30g

MAKE IT GLUTEN-FREE

Use gluten-free pasta, miso paste, breadcrumbs and tamari.

STORAGE

Store for up to 3 days in the refrigerator. Not freezer friendly.

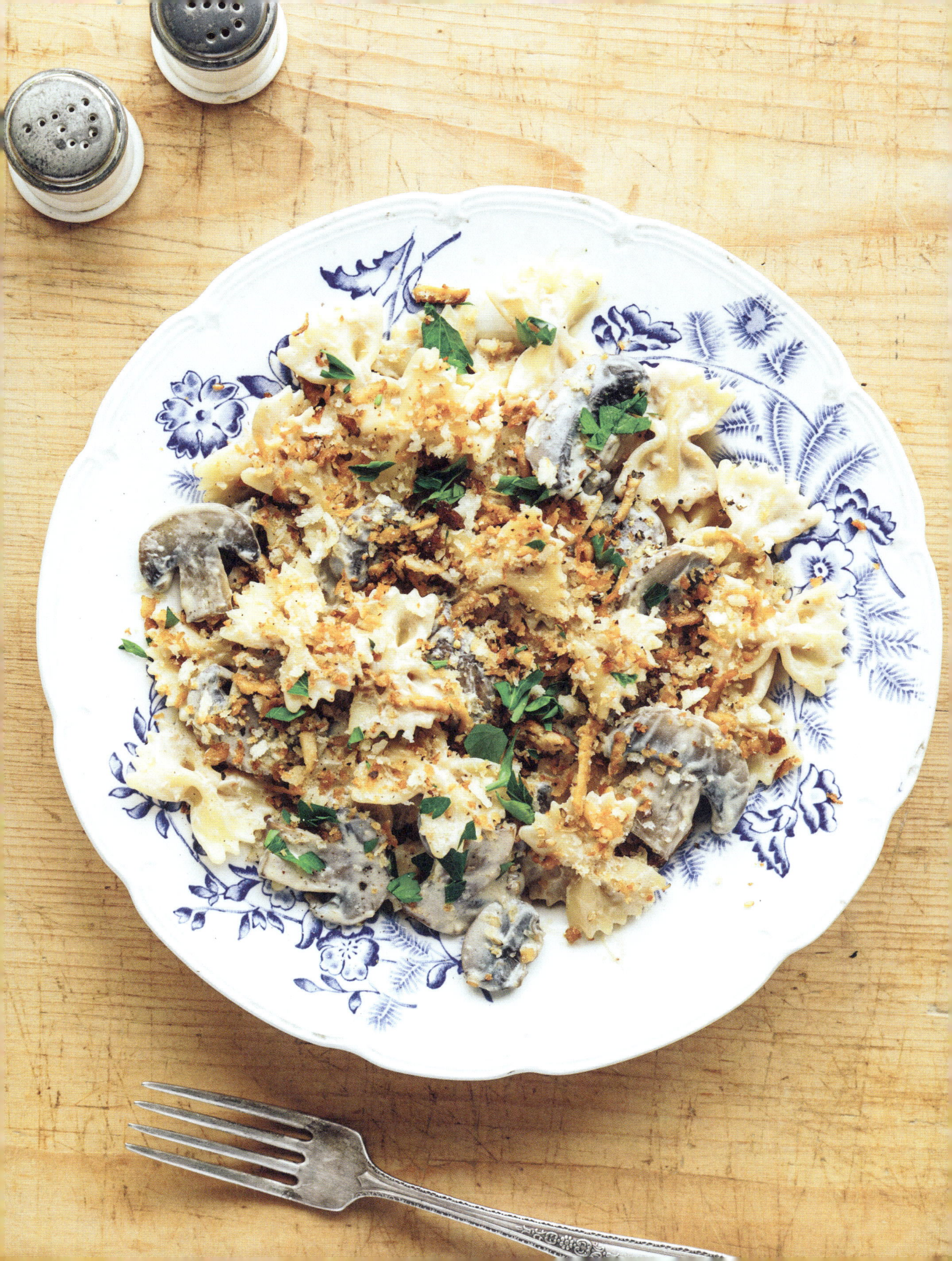

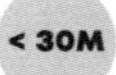

ZINGY SPAGHETTI WITH ASPARAGUS, PISTACHIO AND LEMON PESTO AND EDAMAME

Serves 2–3

When life gives you lemons, find some pistachios and make a pesto! This recipe is like a call to *primavera* (spring in Italian). It's perfect for those transitioning months when it's still a bit chilly outside but hot enough that you start really looking forward to the warm season. The flavours of asparagus, lemon and pistachio complement one another beautifully and also give you a good kick of protein.

250g (9oz) asparagus, woody ends snapped off

200g (7oz) spaghetti

100g (3½oz) cooked edamame beans

50g (1¾oz) lightly salted pistachios, shelled, plus extra to serve

40g (1½oz) nutritional yeast

1 garlic clove

2 tablespoons lemon juice

1 tablespoon lemon zest, plus extra to serve

1 tablespoon tahini

20ml (1½ tablespoons) olive oil

Plant-based Parmesan-style cheese (see page 36, or use shop-bought), to serve

Bring a saucepan of salted water to the boil and cook the asparagus for 5 minutes. They should still be a little crunchy. Remove from the water and dry with a clean dish towel. Do not discard the water.

In the same water, cook the spaghetti according to the packet instructions until al dente. If you're using frozen cooked edamame, throw them in the water a minute before the spaghetti is done.

While the pasta is cooking, put the pistachios into a food processor and pulse briefly until coarsely chopped.

Dice the asparagus, leaving the tops intact for garnishing. Place the chopped stems into the food processor with the pistachios, then add the nutritional yeast, garlic, lemon juice and zest, tahini and olive oil. Blend until a pesto-like paste forms. If it's too dry, add a splash of pasta-cooking water. Season with salt and pepper.

Drain the spaghetti and the edamame once cooked, reserving half a ladle of pasta water.

Place the pasta back into the saucepan and combine it with the asparagus pesto and the pasta water. Stir over a low heat until warmed through.

Serve topped with a small handful of roughly chopped pistachios, lemon zest and plant-based Parmesan-style cheese.

PROTEIN PER SERVING	MAKE IT GLUTEN-FREE	STORAGE
25g	Use gluten-free pasta	Store for up to 3 days in the refrigerator and up to 3 months in the freezer.

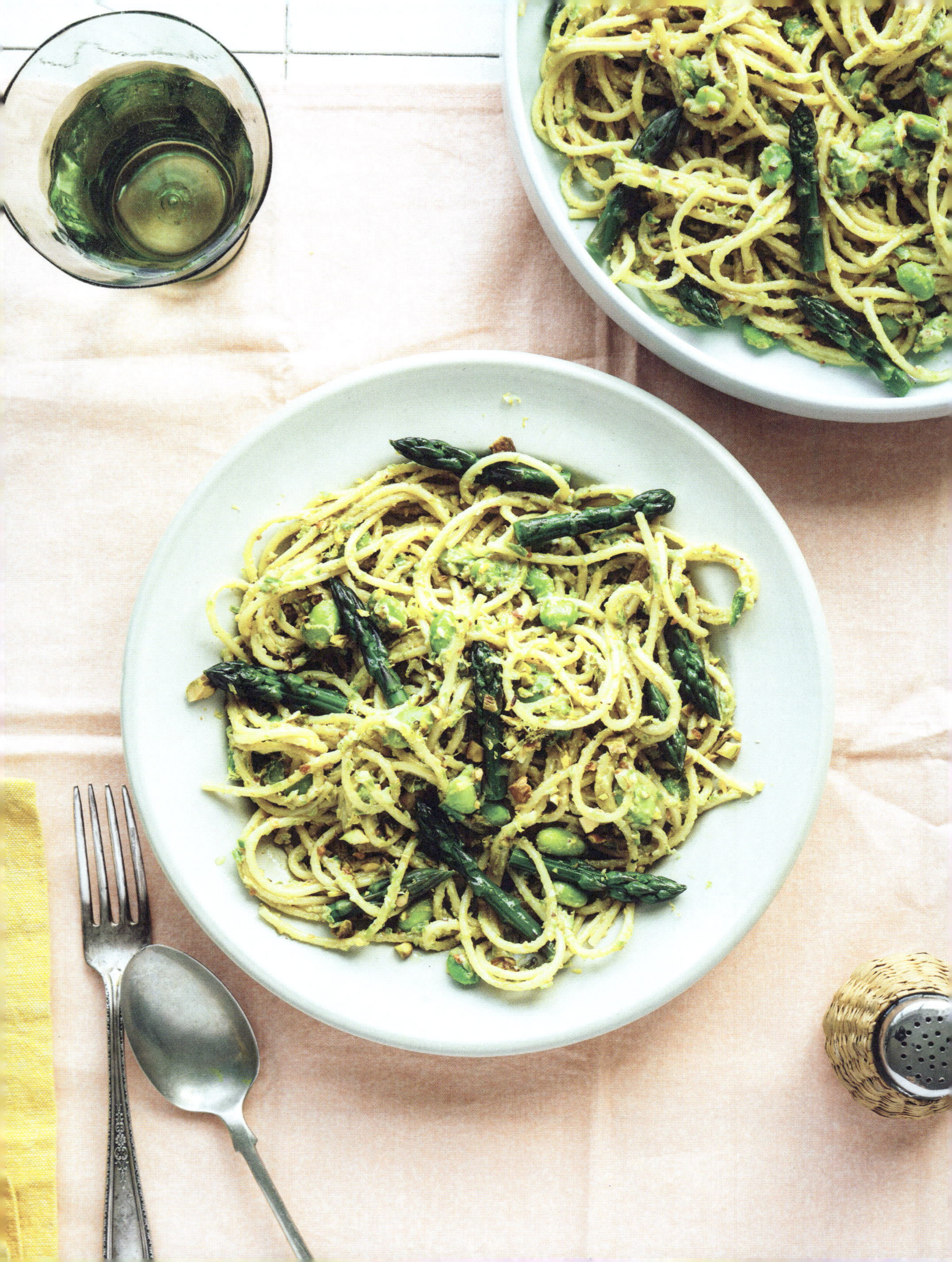

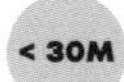

COMFORTING PASTA E CECI

Serves 2–3

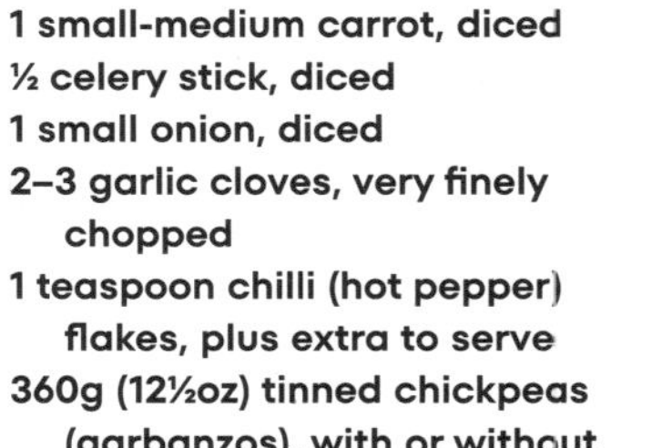

There's nothing as comforting as a steaming bowl of *pasta e ceci* (pasta and chickpeas). Pasta and chickpeas are both very cheap, healthy and filling staple ingredients in Italian cuisine and people have been cooking them in different ways for centuries. My high-protein version features *mezzi rigatoni* (my favourite pasta shape), spinach and a lighter, thinner sauce. This one is super quick and tasty – it will become a staple in your household (as it has been in many households throughout history).

1 small-medium carrot, diced
½ celery stick, diced
1 small onion, diced
2–3 garlic cloves, very finely chopped
1 teaspoon chilli (hot pepper) flakes, plus extra to serve
360g (12½oz) tinned chickpeas (garbanzos), with or without their liquid
180g (6¼oz) mezzi rigatoni pasta
500ml (17fl oz/generous 2 cups) vegetable stock (or more or less as preferred)
Handful of baby spinach
4 tablespoons nutritional yeast
Olive oil, for cooking
Salt and freshly ground black pepper
Plant-based Parmesan-style cheese (see page 36, or use shop-bought), to serve

Heat a good glug of oil in a large saucepan over a medium heat and fry the carrot, celery, onion, garlic and chilli flakes for 5–8 minutes until soft and golden.

Add the chickpeas and the liquid from the tin, if you like. The chickpea liquid creates the broth and has a unique flavour, but you can use more vegetable stock instead if you prefer. Crush about a third of the chickpeas with a fork, then add the pasta. Stir and start adding the stock in small increments. Keep going until the pasta is al dente.

Add the spinach and nutritional yeast and stir well until the spinach is wilted. Taste and season with salt and pepper.

Serve topped with chilli flakes, plant-based Parmesan-style cheese and black pepper.

NOTE

The soffritto base can be batch-cooked and used for many different recipes in this book. See page 34 for my pantry staple recipe.

PROTEIN PER SERVING	MAKE IT GLUTEN-FREE	STORAGE
26g	Use gluten-free pasta.	Store for up to 3 days in the refrigerator and up to 3 months in the freezer.

SMOKY CHICKPEA-LOADED SWEET POTATO WITH AVOCADO AND HERBY SAUCE

Serves 2

  GF

There's so much to love about this dish. Perfectly roasted sweet potatoes are combined with protein-rich crispy chickpeas, a creamy (and secretly protein-rich) avocado topping and a zesty herb-infused sauce to create a nourishing dish that is ready in just a few steps – a winner on all fronts.

2 sweet potatoes
1 x 400g (14oz) tin of chickpeas (garbanzos), drained and patted dry
1 heaped teaspoon smoked paprika
½ teaspoon ground cumin
1 teaspoon onion granules
4 heaped tablespoons tahini
3 tablespoons nutritional yeast
Handful of dill
Juice of 1 lemon, plus zest of ½
1 garlic clove, roughly chopped
1 ripe avocado, peeled and stoned
100g (3½oz/generous ⅓ cup) high-protein plant-based yoghurt
Olive oil, for drizzling
Salt and freshly ground black pepper

TO SERVE
Sesame seeds
Coriander (cilantro)

Preheat the oven to 200°C/180°C fan/400°F/Gas mark 6 and line a baking tray (pan) with baking parchment.

Slice the sweet potatoes lengthwise about halfway through, but do not cut them in half. Drizzle with oil and sprinkle with salt, coating the potatoes evenly using your hands. Set aside.

Put the chickpeas into a bowl with the smoked paprika, cumin, onion granules, 1 tablespoon oil and some salt and pepper. Mix well until evenly coated.

Place the sweet potatoes and chickpeas on the prepared baking tray and roast in the oven for 45–50 minutes until the sweet potatoes are soft and the chickpeas are crunchy. Note that the chickpeas may cook faster, so remove them if they are ready before the sweet potatoes.

Combine the tahini, nutritional yeast, dill, lemon juice and zest, garlic and some salt and pepper in a food processor and blend until creamy, adding a splash of water if the sauce is too thick.

Mash the avocado in a bowl and combine it with the plant-based yoghurt. Season with salt and pepper to taste.

Once the sweet potatoes are soft, prise them open (keeping them intact) and mash the flesh with a fork without removing it from the skin.

Layer the avocado and yoghurt mixture, roasted chickpeas and herby sauce on top of the sweet potato, then finish with sesame seeds and coriander.

PROTEIN PER SERVING	STORAGE
25g	Store for up to 3 days in the refrigerator. Not freezer friendly.

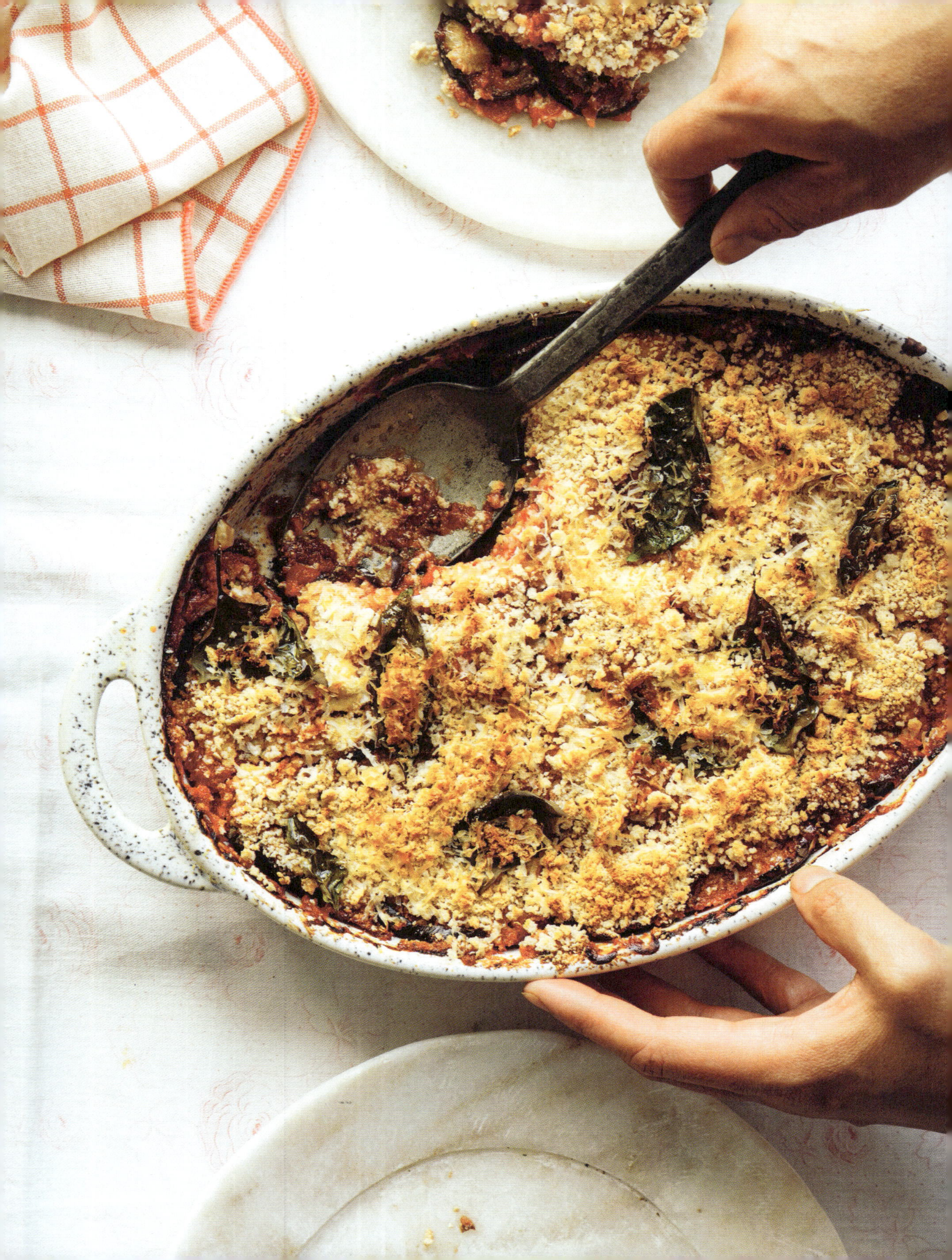

TOFU AUBERGINE PARMIGIANA
Serves 4

Aubergine parmigiana reminds me of my mum. It is a typical Italian dish made with sliced aubergines (eggplants) layered with cheese and tomato sauce, then baked. Sounds amazing, right? Not only was it a hassle-free way to make dinner for two children, it was my absolute favourite. It's a really easy recipe that is perfect for meal prep and for upping your fibre intake. My mum used to make it with mozzarella and Parmesan cheese, but I have tweaked the recipe to make it high-protein and totally plant-based.

3 aubergines (eggplants; about 225–250g/8–9oz each), sliced into 5mm (¼ inch) thick circles
Few big pinches of dried oregano
150g (5½oz) firm tofu
150ml (5fl oz/scant ⅔ cup) soya milk
2 tablespoons nutritional yeast
1 teaspoon cornflour (cornstarch)
Juice of ½ lemon
2 x 400g (14oz) tins of chopped tomatoes
Plant-based Parmesan-style cheese (see page 36, or use shop-bought), to taste
Small handful of basil
Dried breadcrumbs, for coating
Olive oil, for cooking
Salt and freshly ground black pepper
Salad, to serve

Preheat the oven to 220°C/200°C fan/425°F/Gas mark 7 and line two baking sheets with baking parchment.

Arrange the aubergine slices on the prepared baking sheets and drizzle with olive oil, then sprinkle with salt, pepper and oregano. Use a brush to coat both sides.

Roast in the oven for about 35 minutes, or until the aubergines are lightly browned. They should be soft but not fully cooked through.

Meanwhile, put the tofu, soya milk, nutritional yeast, cornflour, lemon juice and a pinch of salt into a food processor and blend until smooth.

Pour the tomatoes into a bowl and lightly crush any large chunks with a fork. Add a drizzle of olive oil and a pinch of salt, pepper and oregano. Stir well to combine.

Spread a thin layer of the tomato sauce over the base of a 28 x 23cm (11 x 9 inch) baking dish. Arrange a layer of aubergine slices on top of the tomato, slightly overlapping them to create a compact layer. Spoon more tomato sauce over the aubergines, then add a light layer of the tofu mixture, plant-based Parmesan-style cheese and a few basil leaves. Repeat this layering process until you have used up the aubergine, finishing with a final layer of tomato sauce, tofu mixture, plant-based Parmesan-style cheese, basil leaves and a generous coating of breadcrumbs.

Bake in the oven for 40 minutes, then turn on the grill (broiler) and grill for 5–8 minutes until the top is crisp and golden and the tomato sauce is bubbling.

Remove from the oven and allow to rest for 10 minutes before scattering some additional basil leaves on top. Slice into squares and serve hot, accompanied by a side salad.

PROTEIN PER SERVING	MAKE IT GLUTEN-FREE	STORAGE
20g	Use gluten-free breadcrumbs.	Store for up to 3 days in the refrigerator and up to 3 months in the freezer.

SHEET PAN CRISPY BLACK PEPPER TOFU, BROCCOLI AND SWEET POTATOES

Serves 2–4

This sweet potato, broccoli and crispy black pepper tofu sheet pan recipe is a delicious way to get my dinner sorted when life gets in the way, especially when paired with a super easy and zingy yoghurt, lime and coriander (cilantro) sauce. The perfect way to get 34 grams of protein on my plate!

300g (10½oz) firm tofu, drained
   and pressed (see page 37),
   cut into cubes
2 tablespoons
   cornflour (cornstarch)
Pinch of salt
1½ teaspoons ground black pepper
1 teaspoon garlic granules
2 sweet potatoes, diced
150g (5½oz) Tenderstem broccoli
   (broccolini), chopped
Olive oil, for drizzling

LIME AND CORIANDER SAUCE

15g (½oz) coriander (cilantro), plus
   extra to serve
3 tablespoons shelled hemp seeds
3 tablespoons nutritional yeast
3 tablespoons high-protein plant-
   based yoghurt
2 tablespoons maple syrup
2 tablespoons olive oil
Juice of 1 lime
Salt and freshly ground
   black pepper

TO SERVE

250g (9oz/1¼ cups) brown rice,
   cooked
Sesame seeds

Preheat the oven to 200°C/180°C fan/400°F/Gas mark 6 and line a baking tray (pan) with baking parchment.

Combine the tofu cubes with the cornflour, salt, pepper and garlic granules in a large bowl. Drizzle with oil, then toss to coat evenly. Transfer the coated tofu to the prepared baking tray and set aside.

In the same bowl, combine the diced sweet potatoes and broccoli. Season with salt, pepper and oil to taste. Toss to coat, then transfer them to the baking tray with the tofu.

Roast in the oven for 40 minutes, or until the sweet potatoes are fork-tender and the tofu is crispy.

Meanwhile, prepare the sauce by combine all the ingredients in a food processor and blending until smooth.

Serve the crispy tofu, sweet potatoes and broccoli with brown rice, sprinkled with coriander and sesame seeds and drizzled with the sauce.

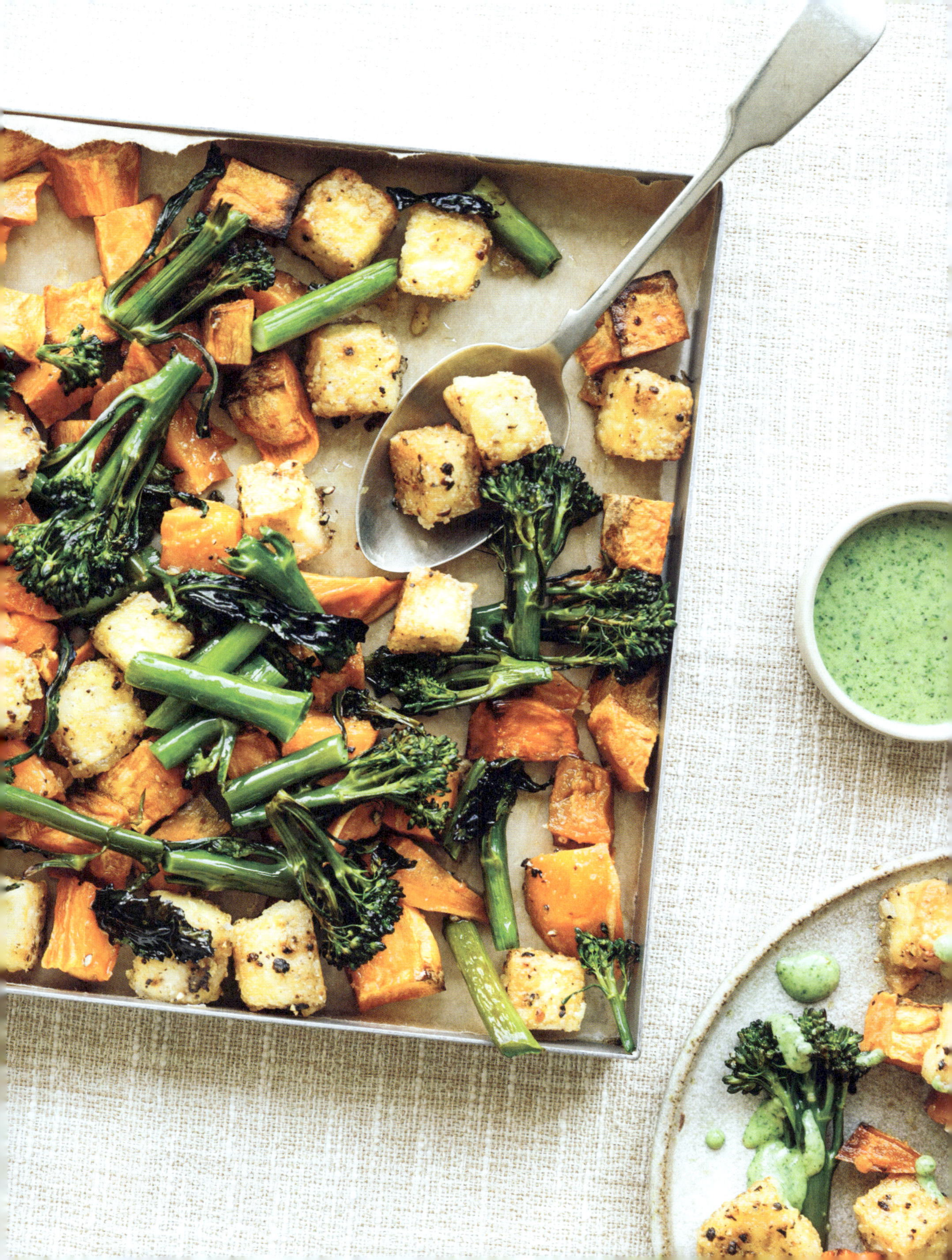

ZUCCHINI SCHIACCIATA

Serves 2–4

  GF

125g (4½oz/generous 1 cup)
  chickpea (gram) flour
1 small courgette (zucchini),
  thinly sliced
1 small red onion, sliced
25ml (scant 2 tablespoon) olive oil
25g (1oz) mixed seeds, such as
  shelled hemp seeds, chia
  seeds, sunflower seeds
  and sesame seeds
Salt and freshly ground
  black pepper
Salad, to serve

A *schiacciata* is a traditional flatbread (sort of like a savoury pancake) from Italy. It seamlessly blends the earthy essence of chickpea (gram) flour with the freshness of courgettes (zucchini) and the subtle sweetness of red onion. It's a simple way to elevate humble ingredients without compromising on taste or balance. Have fun using different vegetables like (bell) peppers, broccoli or leeks! This dish is sure to become a staple in your repertoire.

In a bowl, whisk together the flour and 325ml (11fl oz/1⅓ cups) lukewarm water, making sure there are no lumps or surface bubbles (use a spoon to remove them). Set aside and leave to rest – ideally overnight, but if you are in a hurry you can leave it to rest for 1 hour.

When you're ready to cook, preheat the oven to 200°C/180°C fan/400°F/ Gas mark 6 and line a baking tray (pan) with baking parchment.

Add the courgette and onion to the batter along with the oil and a generous pinch of salt.

Pour the mixture onto the prepared baking tray and level it out with a spatula, ensuring some of the vegetable slices are nicely arranged on top. Sprinkle the seeds on top and sprinkle with pepper, then bake in the oven for 40 minutes, or until the top is golden.

Remove from the oven and allow to cool completely before slicing.

Serve with a side of salad.

PROTEIN PER SERVING

15.5g

STORAGE

Store for up to 3 days in the refrigerator or up to 3 months in the freezer.

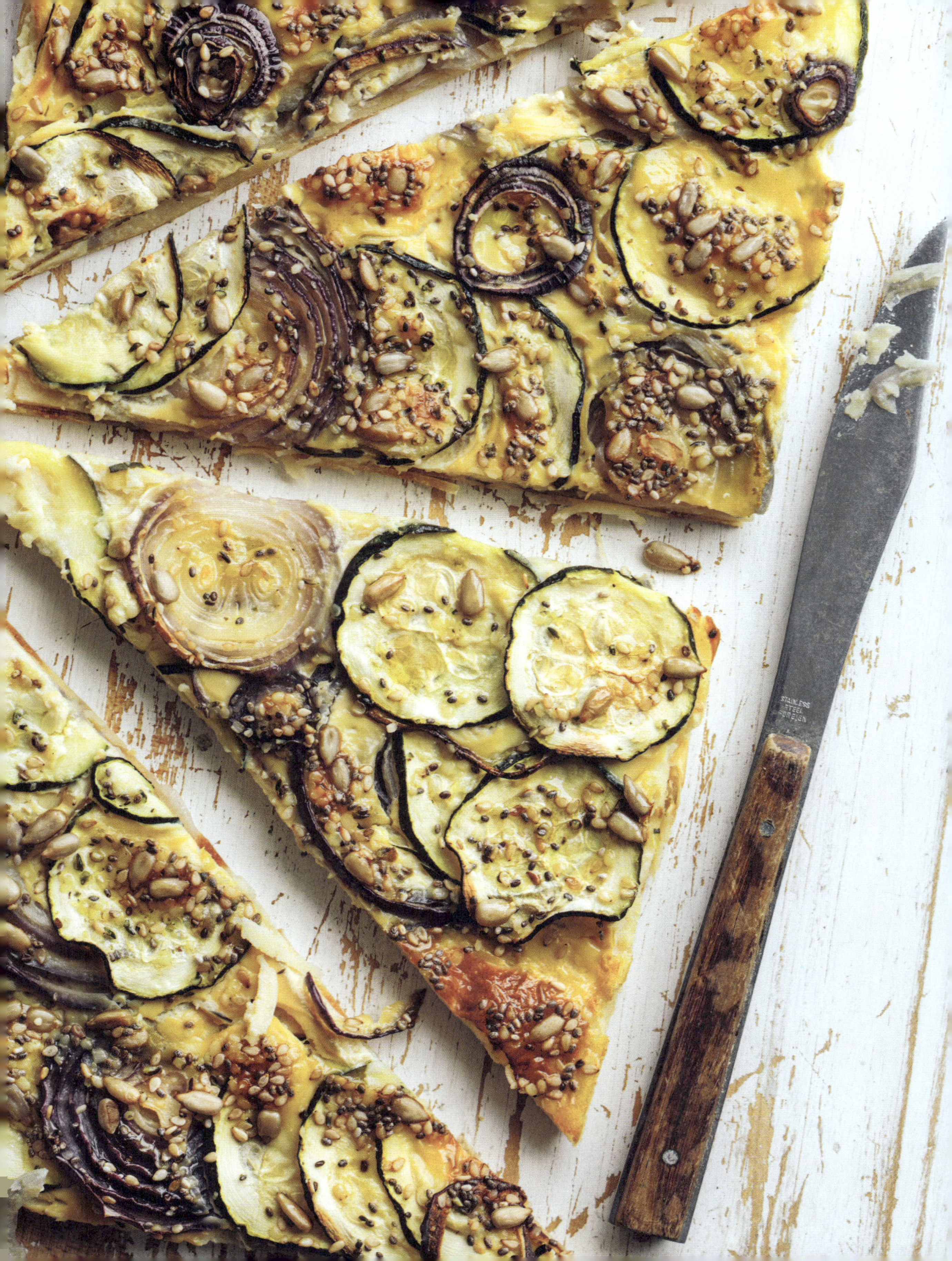

SWEET POTATO COTTAGE PIE

Serves 4–6

This cottage pie is a hearty dish perfect for those chilly evenings when you crave something warming and wholesome. With a velvety layer of creamy sweet potatoes blanketing a filling of tender brown lentils, earthy veggies, walnuts and nutty quinoa, this dish promises to delight with its flavour and nourishing goodness.

SWEET POTATO TOPPING

- 1 kg (2lb 4oz) sweet potatoes, peeled and chopped
- 3 tablespoons plant-based butter
- 40g (1½oz) nutritional yeast
- Salt and freshly ground black pepper

FILLING

- 2 small-medium carrots, chopped
- 1 celery stick, chopped
- 1 onion, chopped
- 2 tablespoons tomato purée (paste)
- 1 sprig of rosemary
- 1 teaspoon thyme leaves
- 50ml (1¾fl oz/3½ tablespoons) red wine
- 100 g (3½oz/⅔ cup) frozen peas
- 200g (7oz) button mushrooms, chopped
- 2 x 400g (14oz) tins of brown lentils, drained
- 50g (1¾oz½ cup) walnuts, chopped
- 1 tablespoon balsamic vinegar
- 300g (10½oz) silken tofu
- 20g (¾oz) nutritional yeast
- 1 teaspoon cornflour (cornstarch)
- Olive oil, for cooking

Preheat the oven to 200°C/180°C fan/400°F/Gas mark 6.

Put the sweet potatoes into a saucepan and cover them with water. Bring to the boil, then cook for 15 minutes, or until the sweet potatoes are fork-tender.

Once ready, drain the potatoes and add them back to the pan along with the plant-based butter, nutritional yeast and a pinch of salt and pepper. Mash with a potato masher or a hand-held electric whisk until smooth and creamy. Set aside.

Meanwhile, heat a good glug of oil in a frying pan (skillet) over a medium heat and fry the carrots, celery, onion, tomato purée, rosemary and thyme for about 10 minutes, or until the vegetables are translucent and soft.

Deglaze with the red wine and allow it to bubble and evaporate, then remove the sprig of rosemary.

Add the peas, mushrooms and lentils and simmer for 8–10 minutes until the liquid has reduced. Finally, add the walnuts and balsamic vinegar.

Put the silken tofu, nutritional yeast and cornflour into a food processor and blend until smooth, then season with salt and pepper. Add to the lentil mixture.

Transfer the lentil mixture to a 23 cm (9 inch) square baking dish, then use a spatula to smooth it and cover with the mashed sweet potatoes. Complete with a last pinch of salt and pepper, then bake for about 25 minutes, or until the potatoes are crisp on top.

PROTEIN PER SERVING

25g

STORAGE

Store for up to 3 days in the refrigerator and up to 3 months in the freezer.

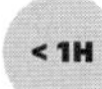

BOLOGNESE PASTA BAKE

Serves 4–5

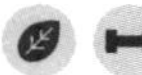

Pasta al forno is a baked pasta dish from Italy. Typically boasting béchamel, tomato sauce, pasta and cheese, this Italian gem has been revamped into a plant-based, high-protein wonder using nutrient-rich lentils. Prepare for unapologetic and satisfying richness, perfect for those nights when only comfort foods will do.

400g (14oz) conchiglie (or another small pasta of your choice)
125g (4½oz) plant-based mozzarella-style cheese (optional)
Plant-based Parmesan-style cheese (see page 36, or use shop-bought), for sprinkling

BOLOGNESE SAUCE

1 small-medium carrot, diced
½ celery stick, diced
1 small onion, diced
2–3 garlic cloves, very finely chopped
2 tablespoons tomato purée (paste)
10 sun-dried tomatoes, chopped
200g (7oz/generous ¾ cup) split red lentils
2 tablespoons light soy sauce
2 tablespoons dried mixed Italian herbs
200g (7oz/generous ¾ cup) passata (sieved tomatoes)
Olive oil, for cooking
Salt and freshly ground black pepper

BÉCHAMEL SAUCE

60ml (2fl oz/¼ cup) olive oil
55g (2oz/½ cup) plain (all-purpose) flour
500ml (17fl oz/generous 2 cups) unsweetened soya milk
1 teaspoon salt
1 heaped teaspoon ground nutmeg

Preheat the oven to 210°C/190°C fan/425°F/Gas mark 7.

First, make the Bolognese sauce. Heat a good glug of oil in a large saucepan over a medium heat and fry the carrot, celery, onion, garlic, tomato purée and sun-dried tomatoes for 5–8 minutes until soft and golden.

Add the lentils, soy sauce and herbs and stir to toast the lentils for 1–2 minutes. Pour in the passata and 400ml (14fl oz/generous 1½ cups) water, season with a pinch of salt and simmer for 7–8 minutes until the lentils are soft. If it looks too dry, add a little more water.

Once the lentils are cooked, remove half of the mixture and blend in a food processor or with a hand-held blender, then return it to the pan and set aside.

Next, make the béchamel sauce. Whisk together the oil and flour in a saucepan over a low heat until well combined. Once the mixture starts to bubble, slowly add the soya milk, stirring continuously for about 10 minutes until the mixture is lump-free and starts to thicken and is silky. Remove from the heat and add the salt and nutmeg.

Finally, bring a large saucepan of salted water to the boil and cook the pasta for 4–5 minutes – it should be very al dente, so you can still feel a crunch when biting it. Drain.

Pour the Bolognese sauce, béchamel (reserving 1 ladle) and pasta into a large baking dish and add the plant-based mozzarella-style cheese (if using). Mix to combine. Pour over the reserved béchamel and sprinkle with plant-based Parmesan-style cheese.

Cover the dish with foil and bake in the oven for 30 minutes, then remove the foil and turn on the grill (broiler). Cook for a further 10 minutes, or until the top is golden brown and bubbling.

Remove from the oven and allow to rest for a few minutes before slicing and serving.

NOTE

The soffritto base for the Bolognese sauce can be batch-cooked and used for many different recipes in this book. See page 34 for my pantry staple recipe.

PROTEIN PER SERVING	MAKE IT GLUTEN-FREE	STORAGE
33g	Use gluten-free flour, pasta and tamari.	Store for up to 3 days in the refrigerator and 3 months in the freezer.

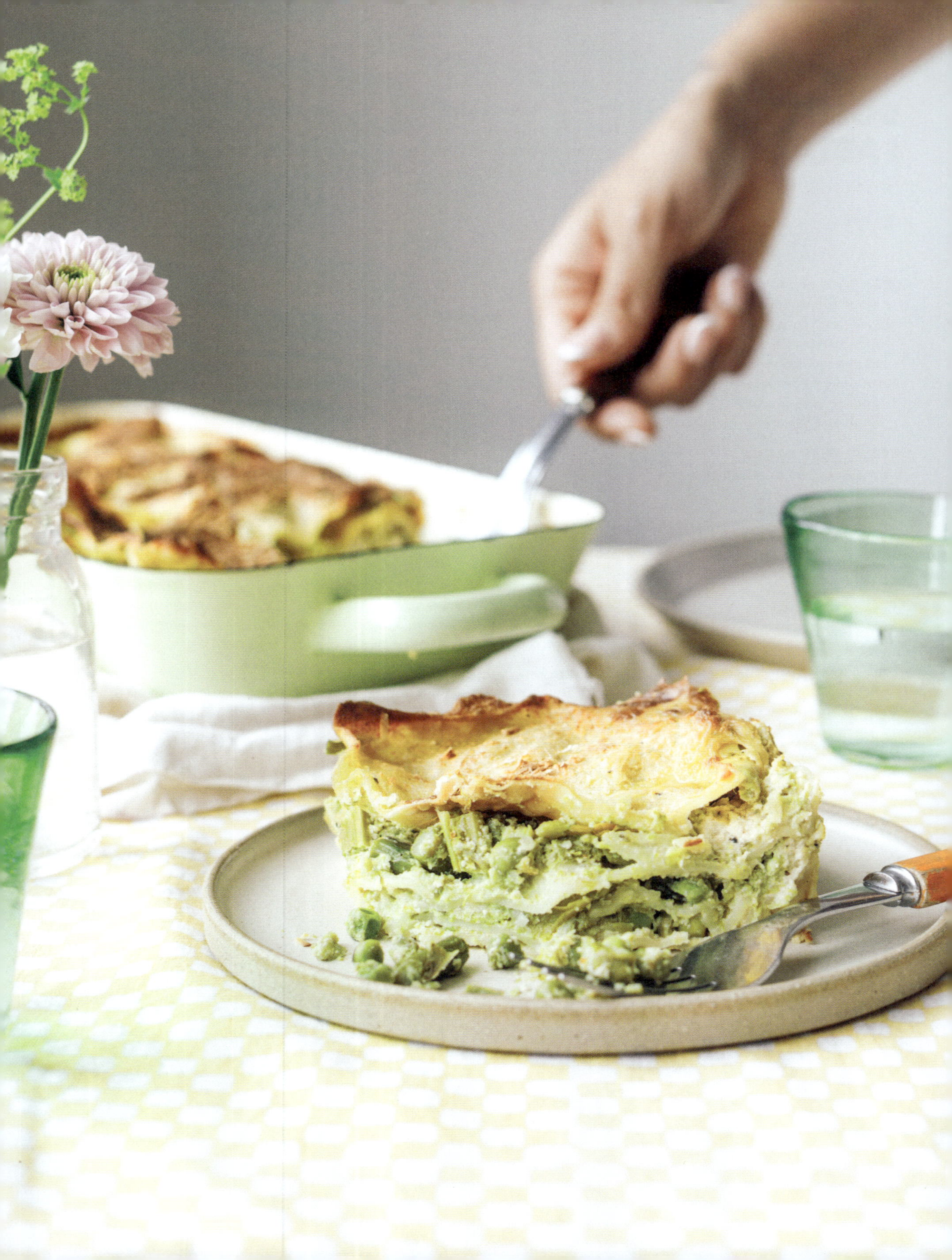

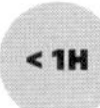

LASAGNE PRIMAVERA

Serves 4

What better way to enjoy the flavours of spring than with a veggie lasagne? This wholesome dish combines layers of tender asparagus, sweet peas and spring onions (scallions) with sheets of delicate lasagne, enveloped in a creamy, homemade béchamel sauce made with tofu. Bursting with freshness and rich with plant-based proteins, this dish will be become a favourite in your kitchen.

6–7 spring onions (scallions;
   or 2 shallots), roughly chopped
300g (10½oz/2 cups) frozen peas
300g (10½oz) asparagus,
   woody ends snapped off
   and spears chopped
250–300g (9–10½oz)
   lasagne sheets
50g (1¾oz) plant-based Parmesan-
   style cheese (see page 36, or
   use shop-bought)
Olive oil, for cooking

BÉCHAMEL SAUCE
200g (7oz) firm tofu
600ml (20fl oz/2½ cups) soya milk
30g (1oz) nutritional yeast
1 teaspoon ground nutmeg
1 teaspoon cornflour (cornstarch)
Salt and freshly ground
   black pepper

Preheat the oven to 220°C/200°C fan/425°F/Gas mark 7.

Heat a good glug of olive oil in frying pan (skillet) over a medium heat and fry the spring onions for about 5 minutes until soft.

Add the peas and the asparagus, cover and cook for 7–8 minutes until softened but still with a nice crunch.

Meanwhile, make the béchamel sauce. Put the tofu, soya milk, nutritional yeast, nutmeg and cornflour into a food processor, season with salt and pepper and blend until smooth. The mixture should be very liquid, so don't worry, it will thicken in the oven. Pour three quarters of the béchamel into a bowl and set aside.

Add roughly one third of the cooked vegetables to the food processor with the remaining béchamel and blend until smooth.

Spread a generous layer of the reserved white béchamel sauce over the bottom of a 28 x 23cm (11 x 9 inch) baking dish, then arrange the some of the lasagne sheets on top. Spread another layer of white béchamel over the top, then spread a layer of the green béchamel sauce over the white béchamel. Scatter some of the cooked vegetables evenly over the sauces, then sprinkle a light layer of plant-based Parmesan-style cheese on top. Repeat the layering process until you've used up all the sauces, vegetables and lasagne sheets, finishing with a layer of sauce and plant-based Parmesan-style cheese on top.

Cover the dish with foil and bake in the oven for 30 minutes, then remove the foil and turn on the grill (broiler). Cook for a further 10 minutes, or until the top is golden brown and bubbling.

Remove from the oven and allow to rest for a few minutes before slicing and serving.

PROTEIN PER SERVING
28g

MAKE IT GLUTEN-FREE
Use gluten-free lasagne sheets.

STORAGE
Store for up to 3 days in the refrigerator and up to 3 months in the freezer.

HARISSA BUTTER BEANS WITH ZINGY YOGHURT SAUCE

Serves 2–4

The perfect weeknight dinner doesn't exist... or does it? Well, picture this: a fragrant blend of red onion, thyme and spicy harissa infusing your kitchen as you cook. Then, add in the savoury tang of kalamata olives, rich tomatoes and finish off with butter (lima) beans. All accompanied by a high-protein flatbread. The result? A protein-packed powerhouse that is so easy it feels like cheating.

1 red onion, diced
1 sprig of thyme
1 tablespoon harissa paste
5–6 chopped kalamata olives
1 x 400g (14oz) tin of chopped
   tomatoes
2 x 400g (14oz) tins of butter (lima)
   beans, drained
4–5 tablespoons nutritional yeast
Handful of spinach
Olive oil, for cooking
Salt and freshly ground
   black pepper
Tofu Flatbread (see page 164),
   to serve

ZINGY YOGHURT SAUCE

150g (5½oz/scant ⅔ cup) high-
   protein plant-based yoghurt
2 tablespoons lemon juice
½ teaspoon ground cumin

Heat a generous glug of oil in a saucepan over a medium heat and fry the onion and thyme for 5–8 minutes until the onion is soft and golden.

Stir in the harissa paste and kalamata olives and cook for a few minutes to let the flavours infuse, then remove the thyme and add the tomatoes. Simmer for 10 minutes, then add the butter beans and nutritional yeast. Mix well, then crush some of the butter beans with a fork for added creaminess. Finally, add the spinach and stir until it has wilted. Taste and adjust the seasoning as needed.

To make the zingy yoghurt sauce, whisk together all the ingredients in a bowl and season to taste.

Serve the beans with the sauce drizzled on top, with flatbreads for dipping.

PROTEIN PER SERVING

26g

MAKE IT GLUTEN-FREE

Serve with gluten-free flatbread

STORAGE

Store for up to 3 days in the refrigerator. The butter beans can be frozen for up to 3 months.

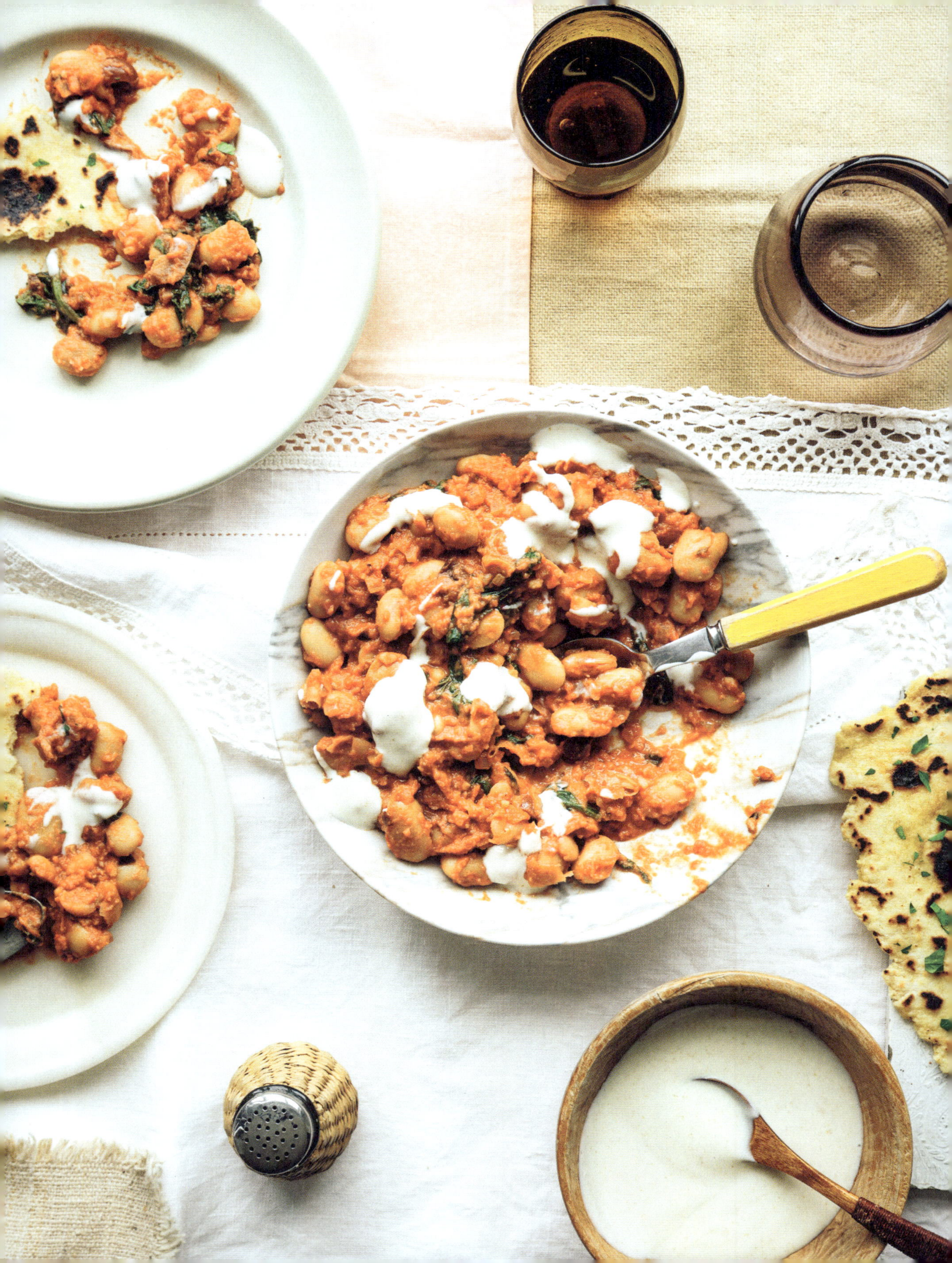

SWEET POTATO AND SPINACH DAHL

Serves 4–6

Dahl can sometimes seem like a difficult dish to tackle, but my easy recipe is here to change that perception. Creamy with a bold and spicy flavour, it's a one-pot dish that not only fills your belly but is also packed with quality protein to nourish your body from the inside out. Serve it alongside fluffy rice and high-protein flatbread for a complete and satisfying feast. The sherpas of Nepal call dahl '24-hour power' for a reason – this dish will show you why!

1 onion, diced
4–5 garlic cloves, very
    finely chopped
1 thumb-sized piece of fresh
    ginger root, peeled and very
    finely chopped
1 tablespoon tomato purée (paste)
1 teaspoon garam masala
1 teaspoon ground cumin
1 teaspoon ground turmeric
½ teaspoon ground coriander
1 teaspoon chilli (hot pepper) flakes
350g (12oz) sweet potato, chopped
    into small chunks
500ml (17fl oz/generous 2 cups)
    vegetable stock
300g (10½oz/1¼ cups) split red
    lentils, washed
1 x 400g (14oz) tin of
    chopped tomatoes
400ml (14fl oz/generous 1½ cups)
    coconut milk
3 tablespoons nutritional yeast
Handful of baby spinach
Olive oil, for cooking
Salt

TO SERVE

Juice of 1 lemon
Small handful of coriander
    (cilantro), chopped
Pickled red onions
Plant-based cream or yoghurt
Tofu Flatbread (see page 164)
    or roti
Fluffy rice or quinoa

Heat a good glug of oil in a saucepan over a medium heat and fry the onion, garlic and ginger for 5–8 minutes until soft and golden.

Add the tomato purée and the garam masala, cumin, turmeric, coriander and chilli flakes. Stir until combined and cook for a couple of minutes until the flavours have infused.

Add the chopped sweet potato and a dash of vegetable stock and stir to combine with the spices. Cook for 10 minutes, adding another splash of stock if the potatoes start to stick to the pan.

Add the lentils, stir and let them toast for a couple of minutes, then add the remaining stock, the tomatoes and the coconut milk. Stir well, then simmer over a medium-low heat for 15 minutes.

Once the sweet potatoes are soft, season with salt and stir in the nutritional yeast and spinach. Remove from the heat and stir until the spinach has totally wilted and the sauce has thickened slightly.

Serve with a squeeze of lemon, topped with coriander, pickled red onions and plant-based cream or yoghurt alongside rice or quinoa and flatbread or roti.

PROTEIN PER SERVING	MAKE IT GLUTEN-FREE	STORAGE
34g	Serve with gluten-free flatbread.	Store for up to 3 days in the refrigerator or up to 3 months in the freezer.

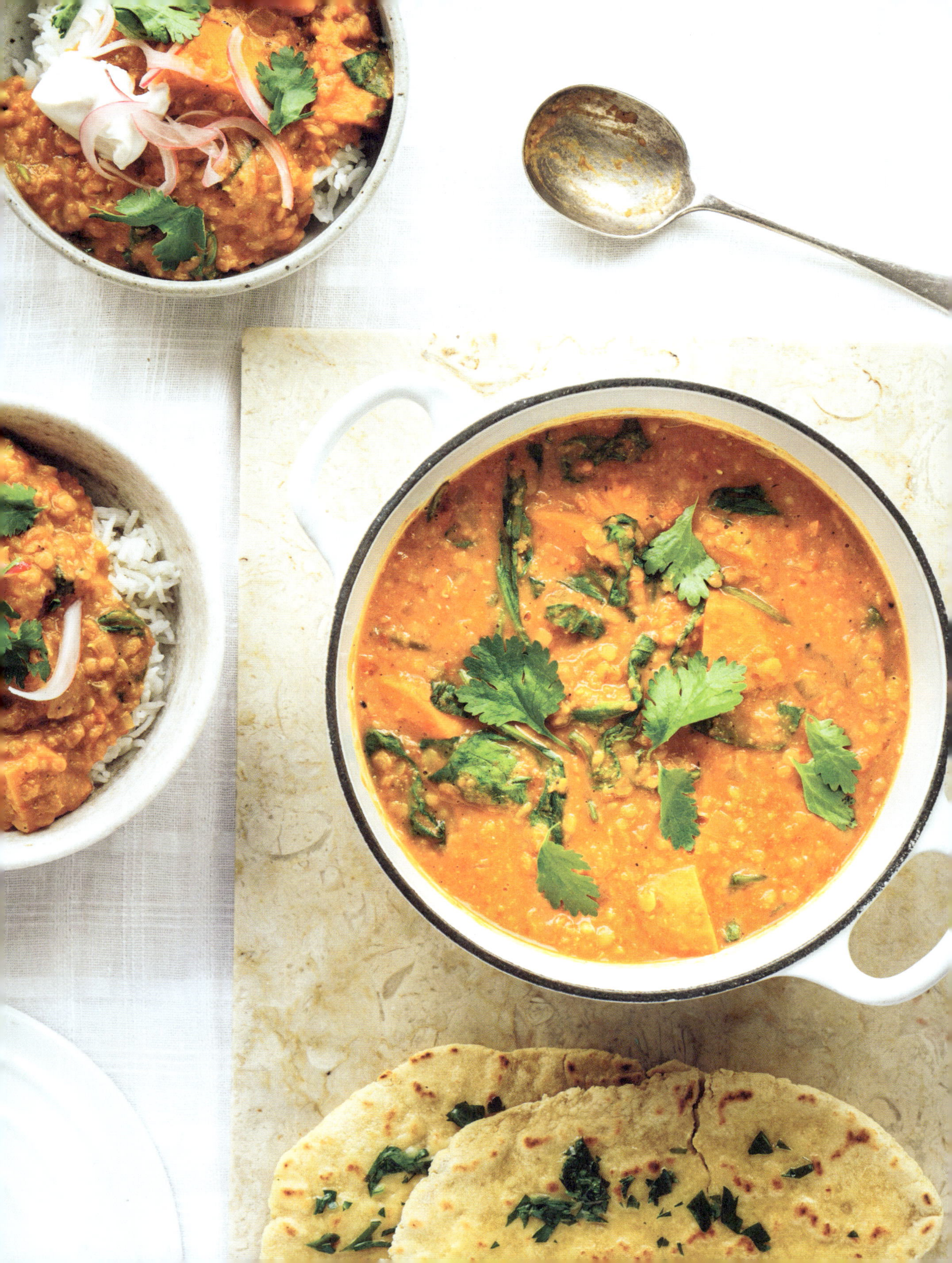

< 1H

ROMESCO CHICKPEAS

Serves 4

Inspired by the Spanish romesco sauce, this protein-packed version brings together the bold flavours of roasted red peppers, tomatoes and garlic in a hassle-free recipe that's as nutritious as it is delicious. With the addition of raw almonds and firm tofu, it becomes a protein-rich powerhouse that quenches hunger and is ideal for both busy weeknights or leisurely dinners with friends.

3 red (bell) peppers, sliced
   (or jarred roasted peppers)
2 tomatoes (or 3–4 sun-dried
   tomatoes), chopped
1 bulb of garlic
1 tablespoon olive oil, plus extra
   for drizzling
200g (7oz) firm tofu
Handful of flat-leaf parsley
3 tablespoons nutritional yeast
85g (3oz/½ cup) whole
   raw almonds
Juice of 1 lemon
Splash of soya milk or
   vegetable stock
1 x 400g (14oz) tin of chickpeas
   (garbanzos), drained
Salt and freshly ground
   black pepper

TO SERVE

Plant-based cream or yoghurt
Chopped flat-leaf parsley
Toasted almonds
Rice or quinoa
Tofu Flatbread (see page 164)

Preheat the oven to 200°C/180°C fan/400°F/Gas mark 6.

If you're using fresh peppers and tomatoes, put them onto a baking tray (pan) with the bulb of garlic, then drizzle with oil and sprinkle with salt and pepper. Roast in the oven for about 25 minutes until tender and juicy. If you're using jarred peppers and sun-dried tomatoes, skip this step (except for roasting the garlic).

Transfer the peppers and tomatoes to a food processor. Squeeze the roasted garlic cloves out of their skins into the food processor too. Add the tofu, 1 tablespoon olive oil, parsley, nutritional yeast, almonds and lemon juice. Season with salt and pepper and add a splash of soya milk or vegetable stock, then blend until smooth, adjusting the liquid to achieve your desired consistency (silkier or more pesto-like).

Pour or scrape the sauce into a saucepan and add the chickpeas. Cook over a medium heat for a couple of minutes to warm though.

Serve topped with plant-based cream or yoghurt, parsley and toasted almonds with a side of rice or quinoa and tofu flatbread.

PROTEIN PER SERVING	MAKE IT GLUTEN-FREE	STORAGE
30g	Serve with gluten-free flatbread.	Store for up to 3 days in the refrigerator and 3 months in the freezer.

LEEK AND MISO LENTILS

Serves 2

I think miso and leeks are a match made in heaven and this recipe proves it! In the blink of an eye, you'll have tender, flavoursome leeks infused with the rich umami taste of miso. A delicious protein-packed dish that supports your body's good health with its wholesome ingredients. Enjoy it solo or alongside buttered toasted sourdough bread, a high-protein flatbread (see page 164) or quinoa for a complete and utterly satisfying meal.

1 onion, finely chopped

1 celery stick, finely chopped

2 garlic cloves, very finely chopped

1 large leek, trimmed and chopped

1 heaped tablespoon white miso paste

1 x 400g (14oz) tin of brown or green lentils, drained

5 heaped tablespoons nutritional yeast

Juice of ½ lemon

Olive oil, for cooking

Salt and freshly ground black pepper

1 teaspoon toasted sesame seeds, to serve

Heat a generous glug of oil in a saucepan over a medium heat and fry the onion, celery and garlic for a couple of minutes until golden, then add the leek and stir to combine.

Dissolve the miso paste in 100ml (3½fl oz/scant ½ cup) hot water, then and pour it into the pan. Cover and cook for 5–7 minutes, adding a splash more water if needed.

Once the leeks are ready, add the lentils and stir well. (If you want to maintain the shape of the leeks for presentation, remove some before stirring in the lentils to prevent them from breaking up.)

Stir in the nutritional yeast and season with salt and pepper, then finish with the lemon juice.

Serve sprinkled with the toasted sesame seeds.

PROTEIN PER SERVING

22.5g

STORAGE

Store for up to 3 days in the refrigerator or up to 3 months in the freezer.

TOMATO AND COCONUT CHICKPEA CURRY

Serves 4–6

1 onion, diced
½ thumb-sized piece of fresh ginger root, peeled and grated
4 garlic cloves, very finely chopped
1 teaspoon ground turmeric
½ teaspoon ground fenugreek
½ teaspoon ground cumin
½ teaspoon chilli powder
1 tablespoon tomato purée (paste)
1 sweet potato, chopped in small chunks
400g (14oz) chopped tomatoes (fresh or tinned)
600g (1lb 5oz) drained tinned chickpeas (garbanzos)
400ml (14fl oz/generous 1½ cups) coconut milk
3–4 tablespoons nutritional yeast
Vegetable stock, as needed
Olive oil, for cooking

TO SERVE
Small handful of coriander (cilantro), chopped
Pickled red onions
Plant-based cream or yoghurt
Tofu Flatbread (see page 164)
Rice or quinoa

If you were to ask me what dish makes my mouth water, I'd answer with this. With each spoonful, you'll experience the comforting warmth of spices, the creamy richness of coconut milk and the sweet tanginess of tomatoes. It satisfies the palate but also nourishes the body, thanks to the protein-packed chickpeas (garbanzos) and the wholesome goodness of sweet potatoes. An ideal dinner option whether you're craving a cosy weeknight meal or looking to impress guests.

Heat a good glug of oil in a saucepan over a medium heat and fry the onion, ginger and garlic for 5–8 minutes until soft and golden.

Add the turmeric, fenugreek, cumin and chilli powder and stir to combine, then add the tomato purée. Stir again and let the flavour infuse for 6–8 minutes (if it starts sticking to the pan, add a splash of vegetable stock or water).

Add the chopped sweet potato, tomatoes and just enough stock to partially cover the potatoes. Cover and simmer for 15–20 minutes until the potato is soft and you can mash it with a fork. If it starts to look dry at any point, add another splash of stock.

Once the potato is soft, add the chickpeas and coconut milk and stir to combine. Bring to a gentle boil, then season with salt and pepper and remove from the heat. Allow to cool for 8–10 minutes, then add the nutritional yeast and stir to combine.

Serve topped with coriander, pickled red onions and plant-based cream or yoghurt alongside rice or quinoa and flatbread.

PROTEIN PER SERVING

33g

MAKE IT GLUTEN-FREE

Serve with gluten-free flatbread.

STORAGE

Store for up to 3 days in the refrigerator and up to 3 months in the freezer.

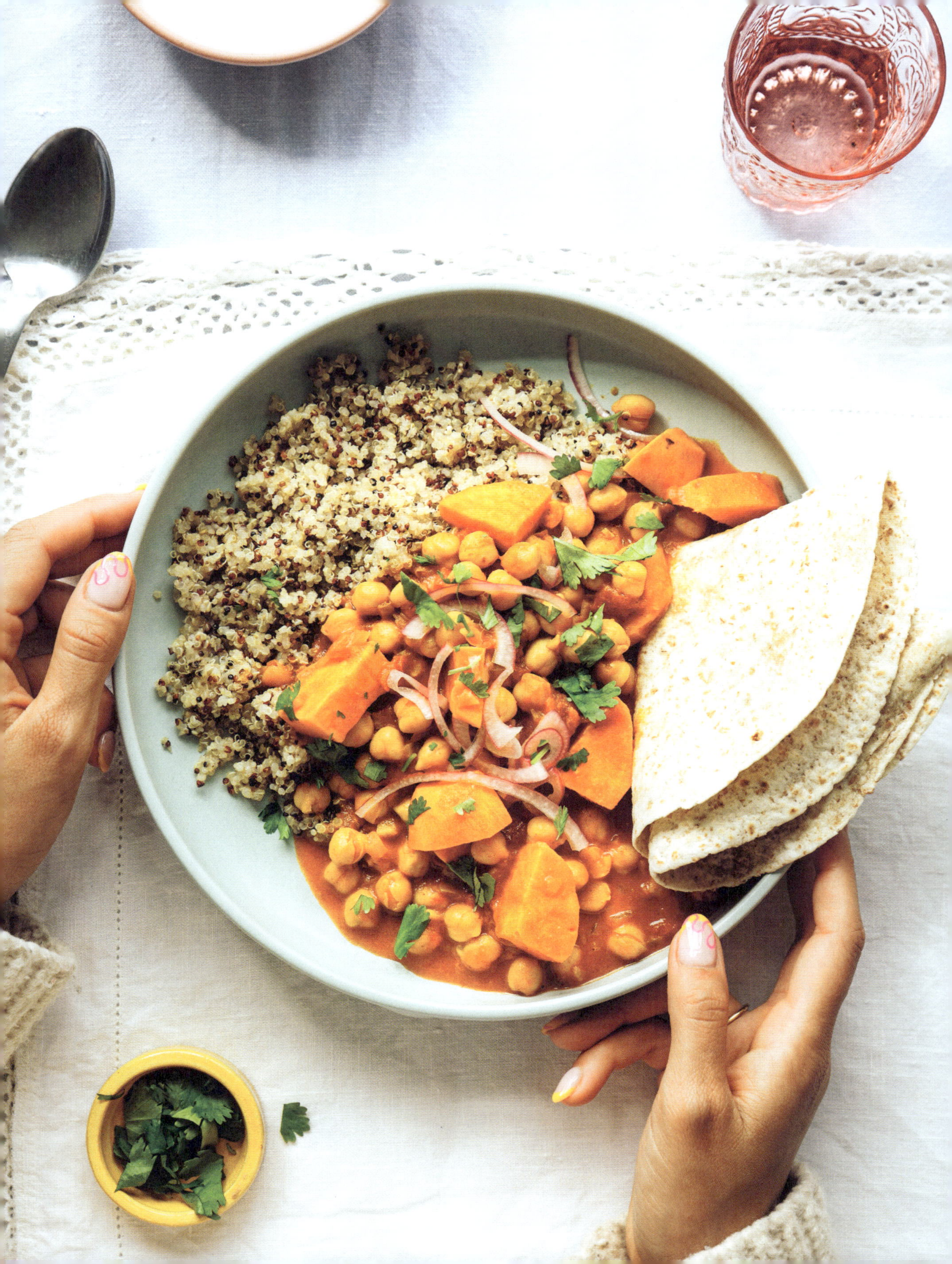

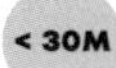

BUTTER TOFU CURRY

Serves 2

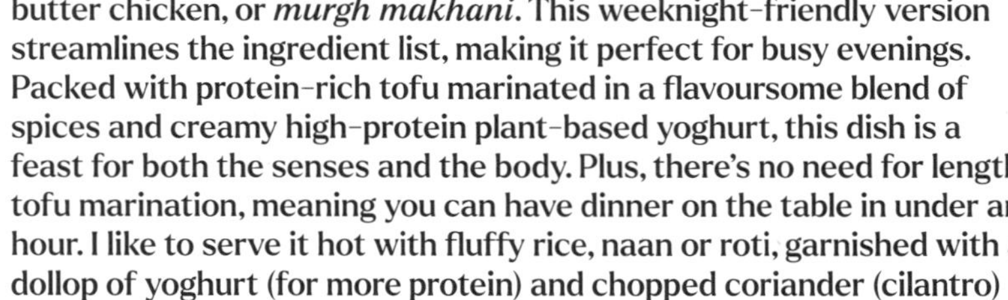

This curry offers a plant-based twist on the classic Indian favourite, butter chicken, or *murgh makhani*. This weeknight-friendly version streamlines the ingredient list, making it perfect for busy evenings. Packed with protein-rich tofu marinated in a flavoursome blend of spices and creamy high-protein plant-based yoghurt, this dish is a feast for both the senses and the body. Plus, there's no need for lengthy tofu marination, meaning you can have dinner on the table in under an hour. I like to serve it hot with fluffy rice, naan or roti, garnished with a dollop of yoghurt (for more protein) and chopped coriander (cilantro) for the perfect finishing touch.

TOFU

- 150g (5½oz/scant ⅔ cup) high-protein plant-based yoghurt
- 1 teaspoon ground cumin
- 1 teaspoon ground turmeric
- 1 teaspoon garam masala
- 1 teaspoon chilli powder
- 2cm (¾ inch) piece of fresh ginger root, peeled
- 3 garlic cloves, peeled
- 300g (10½oz) tofu, drained and pressed (see page 37), crumbled into bite-sized pieces
- 1 tablespoon plant-based butter

BUTTER SAUCE

- 1 tablespoon plant-based butter
- 1 small onion, chopped
- 2 garlic cloves, very finely chopped
- 1 tablespoon tomato purée (paste)
- 1 teaspoon ground cumin
- 1 teaspoon ground turmeric
- 1 teaspoon garam masala
- 1 teaspoon chilli powder
- 400g (14oz/1⅔ cups) passata (sieved tomatoes)
- 400ml (14fl oz/generous 1½ cups) coconut milk
- 4 tablespoons nutritional yeast
- Juice of ½ lemon
- Salt and freshly ground black pepper

TO SERVE

- Naan, roti or basmati rice
- High-protein plant-based yoghurt
- Chopped coriander (cilantro)
- Lemon wedges

First, prepare the tofu. Place the yoghurt, cumin, turmeric, garam masala, chilli powder, ginger and garlic in a food processor and blend until smooth. If needed, add a splash of water to achieve a silky consistency.

Scrape the mixture into a container and add the crumbled tofu, mixing until the tofu is thoroughly coated. Set aside to marinate while you prepare the sauce.

Heat the plant-based butter in a saucepan over a medium heat and fry the onion, garlic and tomato purée for 5–8 minutes until the onion has softened.

Add the cumin, turmeric, garam masala and chilli powder and let the spices toast for a few minutes, then add the passata and coconut milk. Simmer over a low heat for 15–20 minutes until thickened, stirring occasionally. If the sauce starts to dry out, add a splash of water. Season with salt and pepper to taste.

Meanwhile, heat the butter for the tofu in a frying pan (skillet) over a medium heat. Add the marinated tofu, reserving any excess marinade. Fry the tofu for 10–15 minutes until golden, turning frequently to ensure even cooking on all sides.

Add the tofu and the reserved marinade to the sauce, then stir in the nutritional yeast. Squeeze over the lemon juice just before serving.

Serve the curry hot with rice, naan or roti. Garnish with plant-based yoghurt and chopped coriander, with lemon wedges on the side for an extra burst of flavour.

PROTEIN PER SERVING	MAKE IT GLUTEN-FREE	STORAGE
37g	Serve with gluten-free naan or roti.	Store for up to 3 days in the refrigerator and up to 3 months in the freezer.

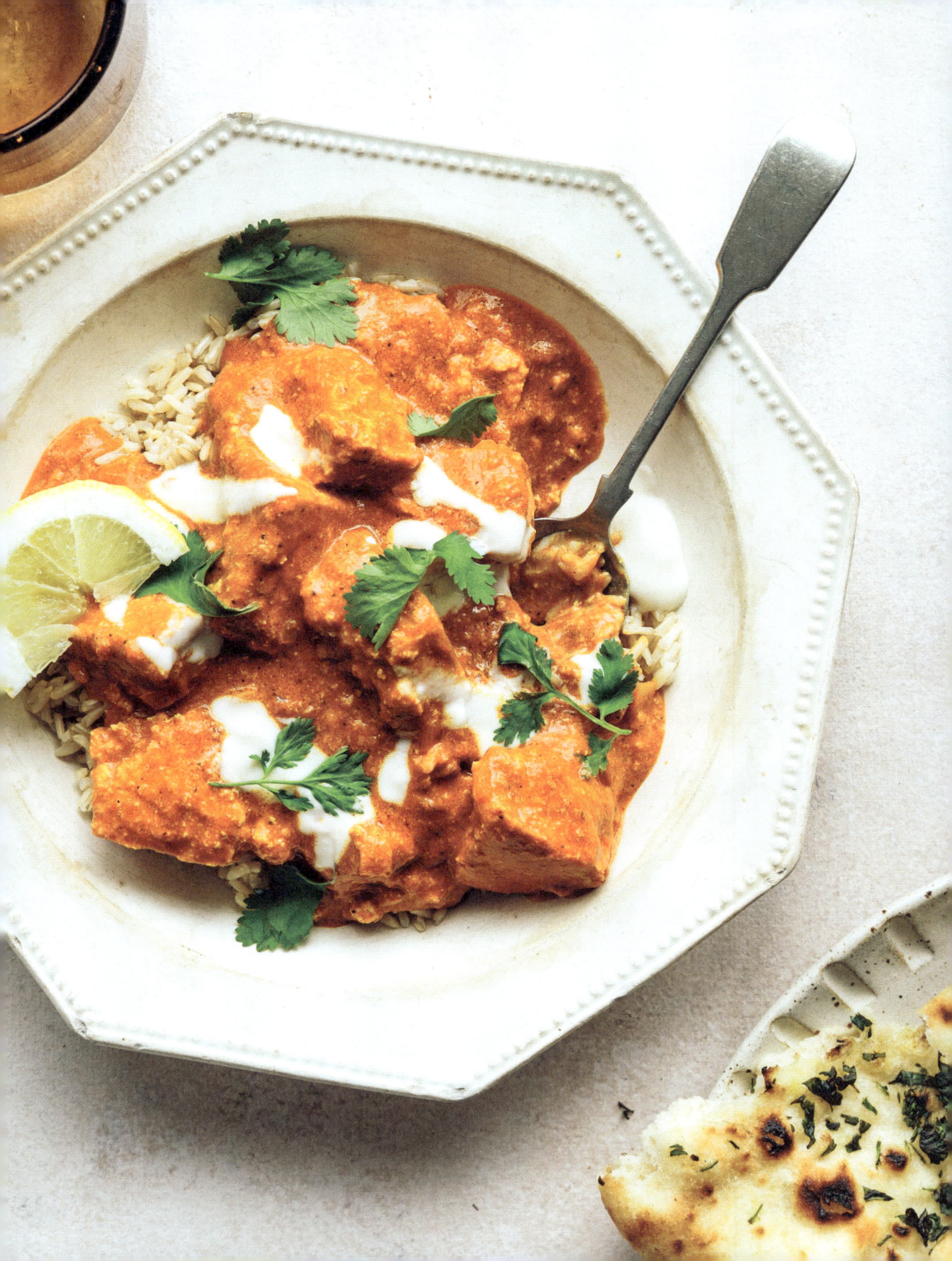

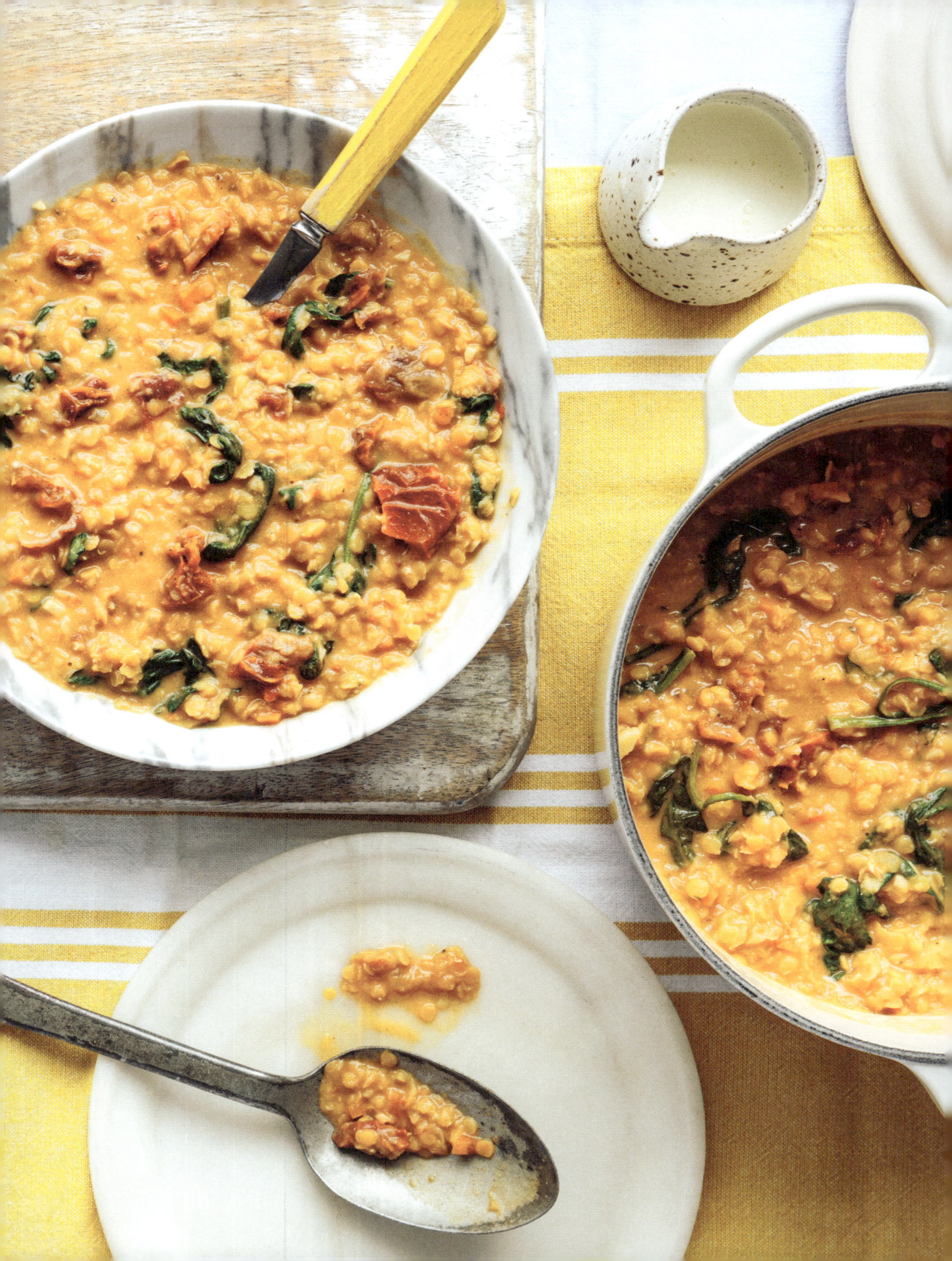

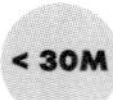

MARRY ME LENTILS

Serves 2–4

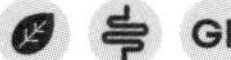

Legend has it that if you make this dish for someone, they'll want to marry you after tasting it! Usually made with chicken, in this version the red lentils soak up and carry the rich flavours of the sun-dried tomatoes and rosemary to create a perfect mouthful. In just 20 minutes, you can have a flavourful, protein-packed dish that I hope will become one of your go-to recipes.

1 small-medium carrot, diced
½ celery stick, diced
1 small onion, diced
2–3 garlic cloves, very
    finely chopped
1 sprig of rosemary
10–12 sun-dried tomatoes,
    chopped, plus extra to serve
1 tablespoon tomato purée (paste)
300g (10½oz/1¼oz) split red
    lentils, washed
700ml (24fl oz/scant 3 cups)
    vegetable stock
200ml (7floz/scant 1 cup) soya milk
4–5 tablespoons nutritional yeast
Handful of baby spinach
Olive oil, for cooking
Salt and freshly ground
    black pepper

TO SERVE

Plant-based cream or yoghurt
Small handful of basil
Plant-based Parmesan-style
    cheese (see page 36, or use
    shop-bought)

Heat a good glug of oil in a saucepan over a medium heat and fry the carrot, celery, onion, garlic, rosemary, sun-dried tomatoes and tomato purée for 5–8 minutes until the onion has softened and the flavours have infused. If it starts to dry out, add a splash of water.

Remove the rosemary and add the lentils, stirring for 1–2 minutes to toast the lentils. Slowly pour in the vegetable stock, stirring frequently, then add the soya milk and simmer for 10 minutes, stirring frequently.

Once the lentils are cooked, season with salt and pepper, then add the nutritional yeast and spinach and stir until the spinach has wilted.

Serve with plant-based cream or yoghurt, more sun-dried tomatoes, basil and plant-based Parmesan-style cheese.

NOTE

The soffritto base can be batch-cooked and used for many different recipes in this book. See page 34 for my pantry staple recipe.

PROTEIN PER SERVING	STORAGE
33.5g	Store for up to 3 days in the refrigerator up to 3 months in the freezer

TEMPEH CACCIATORE

Serves 2–4

 **GF**

Inspired by the traditional chicken cacciatore recipe, this tempeh version has totally won me over. It brings the essence of Tuscany to your table in under 30 minutes, with a rich sauce flavoured with rosemary, black olives and sun-dried tomatoes and crispy cubes of tempeh to add a satisfying crunch. The bicarbonate of soda (baking soda) reduces the acidity in the sauce to create a sweeter flavour. Eat the finished dish with your choice of grains or pasta.

200g (7oz) tempeh, cubed
1 tablespoon cornflour (cornstarch)
½ carrot, diced
½ red onion, diced
½ celery stick, diced
2 garlic cloves, very finely chopped
1 sprig of rosemary
1 teaspoon chilli (hot pepper) flakes
6 sun-dried tomatoes, chopped
30ml (2 tablespoons) red wine
1 x 400g (14oz) tin of plum tomatoes
40g (1½oz) pitted black olives, plus
    extra to serve
½ teaspoon bicarbonate of soda
    (baking soda)
4 tablespoons nutritional yeast
Small handful flat-leaf
    parsley, chopped
3 tablespoons plant-based
    Parmesan-style cheese (see
    page 36, or use shop-bought)
Olive oil, for cooking
Sea salt and freshly ground
    black pepper

TO SERVE

Couscous, quinoa, rice or pasta
Your choice of green vegetables

Put the cubed tempeh into a bowl and add the cornflour, then toss to combine.

Heat a good glug of oil in a saucepan over a medium heat and add the tempeh. Fry for 7–8 minutes until the tempeh is crispy and browned. Remove the tempeh and set aside.

Heat another good glug of oil in the same pan and fry the carrot, onion, celery, garlic, rosemary, chilli flakes and sun-dried tomatoes for 5–8 minutes until softened.

Deglaze with the red wine and allow to bubble for 1 minute, then remove the rosemary and add the tomatoes, olives and tempeh and stir to combine. Add the bicarbonate of soda. You'll see it starts to react. Simmer for 10 minutes over a low heat, or until thickened and creamy.

Stir in the nutritional yeast, parsley and plant-based Parmesan-style cheese and season with salt and pepper.

Serve with a bowl of couscous, quinoa, rice or pasta and a side of greens.

NOTE
Feel free to swap the tempeh for tofu if you prefer.

PROTEIN PER SERVING

28g

STORAGE

Store for up to 3 days in the refrigerator and up to 3 months in the freezer.

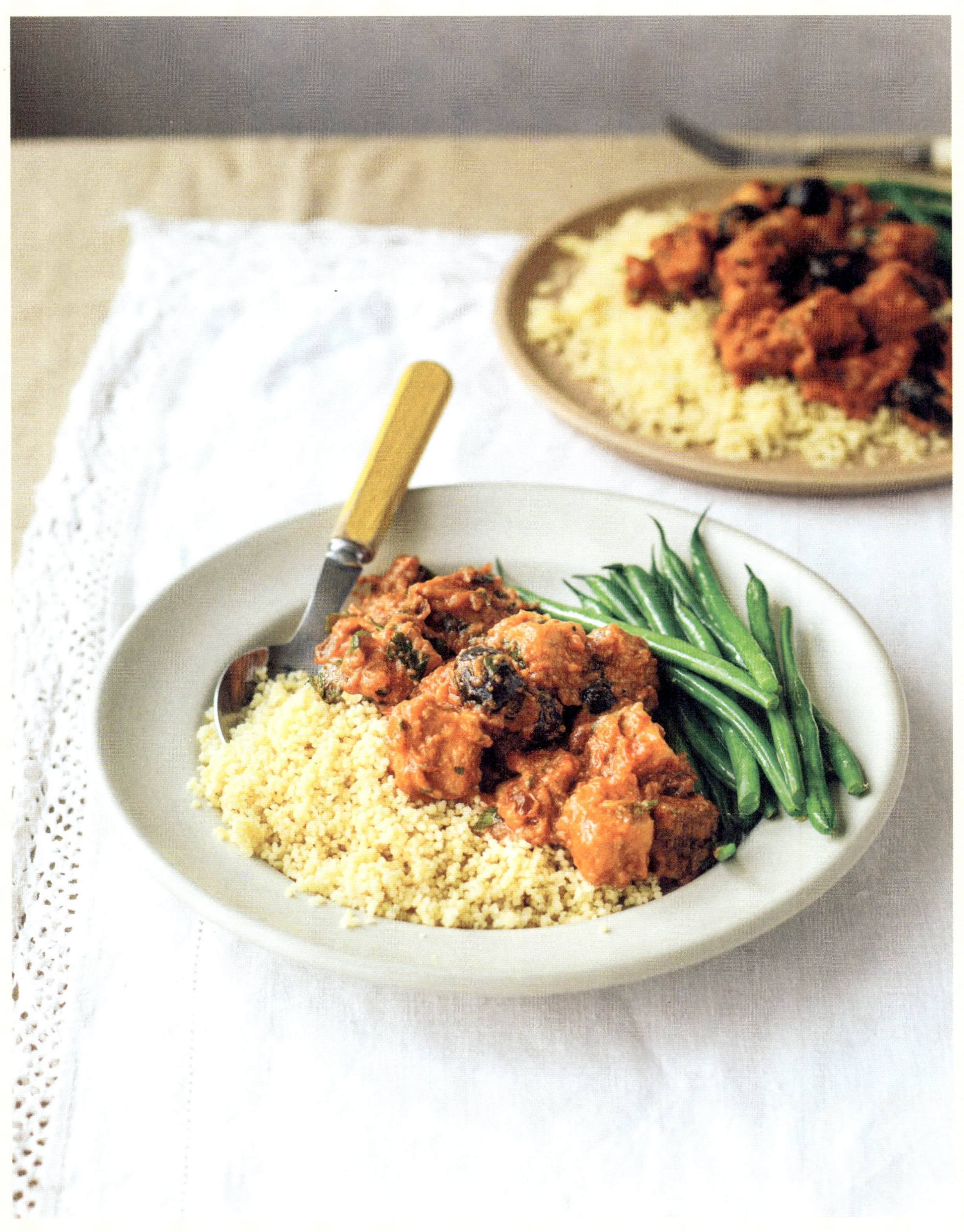

< 1H

SMOKY CHILLI NO CARNE WITH THREE BEANS

Serves 3–4

Is there anything better than a warm, cosy bowl of chilli? This recipe proves that there's not only comfort but also health benefits in every spoonful of this one-pot wonder. With a trio of hearty beans, plum tomatoes and a touch of sweetness from dark (bittersweet) chocolate and cacao powder, this chilli elevates traditional flavours to new heights. Enjoy it topped with avocado, plant-based cream and fresh coriander (cilantro) and paired with rice.

2–3 tablespoons olive oil
1 small-medium carrot, diced
½ celery stick, diced
1 small onion, diced
2–3 garlic cloves, very
    finely chopped
1 teaspoon ground cumin
1 teaspoon chilli powder
1 teaspoon smoked paprika
1 tablespoon dried oregano
30ml (2 tablespoons) red wine
1 red (bell) pepper, diced
1 x 400g (14oz) tin of red kidney
    beans, drained
1 x 400g (14oz) tin of butter (lima)
    beans, drained
1 x 400g (14oz) carlin peas (or
    black-eyed peas), drained
1 x 400g (14oz) tin of plum tomatoes
35g (1¼oz) dark
    (bittersweet) chocolate
2 teaspoons light brown soft sugar
2 teaspoons raw cacao powder
Salt and freshly ground
    black pepper

TO SERVE
Rice
Sliced avocado
Plant-based cream
Sliced red chilli
Coriander (cilantro)

Heat the oil in a saucepan over a medium heat and fry the carrot, celery onion and garlic for 5–8 minutes until soft and golden.

Add the cumin, chilli powder, paprika and oregano, then deglaze the pan with the wine and cook for 3–4 minutes to let the flavours infuse.

Add the red pepper, kidney beans, butter beans, carlin peas and tomatoes, crushing the tomatoes with a fork so they release the juices. Refill the empty tomato tin one-third full with water and add it to the pan. Simmer for 20–25 minutes until thickened, stirring occasionally.

Add the chocolate, brown sugar and cacao powder and stir again until well combined. Season with salt and pepper.

Remove the pan from the heat and allow the chilli to rest for 15 minutes. This is important to ensure the chilli has a velvety consistency.

Serve with rice, topped with avocado, plant-based cream, chilli and coriander.

NOTE
The soffritto base can be batch-cooked and used for many different recipes in this book. See page 34 for my pantry staple recipe.

PROTEIN PER SERVING

25g

STORAGE

Store up to 3 days in the refrigerator and up to 3 months in the freezer

DAN DAN(ISH) NOODLES WITH TEMPEH

Serves 2–4

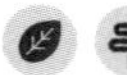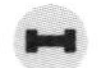

There's nothing in the world quite like Sichuan pepper! It's a little bit spicy, a little bit bitter and a whole lot of delicious! This dan dan(ish) noodle recipe will transport you straight to south-western China and is actually a breeze to prepare, taking just 15 minutes from start to finish (which is way less than waiting for the takeaway to arrive at your door).

NOODLES

200g (7oz) whole-wheat noodles
2 tablespoons smooth peanut
　　butter
2 tablespoons light soy sauce
1 tablespoon chilli oil
1 tablespoon sesame seeds
Sesame oil, for drizzling

TEMPEH

200g (7oz) tempeh, crumbled into
　　small pieces
2 garlic cloves, very finely chopped
2 tablespoons hoisin sauce
2 teaspoons light soy sauce
1 teaspoon rice vinegar
1 teaspoon ground Sichuan pepper
Sesame oil, for frying

TO SERVE

1 pak choi (bok choy), halved and
　　steamed or boiled
4 tablespoons roasted peanuts
Spring onions (scallions), chopped

First, bring a large saucepan of water to the boil and cook the noodles according to the packet instructions, then drain and rinse under cold water. Drizzle with sesame oil and toss to coat, then set aside.

Next, make the tempeh. Heat a good glug of sesame oil in a wok or frying pan (skillet) over a medium heat, then add and all the ingredients and cook for 10–12 minutes until the tempeh is browned. Remove from the pan and set aside.

Prepare the noodle sauce by combining the peanut butter, soy sauce, chilli oil and sesame seeds in a bowl. If it's too thick, add a splash of hot water.

Add the noodles to the wok along with the noodle sauce and cook for a couple of minutes to warm through.

Serve topped with the tempeh, pak choi, peanuts and spring onions.

PROTEIN PER SERVING

31g

MAKE IT GLUTEN-FREE

Use gluten-free noodles, hoisin sauce and tamari.

STORAGE

Store for up to 3 days in the refrigerator and up to 3 months in the freezer.

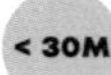

TERIYAKI SOYA STRIPS WITH STIR-FRIED VEGETABLES

Serves 2–4

These teriyaki soya strips are a delightful blend of saucy, sweet flavours that make for a delicious meal. Quick to prepare (just 20 minutes) and far better than your local takeaway spot, they offer a high-protein option for a satisfying weeknight dinner. Serve alongside rice and stir-fried vegetables, they make a perfectly balanced meal.

100g (3½oz) dried soya chunks (or crumbled tempeh if preferred)
400–500ml (14–17fl oz/generous 1½–generous 2 cups) hot vegetable stock
1 garlic clove, very finely chopped
1 teaspoon grated ginger
1 red (bell) pepper, sliced
100g (3½oz) Tenderstem broccoli (broccolini)
Small handful of shiitake mushrooms
2 tablespoons light soy sauce
Sesame oil, for frying

TERIYAKI SAUCE
3 tablespoons light soy sauce
2 tablespoons light brown soft sugar
1 teaspoon rice vinegar
1 teaspoon finely chopped garlic
1 teaspoon finely chopped ginger
1 teaspoon cornflour (cornstarch)
1 teaspoon sesame oil

TO SERVE
160g (5¾oz/¾ cup) basmati or jasmine rice
Small handful of spring onions (scallions), chopped
Sesame seeds

First, bring a large saucepan of water to the boil and cook the rice according to the packet instructions.

Meanwhile, put the soya chunks into a bowl and cover them with the hot vegetable stock. Let them soak for about 10–15 minutes until they are fully rehydrated. Squeeze the soya chunks with your hands to drain any excess liquid.

Next, heat a wok or frying pan (skillet) over a medium-high heat. Add a glug of sesame oil along with the garlic and ginger. Fry for 30 seconds, then add the vegetables and soy sauce. Stir-fry for 2–3 minutes, then add the rehydrated soya chunks and stir-fry for 3–5 minutes until they start to brown slightly.

Meanwhile, whisk together the teriyaki sauce ingredients with 2 tablespoons water in a small bowl.

Pour the teriyaki sauce over the soya chunks and veggies. Stir well to coat evenly with the sauce. Cook for an additional 2–3 minutes, until the vegetables are almost tender but still have a nice crunch and the sauce has thickened.

Divide the rice between plates or bowls and top with the teriyaki soya chunks and vegetables. Sprinkle with spring onions and sesame seeds just before serving.

PROTEIN PER SERVING

30g

MAKE IT GLUTEN-FREE

Swap the soy sauce for tamari.

STORAGE

Store for up to 3 days in the refrigerator. Freeze the soya strips and vegetables separately for up to 3 months.

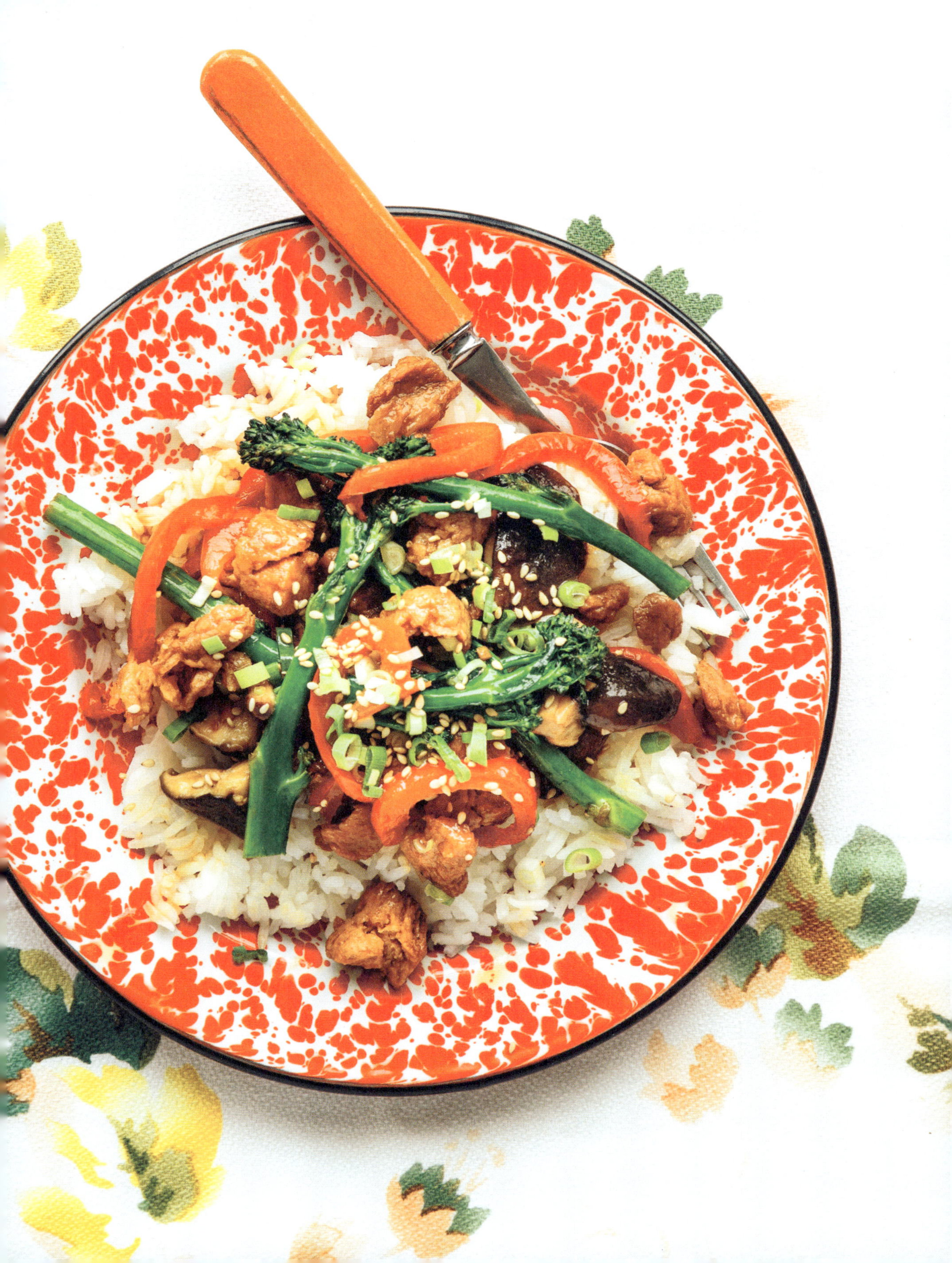

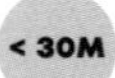

PORK-LESS TEMPEH TACOS
Serves 3

Next time you hear someone say that vegan food is bland, hand them one of these tacos and watch their reaction. Bright, fresh and fun to devour, these pork-less tacos are filled with rich and decadent crispy tempeh, which is balanced by avocado tomato salsa and tangy jalapeños. It's like a nutrient-rich rainbow landing right on your table.

CRISPY TEMPEH
6 tablespoons light soy sauce
4 tablespoons maple syrup
2 tablespoons tomato purée (paste)
½ teaspoon smoked paprika
1 teaspoon liquid smoke (optional)
200g (7oz) tempeh, crumbled
Sesame oil, for cooking

AVOCADO AND TOMATO SALSA
1 ripe avocado, peeled,
    stoned and mashed
80g (2¾oz/scant ⅓ cup) high-
    protein plant-based yoghurt
Juice of ½ lime
150g (5½oz) cherry tomatoes, diced
Salt and freshly ground
    black pepper

TO SERVE
6 mini tortillas
Plant-based sour cream
Small handful of coriander
    (cilantro), chopped
Pickled jalapeños
Lime wedges

First, prepare the tempeh. Combine the soy sauce, maple syrup, tomato purée, smoked paprika and liquid smoke in a container and mix well. Add the tempeh and stir to ensure it is evenly coated with the mixture, then set aside to marinate while you prepare the salsa.

To make the salsa, combine the avocado, yoghurt and lime juice in a bowl. Season with salt and pepper and mix to combine. Alternatively, if you prefer a creamy consistency, you can blend the salsa. Finally, add the chopped tomatoes and stir them through.

Heat a glug of sesame oil in a frying pan (skillet) over a high heat and add the tempeh and its marinade. Be careful, as the tempeh will sizzle, but this is the only way to guarantee a crispy result. Cook for 10–12 minutes until crispy and browned, then transfer to a plate lined with paper towels to absorb the excess oil.

Warm the tortillas in a dry pan over a medium-high heat for 15–30 seconds per side, then layer each tortilla with the avocado and tomato salsa and the crispy tempeh. Top with a dollop of plant-based sour cream, coriander, pickled jalapeños and a squeeze of lime.

Repeat until you can't eat any more!

PROTEIN PER SERVING	MAKE IT GLUTEN-FREE	STORAGE
17g	Use gluten-free tortillas and tamari.	Store for up to 3 days in the refrigerator. The tempeh can be frozen for up to 3 month.

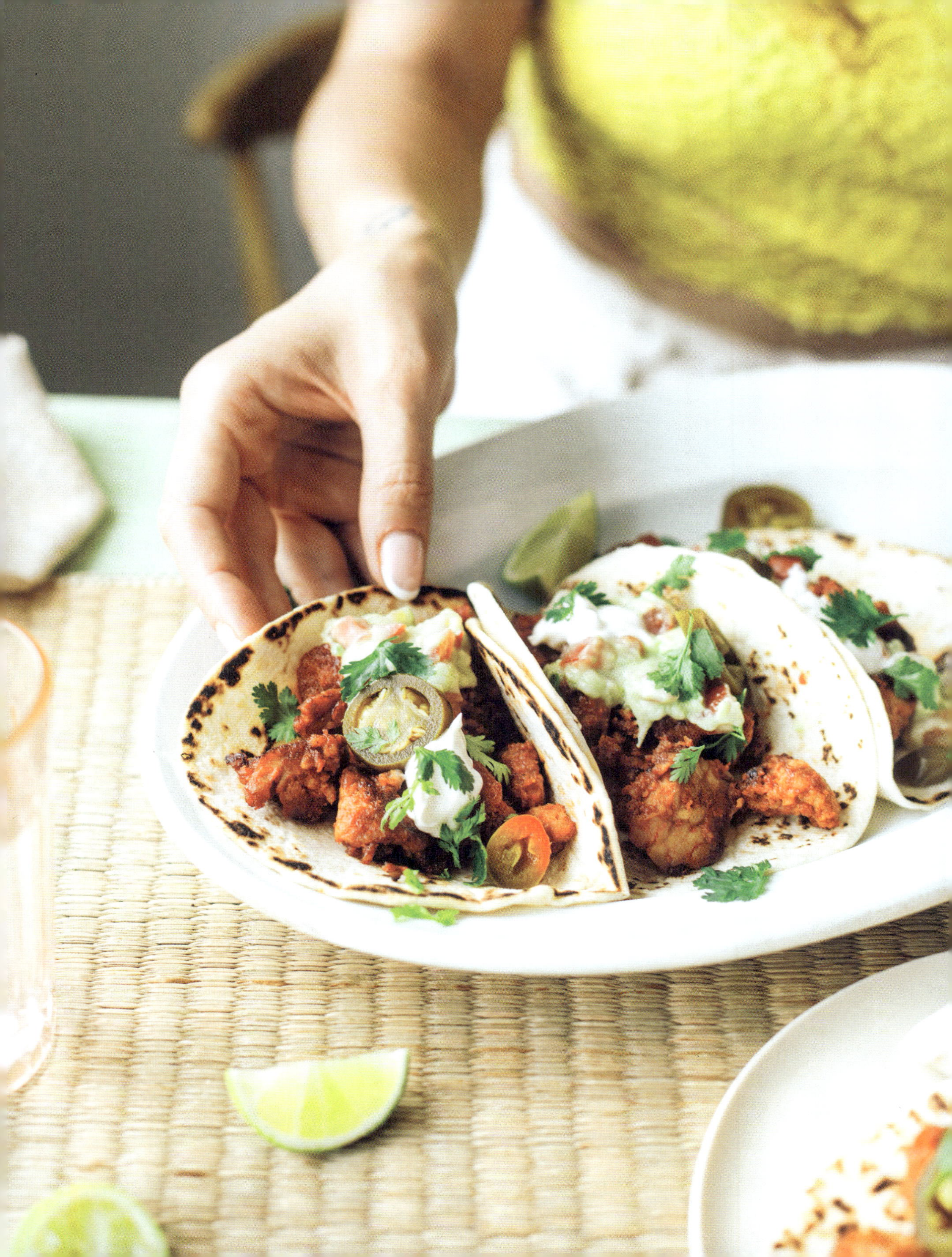

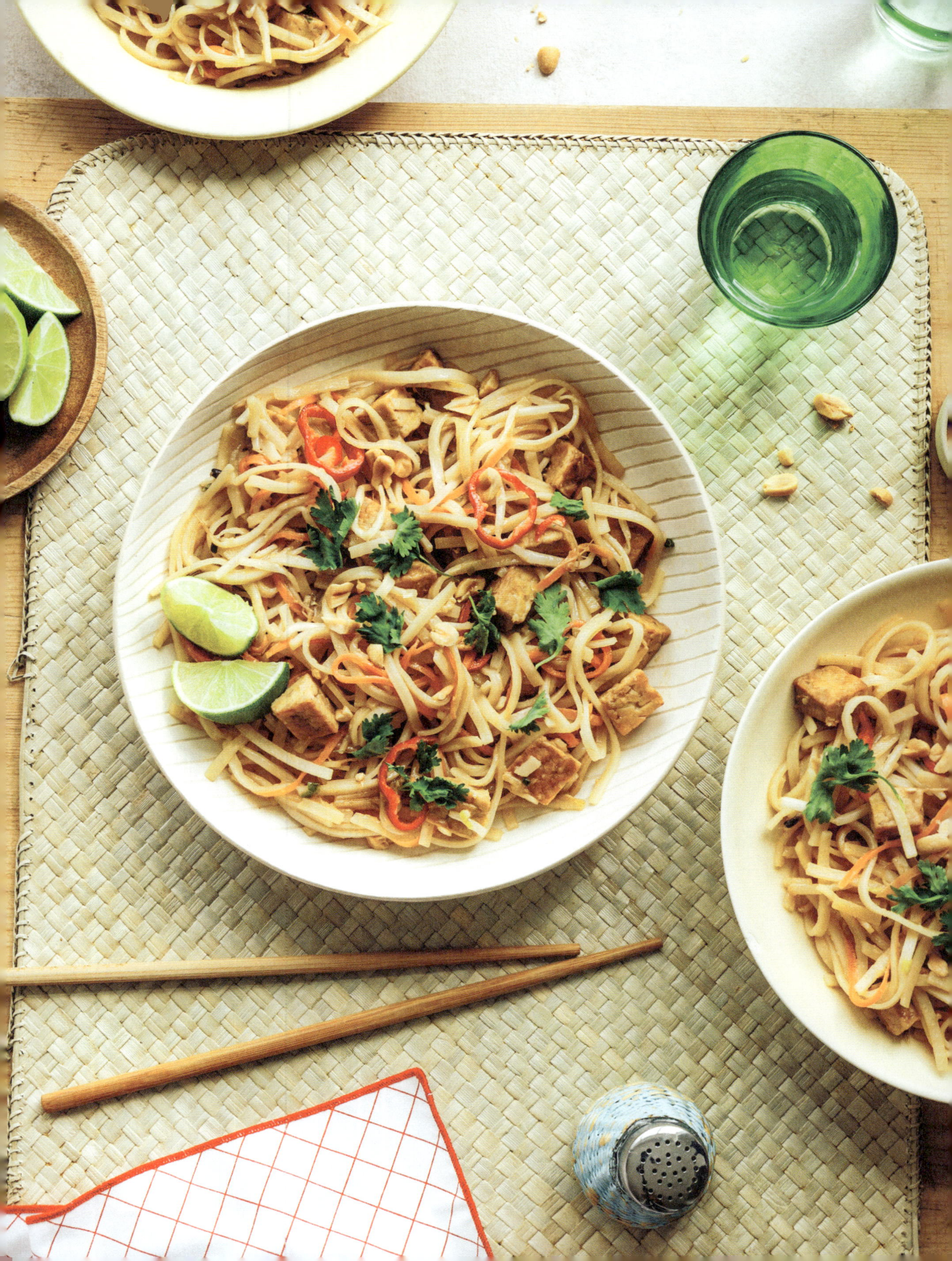

TEMPEH PAD THAI

Serves 2–4

Pad Thai has long been my top pick for a quick takeaway fix, but it's also a breeze to cook at home and turn vegan! Picture this: hearty tempeh meets crisp veggies and velvety rice noodles, which come together in a delicious savoury and sweet sauce. Make sure to top it with a sprinkle of crushed peanuts, a burst of zesty lime some fresh coriander (cilantro), and you'll be licking your lips and craving seconds. I promise!

200g (7oz) flat rice noodles
1 tablespoon vegetable oil
200g (7oz) tempeh, cut into
    bite-sized pieces
2 spring onions
    (scallions), chopped
2 garlic cloves, finely chopped
1 carrot, thinly sliced lengthwise
    (I use a vegetable peeler)
100g (3½oz) beansprouts
Sesame oil, for frying

SAUCE

3 tablespoons light soy sauce
20g (¾oz) coconut sugar
1 tablespoon rice vinegar
1 tablespoon crunchy peanut butter
½ red chilli, sliced (deseeded
    for less heat; optional)

TO SERVE

30g (1oz/scant ¼ cup) lightly
    salted peanuts
15g (½oz) coriander (cilantro),
    leaves roughly chopped
Juice of 1 lime

Prepare the rice noodles according to the packet instructions, then drain and stir through the vegetable oil to prevent sticking. Set aside.

Heat a glug of sesame oil in a non-stick wok or frying pan (skillet) and add the cubed tempeh. Sear for 2–3 minutes per side, then remove and set aside on a plate.

Add another 2 tablespoons sesame oil to the pan, then add the spring onions, garlic, carrot and beansprouts. Stir-fry for 5–10 minutes until the vegetables have softened but still have a nice crunch.

Meanwhile, whisk together the sauce ingredients in a small bowl, adding a splash of water if needed.

Add the noodles, tempeh and sauce to the vegetables and stir-fry over a medium heat to warm through evenly.

Top with the peanuts and coriander and serve with a squeeze of lime.

PROTEIN PER SERVING
24g

MAKE IT GLUTEN-FREE
Swap the soy sauce for tamari.

STORAGE
Store for up to 3 days in the refrigerator and up to 3 months in the freezer.

SWEET POTATO AND BLACK BEAN BURGERS

Serves 6

Sweet potatoes and black beans are a match made in heaven. Sweet, tender, flavourful and super easy to prepare, these burgers can be enjoyed with or without a bread bun. But for the ultimate taste sensation, be sure to pair them with my spicy, zesty sauce.

PATTIES
25g (1oz) ground flaxseed
300g (10½oz) sweet potato, peeled and chopped
1 x 400g (14oz) tin of black beans, drained
½ red onion, diced
1 teaspoon garlic granules
½ teaspoon smoked paprika
1 tablespoon light soy sauce
150g (5½oz/1½ cups) dried breadcrumbs
Salt and freshly ground black pepper

SPICY SAUCE
200g (7oz/generous ¾ cup) high-protein plant-based yoghurt
1 tablespoon sriracha
Juice of ½ lemon

TO SERVE
Burger buns
Your favourite burger toppings (I keep it simple with lettuce, tomato and sliced red onion plus a good plant-based cheese)

Preheat the oven to 200°C/180°C fan/400°F/Gas mark 6 and line a baking tray (pan) with baking parchment.

Mix the ground flaxseeds with 80–90ml (2¾–3fl oz/⅓ cup) water and set aside. This will form a slurry, which will be the binding agent for the burgers.

Bring a large saucepan of salted water to the boil and cook the sweet potato for 15–20 minutes until tender, then drain.

Combine the cooked sweet potato, flaxseed slurry, black beans, red onion, garlic granules, smoked paprika and soy sauce in a food processor. Season with salt and pepper, then blend until smooth and the mixture holds together. Transfer the mixture to a bowl and incorporate the breadcrumbs.

Divide the mixture into six portions and shape them into patties with your hands. It is easier if you wet your hands first to prevent the mixture from sticking to your fingers.

Place the burgers on the prepared baking tray and bake in the oven for 30 minutes, carefully flipping the burgers halfway through.

While the burgers cook, prepare the sauce by whisking together all the ingredients in a bowl and seasoning with salt and pepper to taste.

Serve the burgers in buns with the spicy sauce and your favourite burger toppings.

PROTEIN PER SERVING
14g (patty only)

MAKE IT GLUTEN-FREE
Use gluten-free breadcrumbs, buns and tamari.

STORAGE
Store for up to 3 days in the refrigerator and up to 3 months in the freezer.

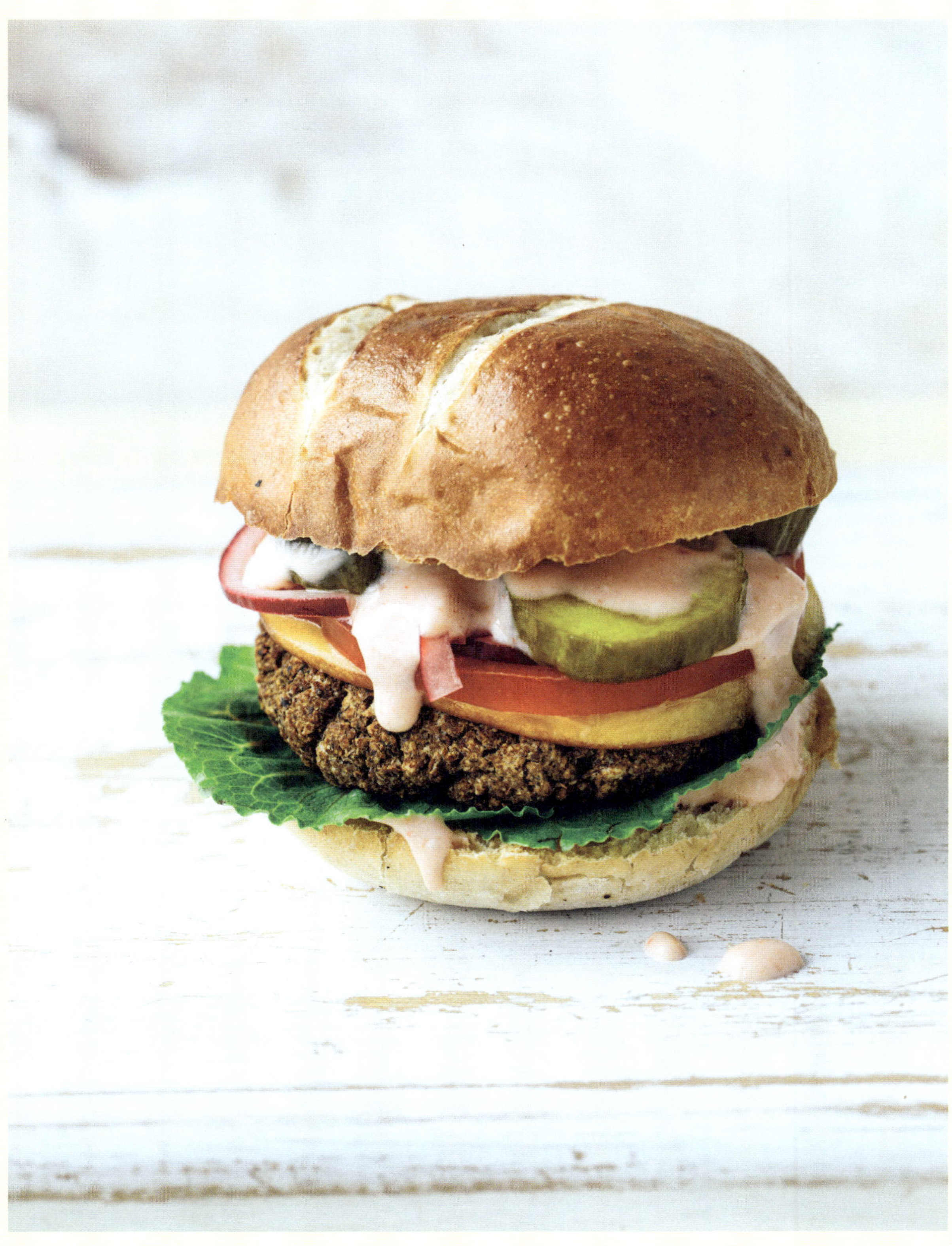

PIZZA PARTY

Serves 2–4

This healthy fakeaway pizza recipe is not only a breeze to prepare but also includes a secret protein-rich ingredient that will leave your taste buds none the wiser. Nobody will suspect the tofu hidden within its crispy, pillowy crust! Actually, you'll find that it disappears quicker than you had expected. Feel free to get creative with the toppings, too. I've added plant-based shredded mozzarella-style cheese, homemade plant-based bacon, roasted (bell) peppers and rocket (arugula), but customize to your heart's content or make it a pizza night and let everyone choose their own.

DOUGH

250ml (8 fl oz/1 cup) lukewarm water
150g (5½oz) firm tofu, drained
7g (¼oz) fast-action dried yeast
550g (1lb 3½oz/4½ cups) '00' flour, plus extra for dusting (or a flour that has a protein content between 12% and 14.5%)
2 teaspoons salt
2 tablespoons olive oil

MARINARA SAUCE

200g (7oz/¾ cup) passata (sieved tomatoes)
Splash of olive oil
Pinch of dried oregano
Salt and freshly ground black pepper

TOFU 'BACON'

170g (6oz) smoked tofu, drained and pressed (see page 37), then diced into 1cm (½ inch) cubes
5 tablespoons light soy sauce
2 tablespoons maple syrup
2 tablespoons tomato purée (paste)
1 teaspoon smoked paprika
Olive oil, for frying

TOPPING

Roasted red (bell) peppers
Shredded plant-based mozzarella-style cheese
Rocket (arugula)

First, make the dough. Combine the water, tofu and yeast in a food processor and blend until smooth and frothy.

Put the flour, salt and oil into a bowl, then slowly add the water-tofu mixture. Mix with a fork, then transfer the dough to a lightly floured surface and knead for 5–8 minutes until stretchy.

Place the dough in a lightly greased bowl, cover with a clean kitchen towel and leave to rise for 2 hours, or until it has doubled in size.

Meanwhile, make the marinara sauce by combining all the ingredients in a bowl.

Next, prepare the bacon. Combine all the ingredients in a bowl and set aside to marinate.

Once doubled in size, halve the dough, place into separate bowls and leave to rise for a further 30–60 minutes, or until doubled in size.

Now cook the bacon. Heat a good glug of oil in a frying pan (skillet) and add the tofu and its marinade. Fry for 5–6 minutes, or until the tofu starts to brown. Set aside.

Preheat the oven to 240°C/425°F/Gas mark 7. If you have a pizza stone, place it in the oven.

Roll out one of the portions of dough into a circle or rectangle on a lightly floured surface as thinly as you can.

Transfer the base to a floured baking sheet or the preheated pizza stone and bake for 5 minutes, or until the edges start to turn golden.

Remove the dough and add your toppings. Start with the marinara sauce, then the bacon and peppers and finally the mozzarella. Bake for a further 15–20 minutes, or until crisp and golden on top. Remove from the oven and top with a handful of rocket.

Repeat with the remaining dough. Serve hot.

NOTE

If you prefer a crusty pizza, divide the dough in four pieces and reduce the baking time from 15–20 to 10 minutes.

PROTEIN PER SERVING	MAKE IT GLUTEN-FREE	STORAGE
43g	Use gluten-free bread and pizza flour and tamari.	Store for up to 4 days in the refrigerator and up to 3 months in the freezer.

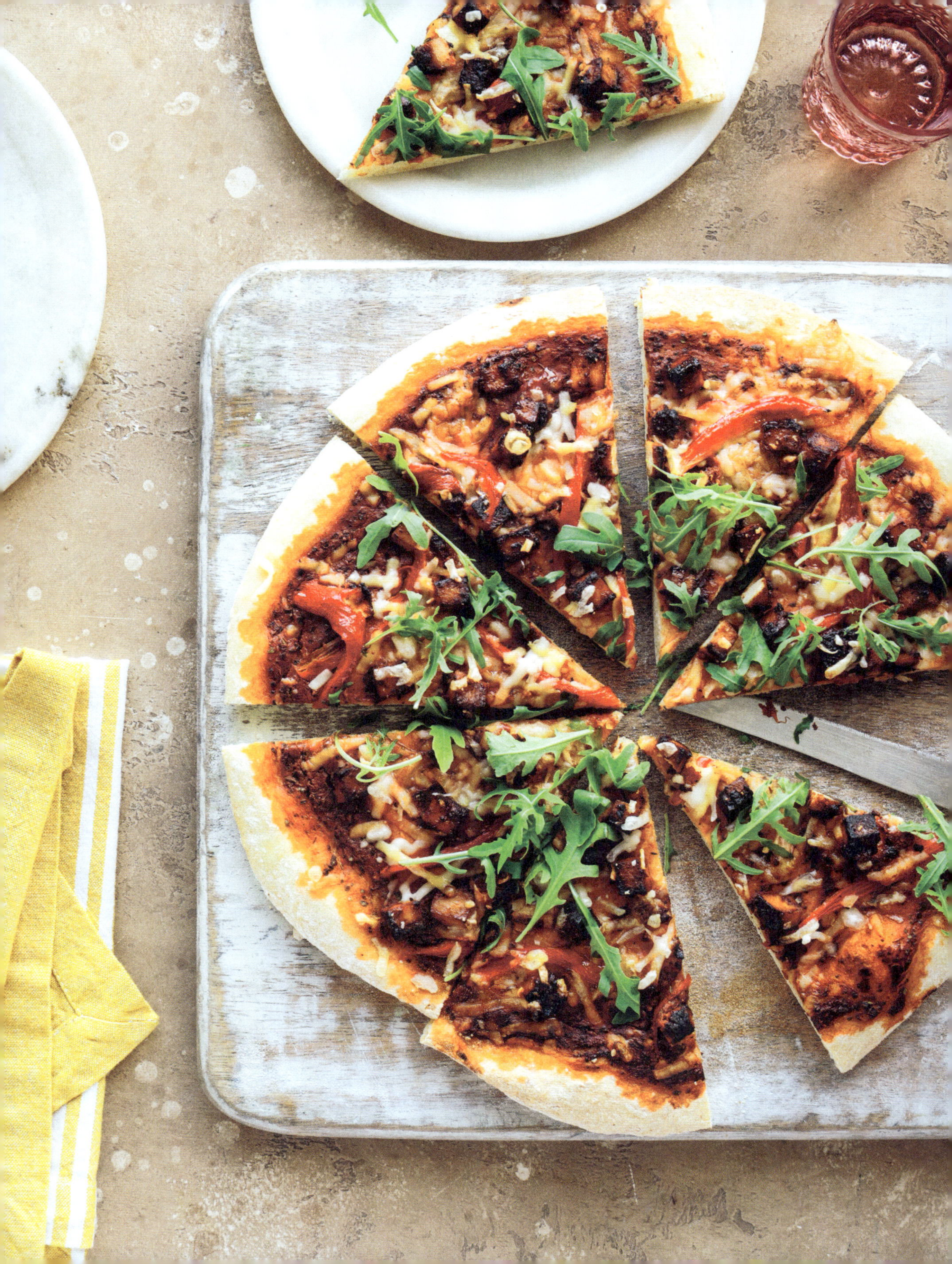

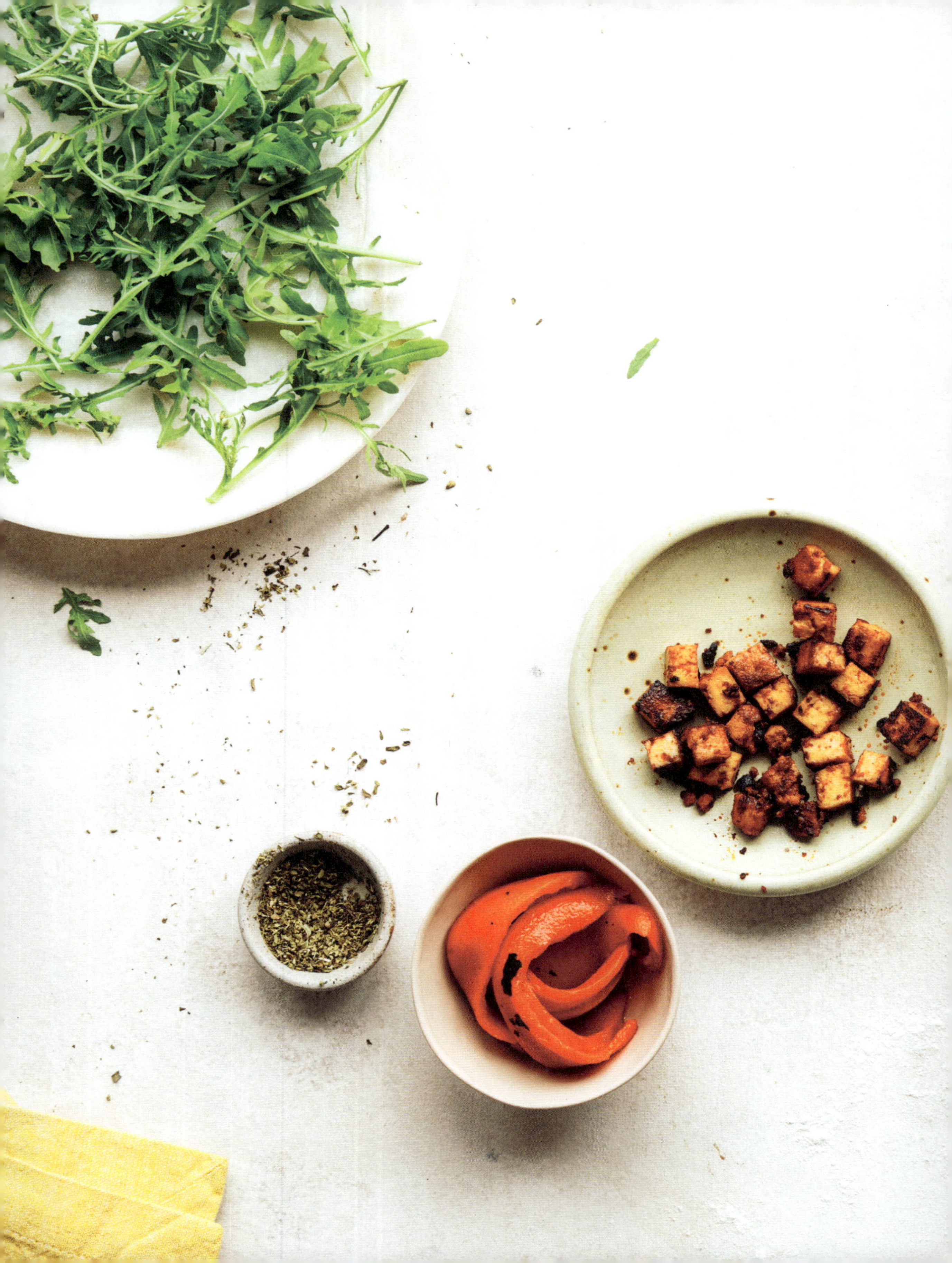

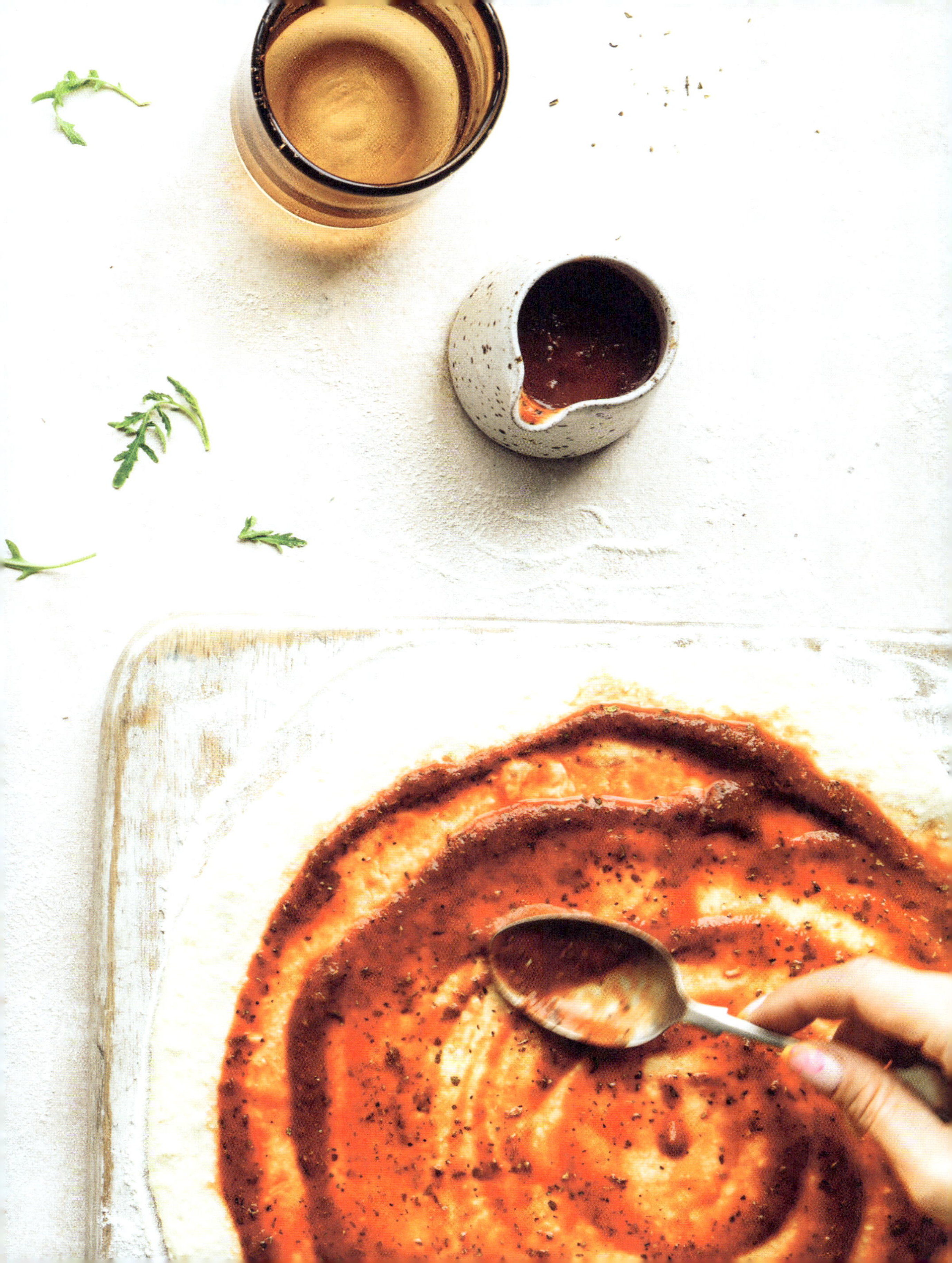

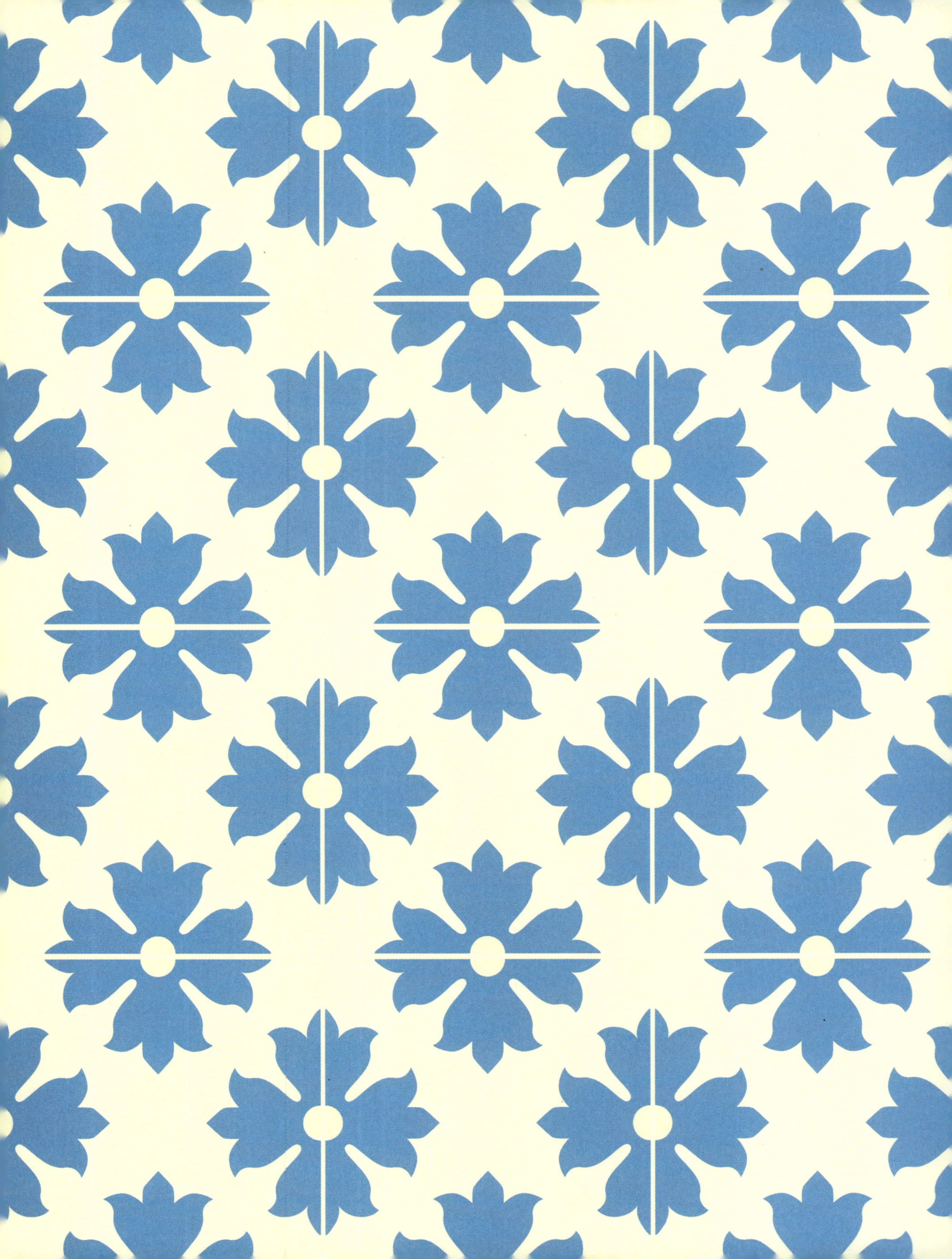

SNACKS

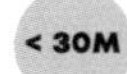

CRUNCHY ASPARAGUS WITH TAHINI LEMON SAUCE

Serves 2–4

I'm constantly seeking inventive ways to savour asparagus, and this recipe takes this versatile vegetable to new heights! With a crispy quinoa and polenta (cornmeal) coating, these asparagus sticks are packed with protein and irresistible flavour and are the perfect finger food for entertaining guests. The zesty tahini lemon sauce that goes with them is a hassle-free delight, too.

400g (14oz) asparagus, woody ends snapped off
30g (1oz/¼ cup) chickpea (gram) flour
Olive oil, for brushing

BATTER
50g (1¾oz/½ cup) chickpea (gram) flour
40g (1½oz/¼ cup) polenta (cornmeal)
100ml (3½fl oz/scant ½ cup) sparkling water

BREADCRUMB MIXTURE
50g (1¾oz/½ cup) chickpea (gram) flour
50g (1¾oz/¾ cup) panko breadcrumbs
20g (¾oz) quinoa
1 teaspoon onion granules
1 tablespoon nutritional yeast
1 tablespoon mixed seeds, such as sesame seeds, flaxseeds, chia seeds and shelled hemp seeds (optional)
Zest of ½ lemon (optional)
Salt and freshly ground black pepper

TAHINI LEMON SAUCE
150g (5½oz/scant ⅔ cup) high-protein plant-based yoghurt
2 tablespoons tahini
1 tablespoon lemon juice
Small handful of coriander (cilantro), chopped
Pinch of salt

Preheat the oven to 200°C/180°C fan/400°F/Gas mark 6 and line a baking tray (pan) with baking parchment).

Brush the asparagus with olive oil and set aside on a plate.

Put the chickpea flour into a shallow dish big enough to hold the asparagus.

In another dish, combine all the ingredients for the batter.

In a third dish, combine all the ingredients for the breadcrumb mixture.

Lightly coat the asparagus in plain chickpea flour first, then dip them in the batter, then evenly coat them with the breadcrumb mixture. Place on the prepared baking tray.

Bake the asparagus in the oven for 25 minutes until golden and crunchy, flipping them halfway through. Alternatively, if you have an air fryer, you can air-fry the asparagus at 180°C (425°F) for 15 minutes.

Meanwhile, combine all the ingredients for the sauce in a bowl and mix well.

Serve the asparagus with the sauce.

PROTEIN PER SERVING	MAKE IT GLUTEN-FREE	STORAGE
26.5g	Use gluten-free panko breadcrumbs.	Best eaten fresh.

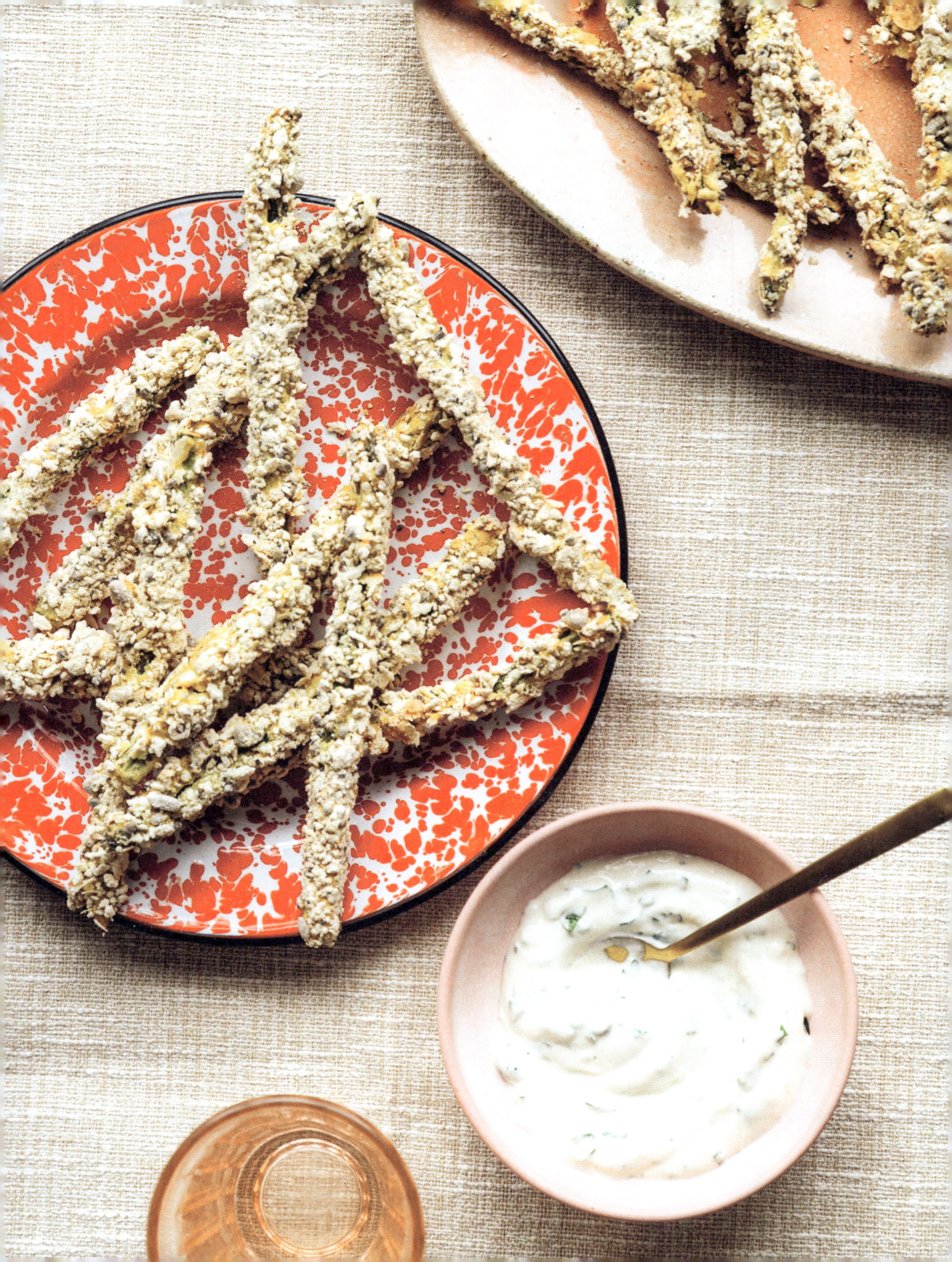

HARISSA RED LENTIL HUMMUS WITH TOFU FLATBREAD

Serves 2–3

Looking for a flavourful and protein-packed snack or starter? This red lentil hummus and high-protein tofu flatbread might be just the thing! This dynamic duo combines the earthy goodness of red lentils with the bold flavours of harissa paste and tahini, creating a creamy and satisfying dip. Paired with homemade tofu flatbread, which is both hearty and light (and amazingly high in protein), this dish is not only delicious and hassle-free to make but is also incredibly good for you too. What's not to like? You can also easily scale up the quantities for the flatbreads and then freeze them once cooked so that you always have a supply to hand!

HARISSA RED LENTIL HUMMUS

200g (7oz/generous ¾ cup) split red lentils
1 tablespoon harissa paste
100g (3½oz) tahini
2 garlic cloves
Juice of 1 lemon
1 teaspoon salt
2 ice cubes (optional, for creaminess)

TOFU FLATBREAD

150g (5½oz) firm tofu, crumbled
45ml (1½fl oz/3 tablespoons) unsweetened soya milk
15g (½oz) nutritional yeast
200g (7oz/1⅔ cups) self-raising (self-rising) flour, plus extra for dusting
Pinch of salt
2 tablespoons olive oil, plus extra to serve

TO SERVE

Chopped garlic
Chopped flat-leaf parsley
Pickled red onions
Pomegranate seeds
Chopped coriander (cilantro)

Bring a large saucepan of water to the boil and cook the lentils for 6–7 minutes until softened.

Transfer the lentils to a food processor along with the harissa paste, tahini, garlic, lemon, salt and ice cubes (if using). Blend until creamy, then scrape out and set aside.

For the flatbread, put the tofu, soya milk and nutritional yeast into a clean food processor and blend until creamy. Add the flour, salt and oil and blend again until a dough forms.

Tip out the dough onto a lightly floured work surface and divide it into three or four pieces. Roll out each piece to 5mm (¼ inch) thick using a rolling pin sprinkled with flour.

Heat a dry frying pan (skillet) over a medium heat and cook the flatbreads for 3–4 minutes on each side until golden. Brush with a little oil and sprinkle over a little garlic and parsley before serving.

Transfer the hummus to a plate and top with a drizzle of oil, pickled red onions, pomegranate seeds and chopped coriander.

PROTEIN PER SERVING	MAKE IT GLUTEN-FREE	STORAGE
36g	Use gluten-free flour.	Store for up to 3 days in the refrigerator. Freeze the hummus and flatbreads separately for up to 3 months.

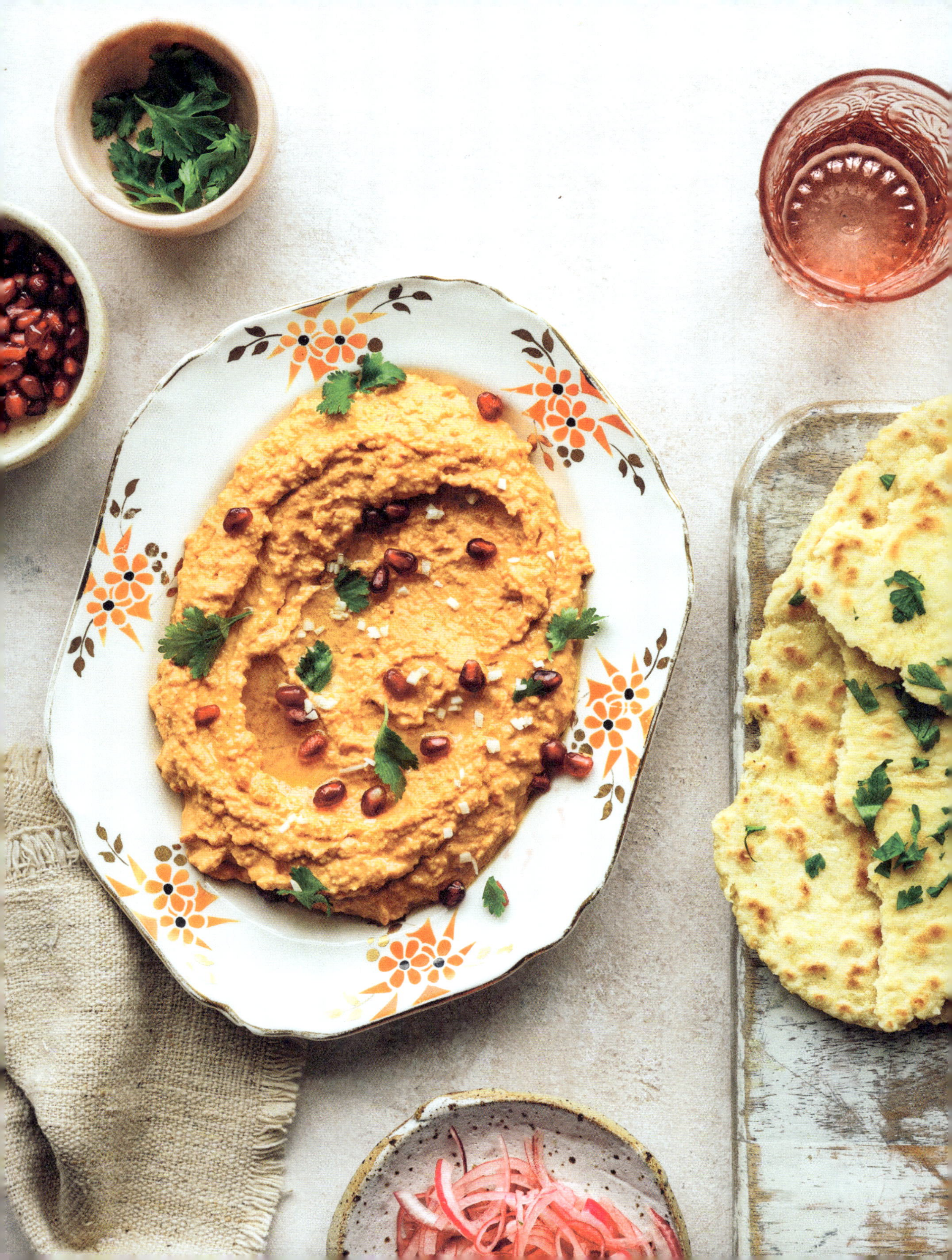

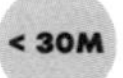

HARISSA-ROASTED CRUNCHY BUTTER BEANS

Serves 1–2

Ditch the crisps (chips), because there's a new snack in town – harissa-roasted butter (lima) beans! These crispy, flavour-packed beans are about to become your new favourite healthy indulgence. With just a handful of ingredients and a simple method, you'll have a protein-packed snack ready in no time. Whether you're craving a spicy treat or need a crunchy side dish, these roasted beans are the perfect solution. Goodbye bland and unhealthy snacks – you won't be missing them!

1 x 400g (14oz) tins of butter (lima) beans, drained
1 tablespoon olive oil
½–1 tablespoon harissa paste (according to spice preference)
1 teaspoon garlic granules
Pinch of salt

Preheat the oven to 220°C/200°C fan/425°F/Gas mark 7 and line a baking tray (pan) with baking parchment.

Place the butter beans on a clean dish towel and pat them dry. This step is crucial to ensure the beans turn crispy.

Pur the beans into a bowl and add the olive oil, harissa paste, garlic granules and salt. Mix until well combined.

Transfer the beans to the prepared baking tray, spreading them out evenly and ensuring they have as much space as possible between them. Roast in the oven for 35–40 minutes, stirring halfway through to ensure an even crisping. Alternatively, if you have an air fryer, you can air-fry the beans at 200°C (400°F) for 20 minutes, shaking them halfway through.

Enjoy hot or cold.

PROTEIN PER SERVING

12g

STORAGE

Store for up to 3 days in an airtight container. Not freezer friendly.

TOFU PUFFS
Serves 1–2

Crispy on the outside, soft on the inside and bursting with flavour, these tofu puffs will be your new favourite snack! They come together in less than 30 minutes and they'll disappear in even less time! Pair them with your favourite dips for an extra flavour punch. I've included a simple recipe for a high-protein spicy dip to kick things up a notch, but feel free to get creative and experiment with your own delicious dips!

300g (10½oz) extra-firm smoked tofu, drained and pressed (see page 37)
40g (1½oz) nutritional yeast
½ teaspoon garlic granules (optional)
½ teaspoon onion granules
½ teaspoon smoked paprika
Golden breadcrumbs, for coating
Sesame seeds, for coating

SPICY DIP
100g (3½oz/generous ⅓ cup) high-protein plant-based yoghurt
1 tablespoon sriracha
Juice of ½ Lemon

Put the tofu, nutritional yeast, garlic and onion granules and smoked paprika into a food processor and blend to a thick paste. Depending on how much water you drained from the tofu it'll be softer or denser, but it'll work either way.

Pour some breadcrumbs onto a plate and stir through some sesame seeds.

Scoop out walnut-sized pieces of the mixture and, if it's firm enough, roll them in your hands to shape into balls. Place the balls on the plate of breadcrumbs and roll to coat them in the breadcrumbs.

Air-fry the balls at 200°C (400°F) for 20–25 minutes until golden. Alternatively, place the balls on a baking tray (pan) lined with baking parchment and bake in the oven at 200°C/180°C fan/400°F/Gas mark 6 for 20–25 minutes.

Meanwhile, mix together the ingredients for the dip in a small bowl.

Serve the tofu puffs with the dip.

PROTEIN PER SERVING

33g

MAKE IT GLUTEN-FREE

Use gluten-free breadcrumbs.

STORAGE

Best eaten fresh.

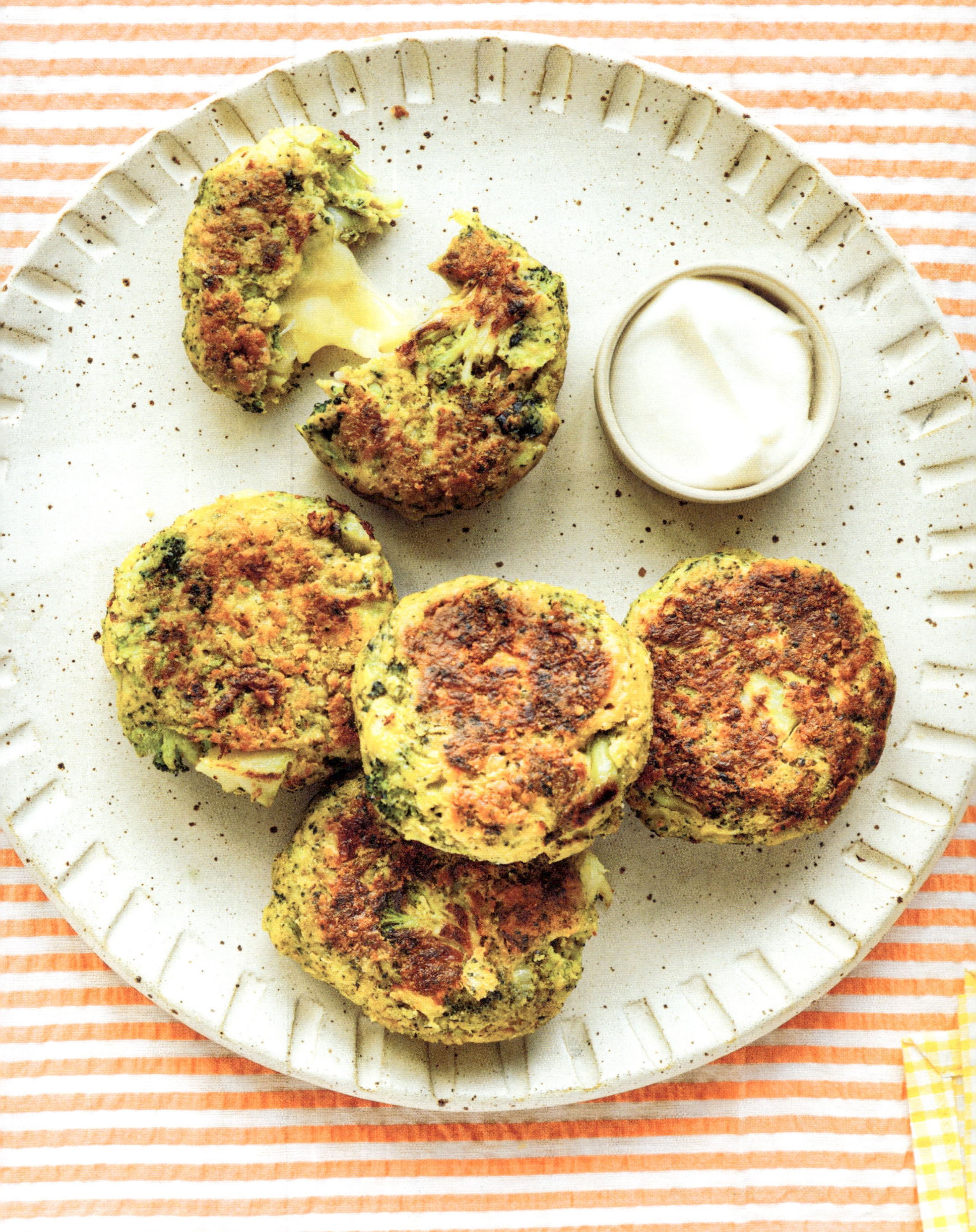

BROCCOLI BITES

Makes 5–6 bites

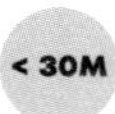

If you're looking for a way to get your little ones (or grown ones) to gobble up their greens, then these broccoli bites might be just the ticket! They are not only bursting with flavour but are also incredibly simple to whip up. With just a handful of simple ingredients, including nutrient-packed broccoli, nutritional yeast, chickpea flour and plant-based cheese, you'll be surprised to see how quickly they disappear! Why not pair them with vegan mayo (see page 170) or a cannellini bean and garlic dip (see page 174) for an extra tasty treat?

300g (10½oz) broccoli (see Note)
1 teaspoon onion
    granules (optional)
1 teaspoon garlic
    granules (optional)
80g (2¾oz/¾ cup) chickpea
    (gram) flour
40g (1½oz) nutritional yeast
5–6 slices of plant-based
    mozzarella-style cheese or
    plant-based hard cheese
Salt and freshly ground
    black pepper
Your favourite dip, to serve

Steam or boil the broccoli until it is very soft – it has to be so soft that you can easily mash it with a fork.

Put the cooked broccoli into a bowl and add a pinch of salt and pepper and the onion and garlic granules (if using). Mash it with a fork until mostly smooth.

Add the chickpea flour and nutritional yeast and mash again. The texture should be soft but consistent enough to form patties. If it's too loose, add more flour. If it's too dry, sprinkle it with some water and press to see if the mixture sticks.

With wet hands, shape the mixture into 5–6 patties, placing a piece of cheese in the middle of each one.

Heat a dry non-stick frying pan (skillet) over a medium heat and cook the patties for 5 minutes on each side, or until golden. If the pan is not the best quality, you may need to add a bit of oil, otherwise the patties will stick to the pan.

Enjoy with your favourite dip.

NOTE
If your broccoli is bigger than the quantity stated, don't waste it. Cook it all and simply add more flour and nutritional yeast until you have the right consistency.

PROTEIN PER SERVING

9.5g

STORAGE

Store for up to 3 days in the refrigerator and up to 3 months in the freezer.

CRUNCHY SOYA-FREE LENTIL TOFU BITES WITH VEGAN MAYO

Serves 2–4

If you're on the hunt for a soy-free snack option that doesn't skimp on protein, these lentil bites are a must-try! With just a touch of patience, you'll be rewarded with a satisfying crunch and a boost of fibre. And let's talk flavour – these bites deliver! Personally, I love pairing them with a quick and effortless homemade garlic mayo, but the beauty lies in your freedom to experiment with your favourite dip.

LENTIL TOFU

125g (4½oz/½ cup) split red
 lentils, washed
375ml (121/2floz/11/2 cups) hot
 water
1 teaspoon paprika
½ teaspoon ground black pepper
Pinch of salt

VEGAN MAYO

125ml (4½fl oz/½ cup) unsweetened
 soya milk
1 teaspoon apple cider vinegar
½ teaspoon sea salt
2 teaspoons onion granules
240ml (8¼fl oz/1 cup) vegetable oil

Put the lentils into a bowl and cover them with the hot water. Leave to soak for at least 1 hour. This softens the lentils and makes them easier to blend.

Put the lentils and their soaking liquid into a blender along with the paprika, pepper and salt. Blend until smooth, then transfer the lentil batter to a large saucepan. Cook over a medium heat for 5–8 minutes, stirring constantly to avoid lumps, until the mixture is very thick.

Line a 12 x 12cm (5 x 5 inch) baking dish with baking parchment and scrape the batter into it, smoothing the top. Refrigerate the lentil tofu, uncovered, for at least 2 hours (or more for firmer tofu).

Once set, slice the lentil tofu into cubes or any desired shape and air-fry at 180°C (350°F) for 15–20 minutes. Alternatively, bake in the oven at 180°C/160°C fan/350°F/Gas mark 4 for 35–40 minutes.

Meanwhile, make the mayo. Combine the soya milk, apple cider vinegar, sea salt and onion granules in a jar or the beaker of your hand-held blender.

Slowly pour in the oil in a thin stream, blending constantly. It is crucial for the emulsification process for the oil to be added slowly. Keep adding the oil even when the mixture starts to thicken. Taste the mayo and adjust the seasoning as needed.

Serve the lentil tofu bites with the mayo.

You can store the mayo in an airtight container in the refrigerator for up to 3 weeks. It will thicken with time, so if you see this happening, add a bit more oil to soften it.

PROTEIN PER SERVING	STORAGE
15g	Store before cooking for up to 3 days in the refrigerator and up to 3 months in the freezer.

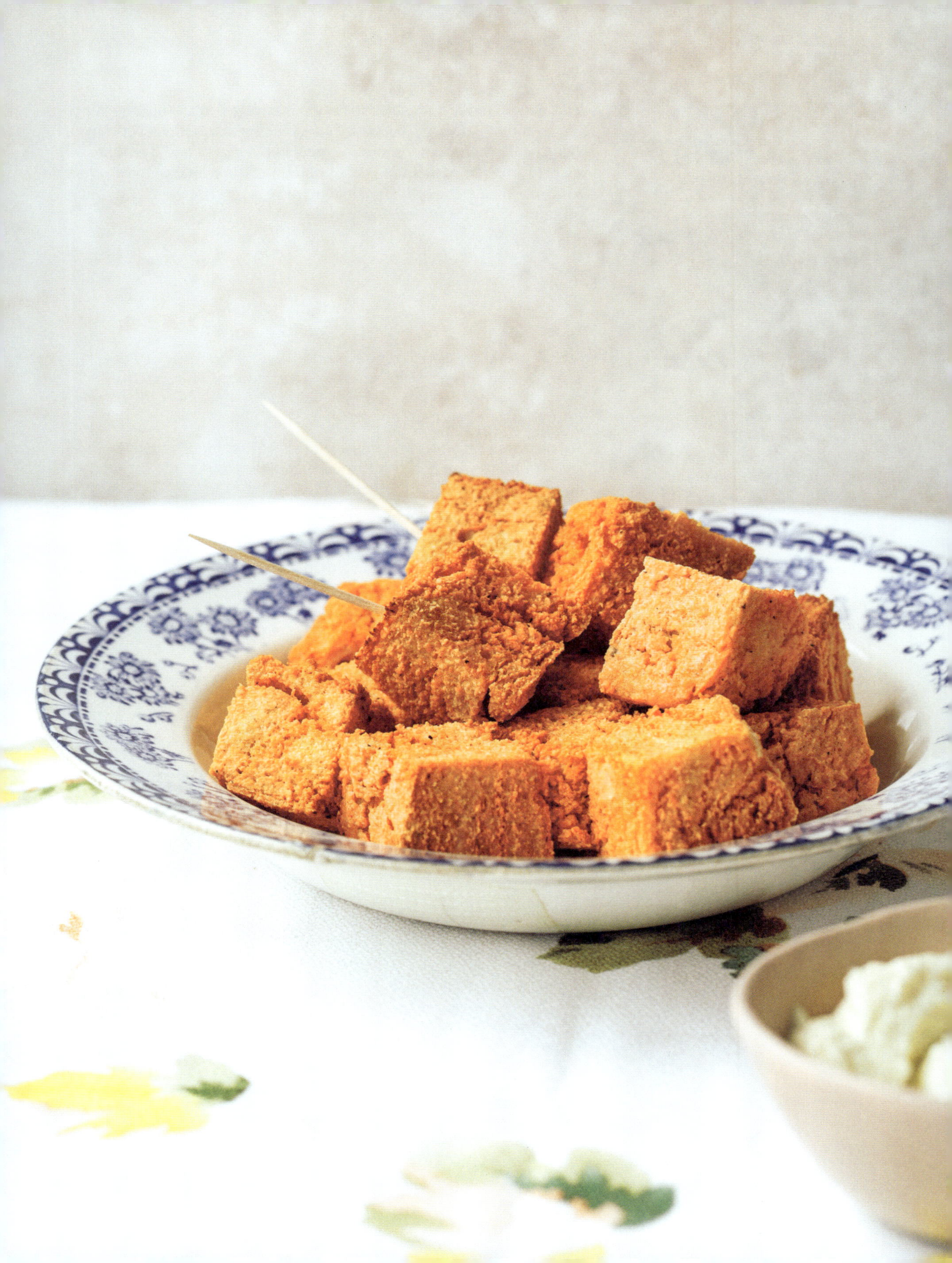

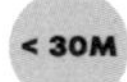

TOMATO BRUSCHETTA WITH TOFU RICOTTA

Serves 2

4–6 slices heirloom tomato
1 teaspoon baby capers
200g (7oz) firm tofu
3 tablespoons nutritional yeast
Juice of ½ lemon
1 tablespoon dried Italian herbs
2 slices of sourdough bread
1 small garlic clove, peeled
Olive oil, for drizzling
Salt and freshly ground
    black pepper

TO SERVE
Balsamic glaze (optional)
Fresh basil leaves (optional)

This simple tomato bruschetta recipe is a high-protein alternative to the traditional dish, perfect for those seeking a nutritious yet flavourful snack. Juicy heirloom tomatoes, tangy baby capers and a creamy tofu 'ricotta' infused with Italian herbs come together on toasted sourdough to create a pleasing bite. Drizzle with olive oil and, if desired, a touch of balsamic glaze for added depth of flavour.

Put the sliced tomato into a container with the capers, then drizzle with olive oil and add a pinch of salt and pepper. Using a brush or with your hands, spread the oil marinade evenly over the tomatoes. Set aside to marinate.

Put the tofu into a food processor with the nutritional yeast, lemon juice, Italian herbs and a splash of water. Blend until smooth and well combined.

Toast the sourdough, then rub the garlic clove on both sides. Drizzle the toast with olive oil and add a pinch of salt.

Spread the tofu mixture evenly on one side of the bread slices, then top with the marinated tomatoes and capers.

If desired, drizzle with balsamic glaze and scatter some basil leaves on top to finish. Cut in half to serve.

PROTEIN PER SERVING

15g

MAKE IT GLUTEN-FREE

Use gluten-free bread.

STORAGE

Store the ingredients separately for up to 3 days in the refrigerator. Not freezer friendly.

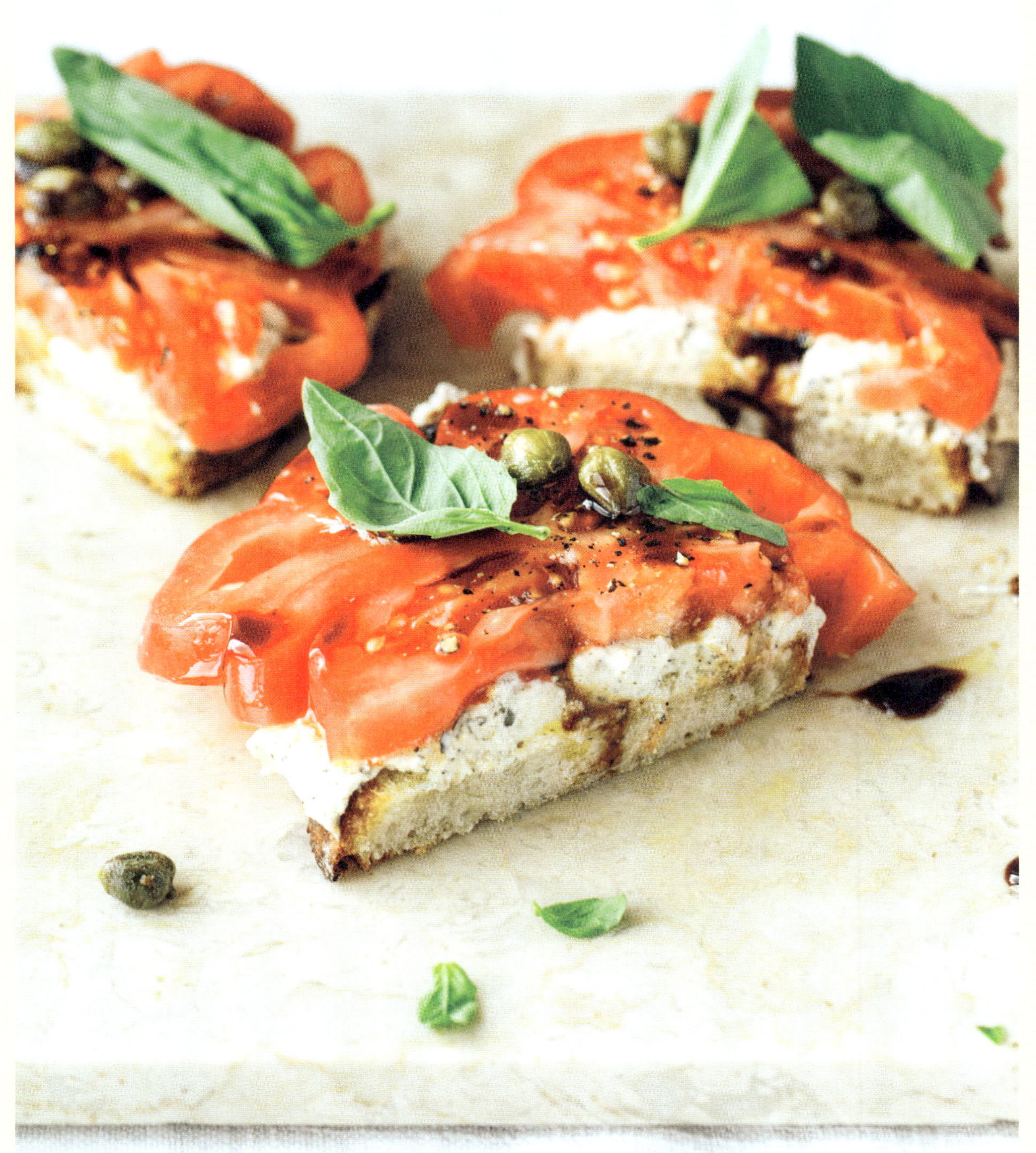

< 1H

POLENTA CHIPS WITH CANNELLINI BEAN AND GARLIC DIP

Serves 2–4

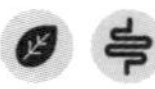

Crispy on the outside and tender on the inside, these golden polenta chips (fries) are packed with savoury goodness that'll surely please your taste buds. But why not take it up a notch? Pair them with a simple yet delightful creamy dip, boasting subtle hints of garlic and nutty richness. Together, they create a comforting and perfectly balanced treat that's easy to whip up in no time.

POLENTA CHIPS

600ml (20fl oz/2½ cups) vegetable stock (or water)
30g (1oz) nutritional yeast
1 teaspoon onion granules
170g (6oz/scant 1¼ cups) instant (quick-cook) polenta (cornmeal)
30g (1oz/½ cup) panko breadcrumbs
40g (1½oz/scant ¼ cup) tricolour quinoa
15g (½oz) plant-based Parmesan-style cheese (see page 36, or use shop-bought)
2 teaspoon dried oregano
2 teaspoon dried rosemary
3 tablespoons olive oil, plus extra for greasing
Salt and freshly ground black pepper

CANNELLINI BEAN AND GARLIC DIP

1 bulb of garlic
2 tablespoons olive oil, plus extra for drizzling
2 x 400g (14oz) tins of cannellini beans, drained
2 tablespoons lemon juice
4 tablespoons tahini
Chopped chives, to serve

Preheat the oven to 200°C/180°C fan/400°F/Gas mark 6 and grease a 20 x 20cm (8 x 8 inch) baking dish.

First, roast the garlic for the dip. Slice the top off the bulb of garlic to expose the cloves, then drizzle it with a little olive oil, wrap it in foil and roast in the oven for 30–40 minutes, or until the cloves are soft and golden brown. Remove the garlic and set aside.

Next, make the polenta chips. Pour the stock into a saucepan and bring to the boil, then reduce the heat to medium and add the nutritional yeast, onion granules and a pinch of salt and pepper.

Slowly pour in the polenta, stirring continuously until the mixture thickens (it will happen almost instantly). Remove the pan from the heat and pour the mixture into the prepared baking dish. Smooth out the surface with a spatula and allow it to cool completely.

When you're ready to cook, preheat the oven to 200°C/180°C fan/400°F/Gas mark 6 again and line two baking trays (pans) with baking parchment.

Combine the panko breadcrumbs, quinoa, plant-based Parmesan-style cheese, oregano, rosemary and olive oil in a bowl and season with salt and pepper. Mix until well combined.

Flip the baking dish upside down and carefully remove the polenta. Cut the polenta into rectangles, about 8cm (3 inches) long, then gently coat the polenta chips with the quinoa and breadcrumb mixture.

Place the chips on the prepared baking trays and bake in the oven for 40 minutes, flipping them halfway though.

While the chips are baking, prepare the dip. In a food processor, combine the beans, roasted garlic cloves, olive oil, lemon juice, tahini and some salt and pepper. Blend until smooth and creamy. If the mixture is too thick, add water a tablespoon at a time.

Transfer the dip to a bowl and garnish with chives. Serve with the chips.

PROTEIN PER SERVING	MAKE IT GLUTEN-FREE	STORAGE
30g	Use gluten-free breadcrumbs.	The polenta chips are best eaten fresh. The dip can be stored for up to 3 days in the refrigerator or up to 3 months in the freezer.

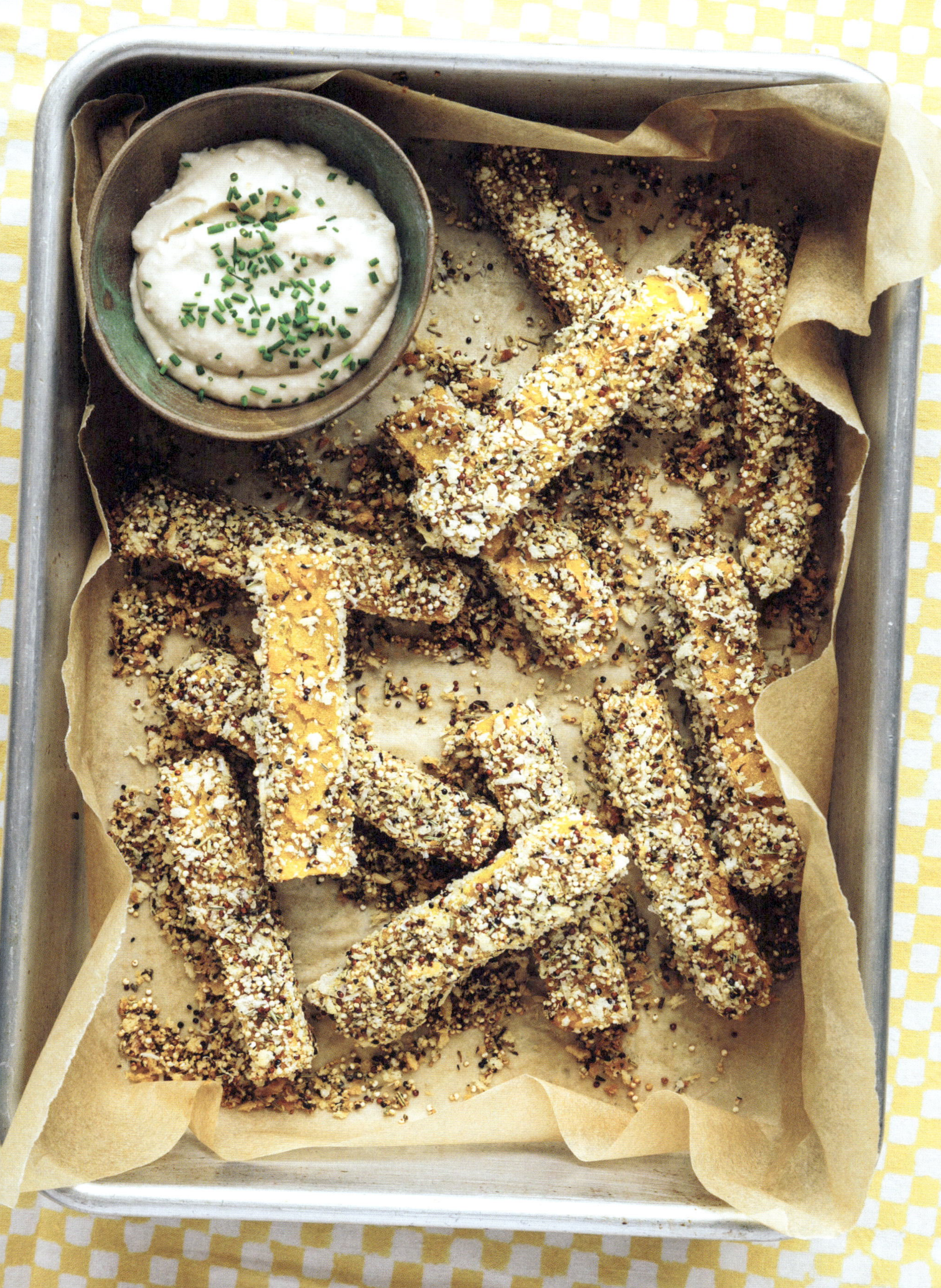

CHOCOLATE CRISPY CHICKPEAS

Serves 5–6

GF

We all agree that crispy chickpeas (garbanzos) are good, but have you tried covering them in chocolate? I have been making this snack for years and I never get tired of it! Packed with protein-rich chickpeas and coated in luscious dark (bittersweet) chocolate, these treats are as satisfying as they are indulgent. Plus, they're hassle-free to make, whether you opt for air frying or baking. A crunchy, chocolatey snack that's perfect for satiating your sweet cravings.

1 x 400g (14oz) tin of chickpeas
   (garbanzos), drained
130g (4½oz) dark
   (bittersweet) chocolate
2 teaspoons coconut oil
20g (¾oz) chocolate protein
   powder (optional)
Sea salt flakes

Preheat the oven to 200°C/180°C fan/400°F/Gas mark 6 and line a baking tray (pan) with baking parchment.

Place the chickpeas on a clean dish towel and pat them dry. This step is crucial to ensure the chickpeas turn crispy.

Transfer the chickpeas to the prepared baking tray and bake in the oven for 30 minutes, or until crunchy. Alternatively, if you have an air fryer, you can air-fry the chickpeas at 200°C (400°F) for 15 minutes.

Meanwhile, put the chocolate and coconut oil into a microwave-safe bowl and microwave at medium power until melted, stirring at 10-second intervals to avoid burning.

Put the crispy chickpeas and protein powder (if using) into a bowl and mix together, then pour over the melted chocolate and mix until well combined.

Pour the chocolate chickpea mixture onto a baking tray lined with baking parchment, flattening the surface with a spatula, and leave it to set in the refrigerator for a couple of hours.

Once ready, slice it into portions and store in the refrigerator in an airtight container.

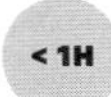

SWEET POTATO AND OAT PROTEIN BARS

Makes 4 bars

Say goodbye to spending money on overpriced protein bars now that you can make your own! Packed with wholesome ingredients like sweet potato, oats, peanut butter and ground flaxseed, these bars are a powerhouse of nutrition and protein. Plus, they're hassle-free to make, requiring just a few simple steps and minimal ingredients.

320g (11¼oz) sweet potato
10g (½oz) ground flaxseeds
100g (3½oz/1 cup) rolled oats
100g (3½oz/⅓ cup) smooth
   peanut butter
30g (1oz) vanilla protein powder or
   ground almonds (almond meal)
20ml (1½ tablespoons) maple syrup
   (or more to taste)

TOPPING

80g (2¾oz) dark (bittersweet)
   chocolate
1 teaspoon coconut oil
Smooth peanut butter

Preheat the oven to 180°C/160°C fan/350°F/Gas mark 4 and line a 15 x 20cm (6 x 8 inch) baking tin (pan) with baking parchment.

Pierce the sweet potato with a fork, place it on a microwave-safe plate and microwave for 5–8 minutes. If the sweet potato isn't fork-tender after 5–8 minutes, microwave at 30 seconds intervals until it becomes soft. If you don't have a microwave, you can steam the sweet potato or bake it in the oven at 200°C/180°C fan/400°F/Gas mark 6 for 30–40 minutes.

Combine the ground flaxseeds and 50ml (1¾fl oz/3½ tablespoons) water in a small bowl and stir to combine, then set aside to rest for 5 minutes. With time it will form a slurry.

Peel the sweet potato and put the cooked flesh into a bowl with the oats, peanut butter, protein powder or ground almonds, maple syrup and flaxseed slurry. Mix until well combined.

Transfer the mixture to the prepared baking tin and bake in the oven for 30 minutes. Remove from the oven and allow to cool completely.

Meanwhile, combine the chocolate and coconut oil in a microwave-safe bowl and microwave at medium power until melted, stirring at 10-second intervals to prevent burning.

Spread the chocolate evenly over the sweet potato base, then add dollops of peanut butter and create swirls with a cocktail stick (toothpick). Allow the bars to set in the refrigerator, then cut into portions.

PROTEIN PER SERVING

17g

MAKE IT GLUTEN-FREE

Use certified gluten-free oats.

STORAGE

Store for up to 3 days in the refrigerator and 3 months in the freezer.

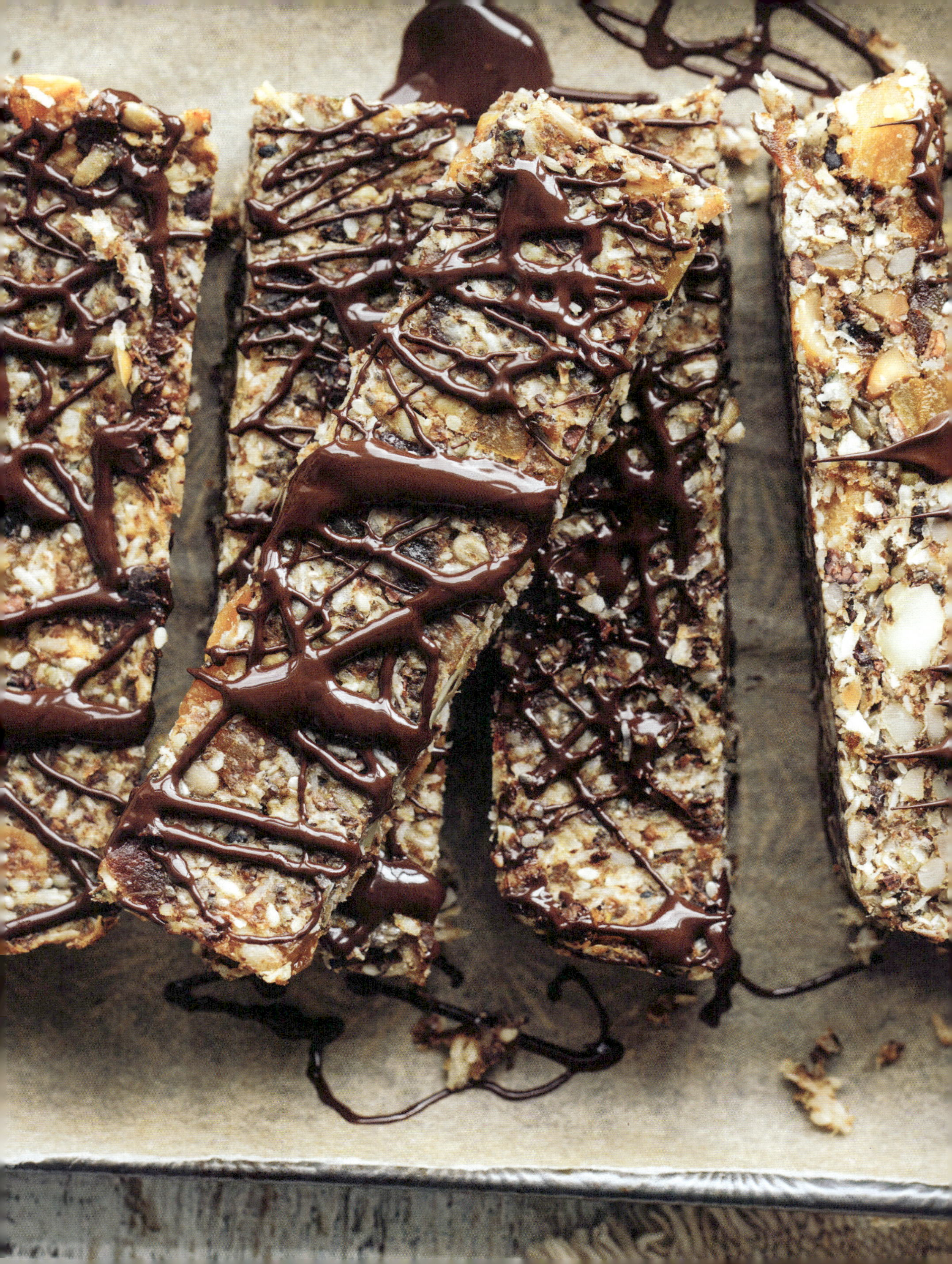

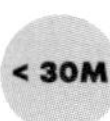

CHEWY GRANOLA BARS

Makes 5 bars

  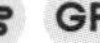

These homemade granola bars are so much better than any kind you'd buy in the shops. Packed with nutritious ingredients like tahini, nuts, seeds, dried fruits and cacao nibs, these bars are not only packed full of protein, but are also loaded with fibre and essential nutrients to keep you fuelled throughout the day. Make them once and trust me, you are going to go bananas for them!

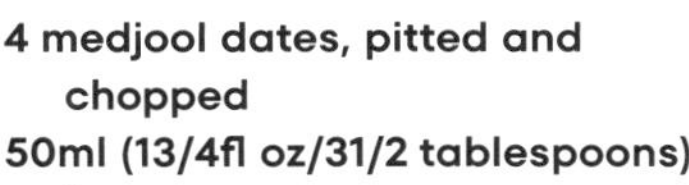

4 medjool dates, pitted and chopped
50ml (13/4fl oz/31/2 tablespoons) hot water
½ banana, mashed
2 tablespoons tahini
60g (2oz) mixed nuts, such as peanuts, walnuts, hazelnuts and pecans, roughly chopped
20g (¾oz) ground flaxseeds
60g (2oz) mixed seeds, such as pumpkin seeds, chia seeds, shelled hemp seeds and sesame seeds
60g (2oz) dried fruits, such as apricots and cranberries, chopped
20g (¾oz) cacao nibs
45g (12/oz/½ cup) desiccated (dried shredded) coconut
Pinch of salt
30g (1oz) dark (bittersweet) chocolate
½ teaspoon coconut oil (optional)

Preheat the oven to 180°C/160°C fan/350°F/Gas mark 4 and line a 15 x 20cm (6 x 8 inch) baking tin (pan) with baking parchment.

Put the dates into a bowl and cover with the hot water, then set aside for 10 minutes. Once softened, mash with a fork.

Add the mashed banana and tahini to the dates and mix until well combined. It will form a paste.

Incorporate the nuts, ground flaxseeds, mixed seeds, dried fruits, cacao nibs and coconut and mix until combined.

Place the mixture in the prepared baking tin and bake for 15–20 minutes.

Allow to cool completely, then cut into bars.

Put the chocolate and coconut oil into a microwave-safe bowl and microwave at medium power until melted, stirring at 10-second intervals to avoid burning. Coat one side of the bars with the melted chocolate, then turn them over and drizzle the other side with chocolate. Place them on their shorter side and refrigerated until set.

PROTEIN PER SERVING

10g

STORAGE

Store for up to 3 days in the refrigerator or up to 3 months in the freezer.

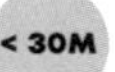

RED BEAN AND CHOCOLATE COOKIES

Makes 8 cookies

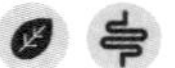

5g (¼oz) ground flaxseeds
1 x 400g (14oz) tin of kidney beans, drained
80g (2¾oz/scant ⅓ cup) smooth peanut butter
60ml (2fl oz/¼ cup) maple syrup
5g (¼oz) baking powder
30g (1oz) raw cacao powder
80g (2¾oz) dark (bittersweet) chocolate chips, plus extra for topping
Sea salt flakes (optional)

Red bean and chocolate cookies. Unconventional? Maybe. Irresistible? Absolutely. Just wait until you sink your teeth into one – you'll be clamouring for more.

Preheat the oven to 180°C/160°C fan/350°F/Gas mark 4 and line a baking sheet with baking parchment. (Avoid using the fan option if possible, as it may dry out the cookies too much.)

In a small bowl, whisk together the ground flaxseeds and 4–5 tablespoons water and set aside for 5–10 minutes to form a slurry.

Combine the kidney beans, peanut butter, maple syrup, baking powder, cacao powder and flaxseed slurry in a food processor and blend until a dough forms. Stir in the chocolate chips.

Using an ice cream scoop or two spoons, portion out the dough into eight cookies and place them on the prepared baking sheet. If you like, top the cookies with more chocolate chips and some sea salt flakes.

Bake in the oven for 15 minutes, then remove from the oven and allow to cool completely before enjoying.

PROTEIN PER SERVING

8g

STORAGE

Store for up to 4 days in an airtight container and up to 3 months in the freezer.

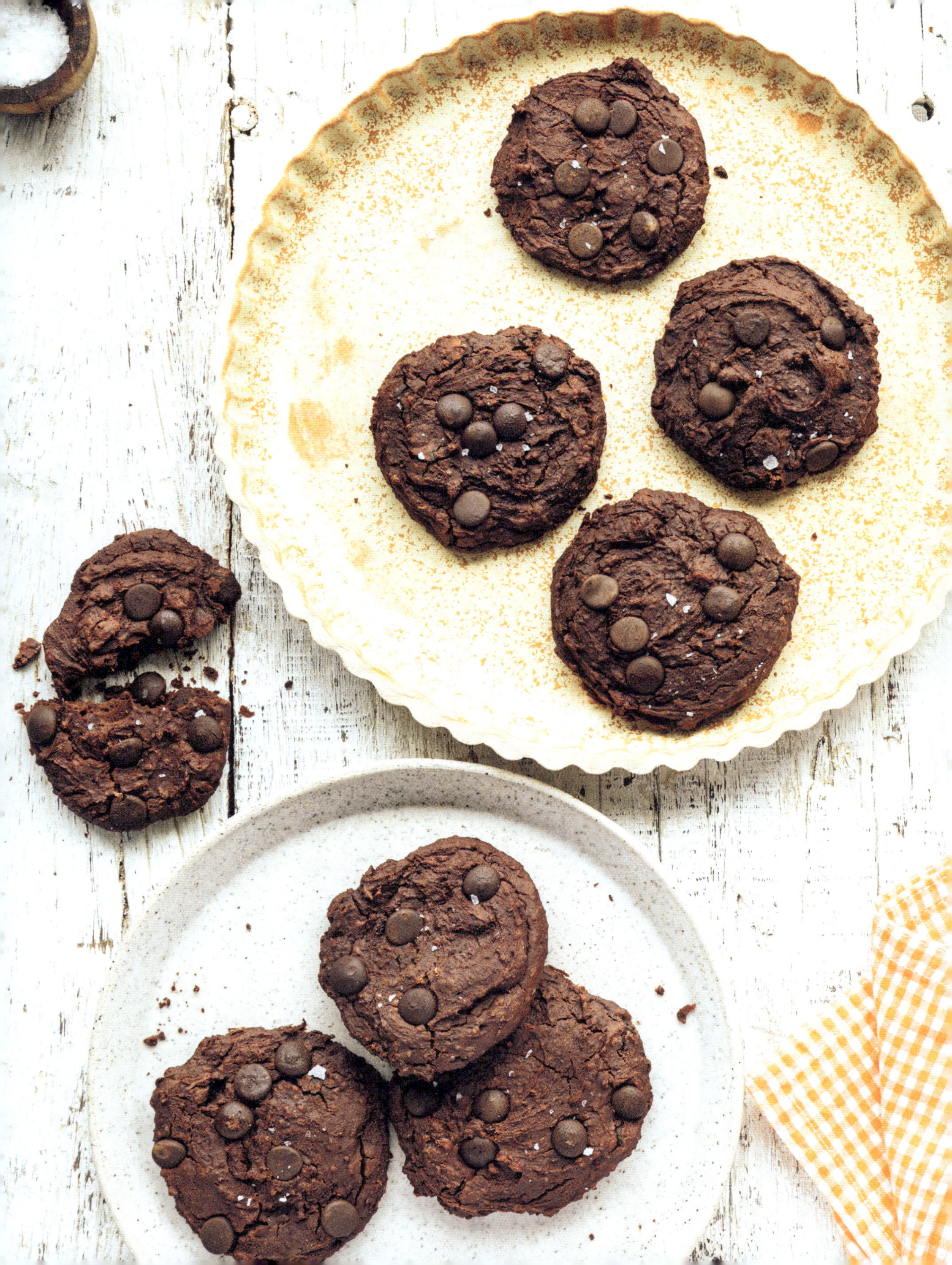

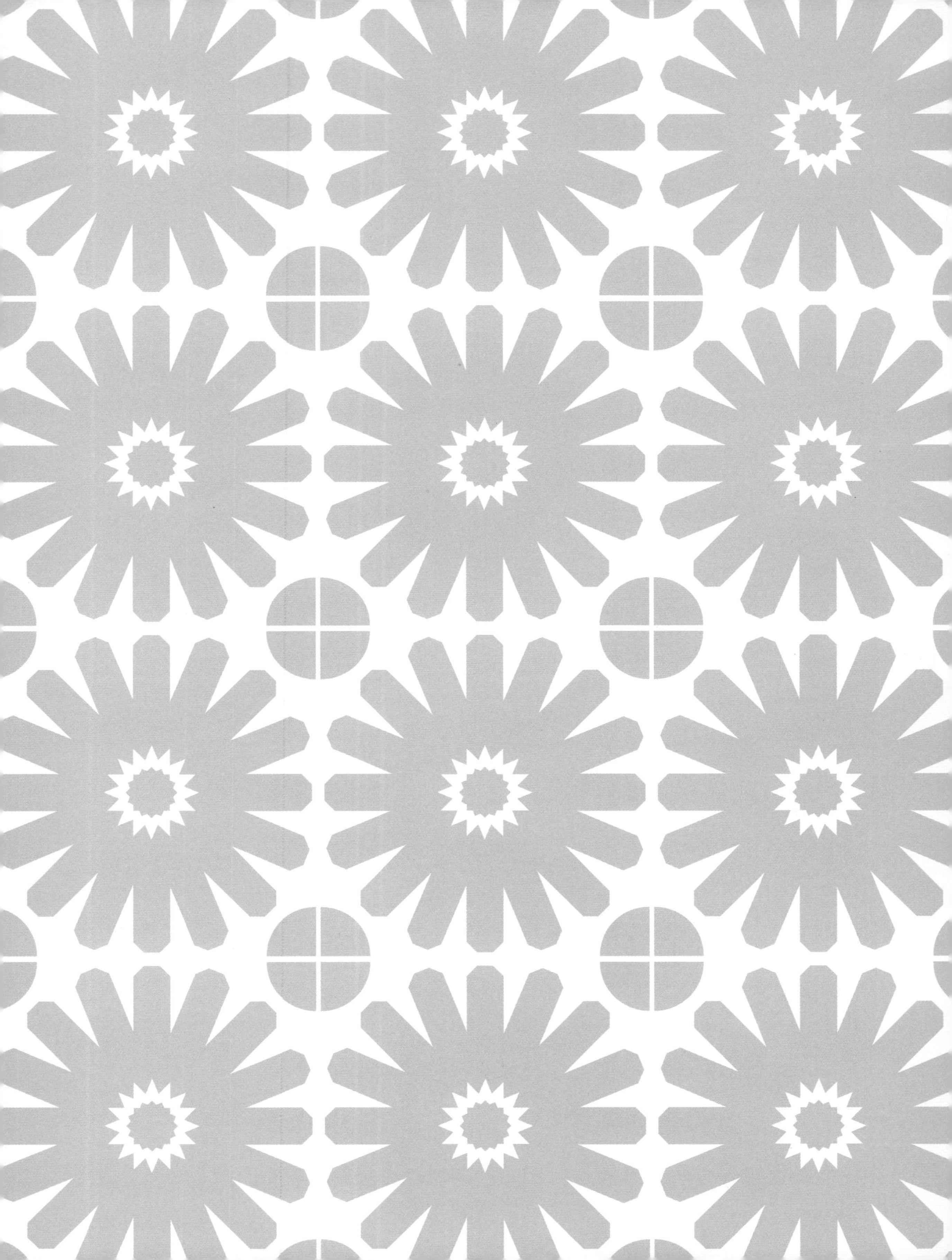

SWEET TREATS

QUINOA PROTEIN BROWNIES

Serves 6

These brownies are perfect or those seeking a wholesome indulgence. Bursting with plant-based protein from quinoa, peanut butter and yoghurt, naturally sweetened with banana and maple syrup and enriched with cacao powder, they're a protein-packed treat perfect for any time of day. I love changing the toppings depending on my mood! Chocolate chips? Peanut butter swirls or dried raspberries? What's it going to be next time?

120g (4oz/scant ⅔ cup) tricolour quinoa

10g (½oz) ground flaxseeds

100g (3½oz/generous ⅓ cup) high-protein plant-based yoghurt

90g (3¼oz) overripe banana

40g (4½oz) raw cacao powder

40ml (1½fl oz/3 tablespoons) maple syrup

1 teaspoon vanilla extract

50g (1¾oz/scant ¼ cup) smooth peanut butter

1 teaspoon baking powder

Handful of dark (bittersweet) chocolate chips

Put the quinoa into a bowl and pour over enough hot water to fully cover it. Leave to soak for at least 1 hour.

Preheat the oven to 200°C/180°C fan/400°F/Gas mark 6 and line a 15 x 20cm (6 x 8 inch) baking tin (pan) with baking parchment.

In a small bowl, combine the ground flaxseeds with 40ml (1½fl oz/ 3 tablespoons) water. Stir and set aside to rest for 10 minutes. With time it will form a slurry.

Drain the quinoa and put it into a food processor with the yoghurt, banana, cacao powder, flaxseed slurry, maple syrup, vanilla extract, peanut butter and baking powder and blend until smooth. Stir in some chocolate chips.

Transfer the batter to the prepared baking tin and top with more chocolate chips. Bake in the oven for 20–25 minutes, or until a skewer inserted into the centre comes out with just a little crumb on it (it should be cooked but still moist).

Remove from the oven and allow to cool completely before slicing and serving.

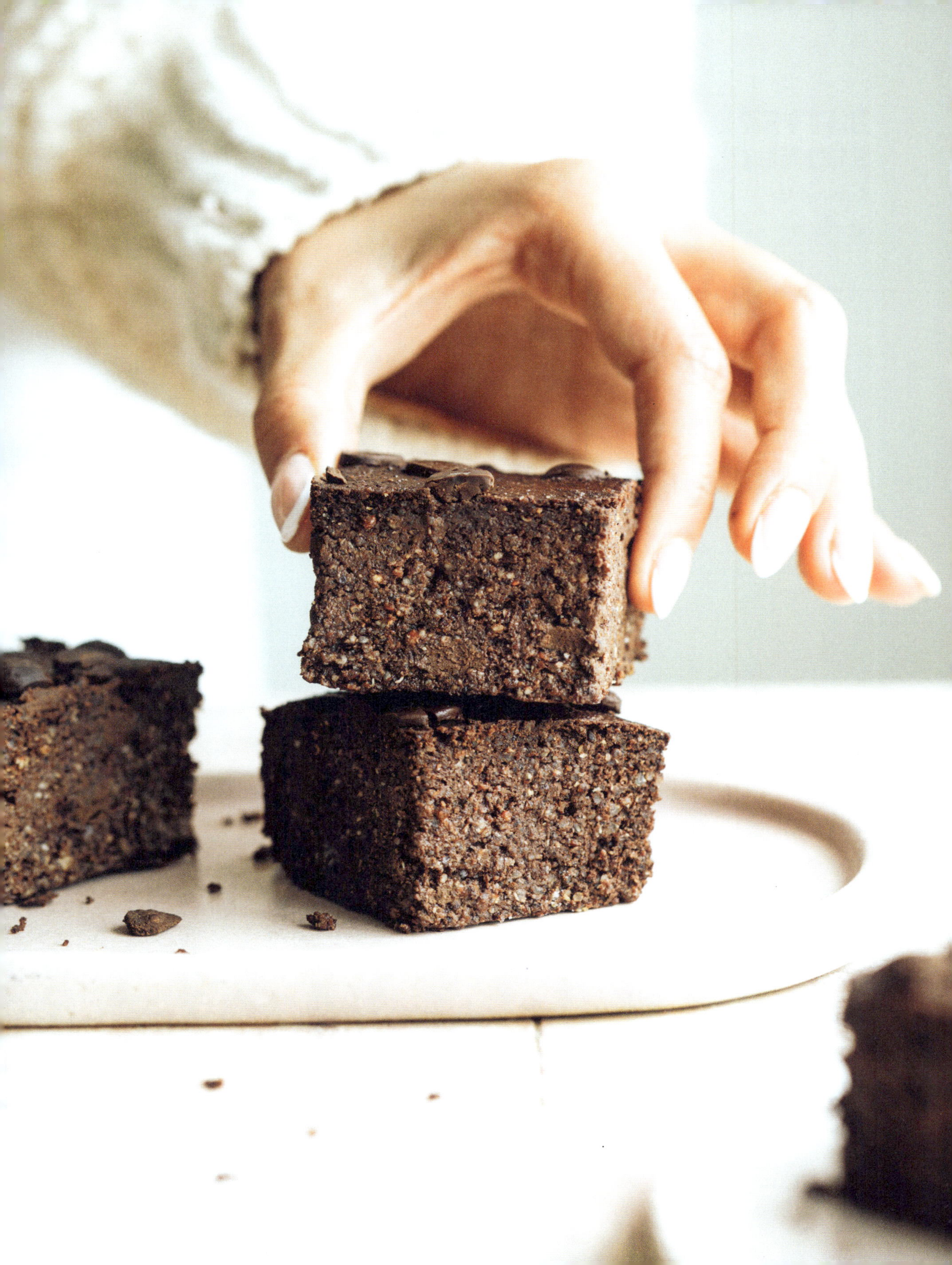

BUTTER BEAN BLONDIES

Serves 6

Imagine the face of your friends when you tell them that these blondies are made with butter (lima) beans! Truth is, butter beans are the perfect secret ingredient, lending a delectably chewy texture to this bake while preserving every bit of flavour and packing a serious protein punch!

10g (½oz) ground flaxseeds
1 x 400g (14oz) tin of butter (lima) beans, drained
100ml (3½fl oz/scant ½ cup) plant-based milk (I used soya)
100g (3½oz/generous ⅓ cup) almond butter
80ml (2¾oz/⅓ cup) maple syrup
2 teaspoons vanilla extract
100g (3½oz/1 cup) ground almonds (almond meal)
5g (¼oz) baking powder
Pinch of salt
50g (1¾oz) dark (bittersweet) chocolate chips, plus extra for topping

Preheat the oven to 200°C/180°C fan/400°F/Gas mark 6 and line a 15 x 20cm (6 x 8 inch) baking tin (pan) with baking parchment.

In a small bowl, combine the ground flaxseeds with 40ml (1½fl oz/ 3 tablespoons) water. Stir and set aside to rest for 10 minutes. With time it will form a slurry.

Put the butter beans, milk, almond butter, maple syrup, flaxseed slurry and vanilla extract into a food processor and blend until smooth. It'll be very liquid, but don't worry that's how it's meant to be.

Transfer the mixture to a bowl and sift in the ground almonds, baking powder and salt, then stir until well mixed. Stir through the chocolate chips, then transfer the batter to the prepared baking tin.

Top with more chocolate chips, then bake in the oven for 30 minutes.

Removed from the oven and allow to cool completely before slicing.

PROTEIN PER SERVING

15g

STORAGE

Store for up to 3 days in the refrigerator. and up to 3 months in the freezer.

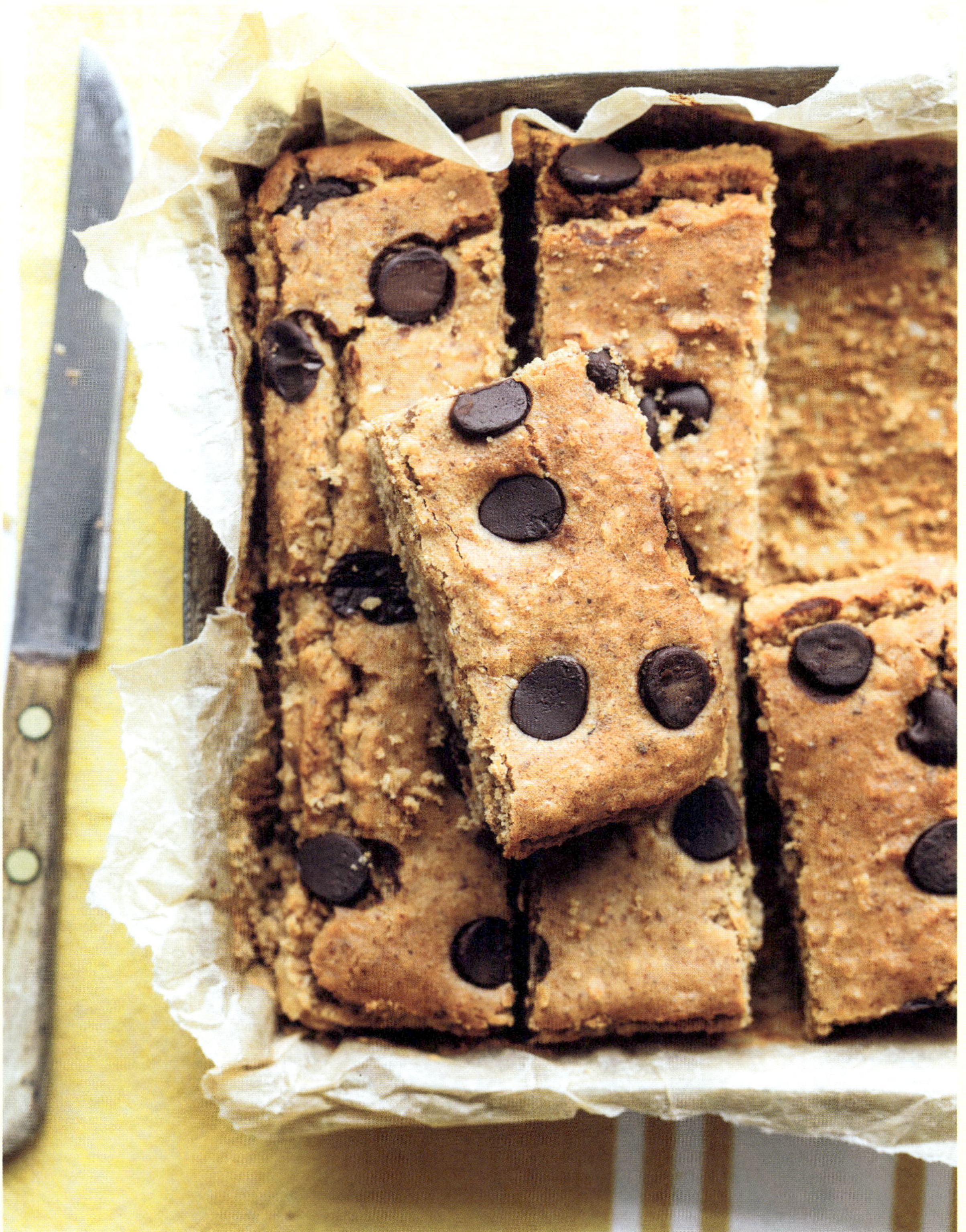

SNEAKY PROTEIN COFFEE AND CHOCOLATE MOUSSE

Serves 2

This mousse offers a delightful twist on the classic French *mousse au chocolat*. It requires just 10 minutes of prep time and also provides a nutritious boost of protein, while maintaining the original French dish's decadence and velvety smooth texture. Before serving, adorn it with chocolate flakes and cacao powder for an extra touch of luxury. I also like serving this with fresh raspberries.

90g (3¼oz) dark (bittersweet) chocolate, melted
½ teaspoon coconut oil
300g (10½oz) shelf-stable silken tofu, drained
5g (¼oz) instant coffee granules
2 tablespoons maple syrup

TO SERVE
Dark (bittersweet) chocolate flakes
Cacao powder

Put the chocolate and coconut oil into a microwave-safe bowl and microwave at medium power until melted, stirring at 10-second intervals to avoid burning.

Combine the silken tofu, coffee, maple syrup and melted chocolate in a food processor and blend until smooth.

Pour the mixture into jars or cups and refrigerate for at least 2 hours, or ideally overnight.

Top with chocolate flakes and cacao powder before serving, if liked.

<table>
<tr><td>PROTEIN PER SERVING</td><td>STORAGE</td></tr>
<tr><td>19g</td><td>Store for up to 4 days in the refrigerator. Not freezer friendly.</td></tr>
</table>

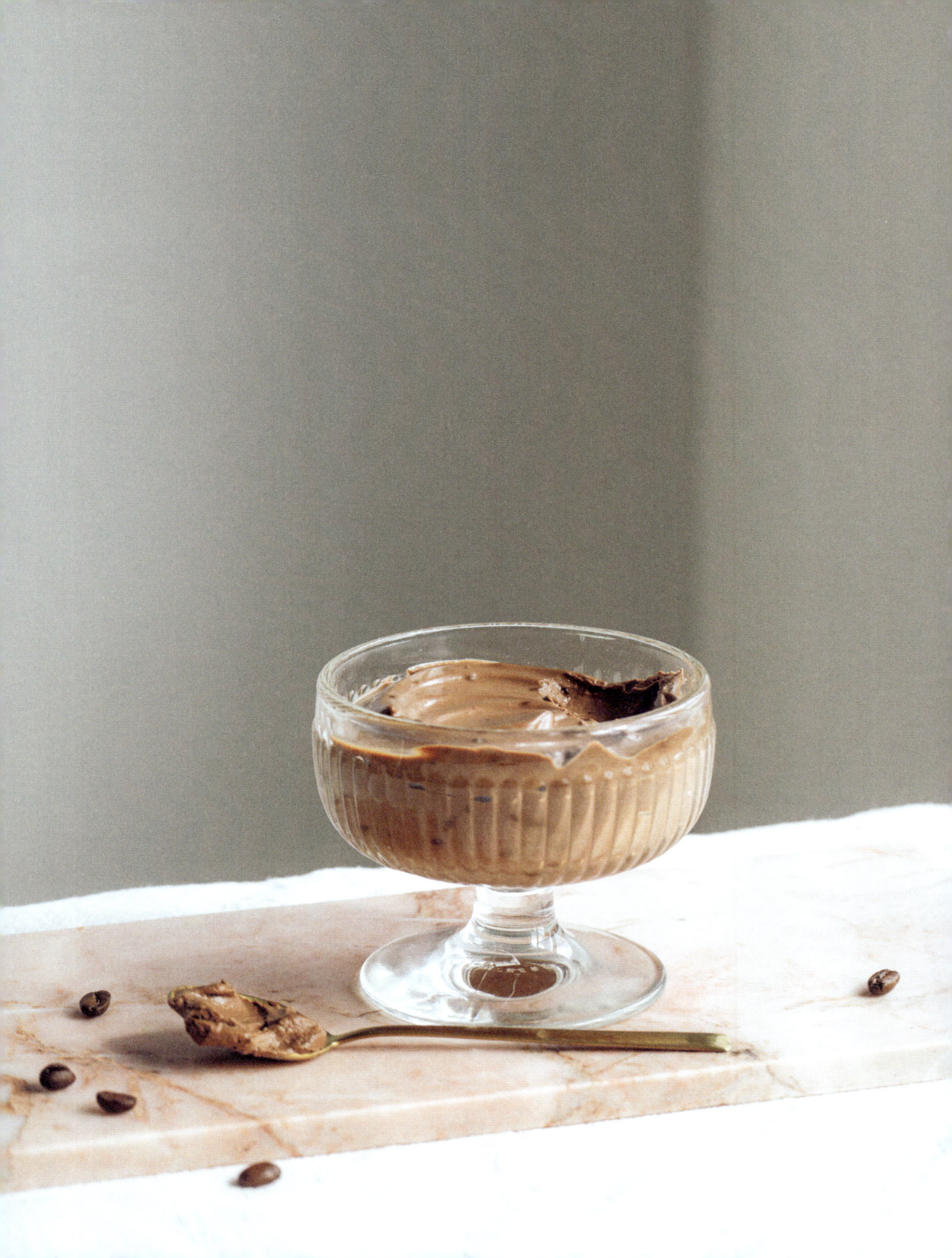

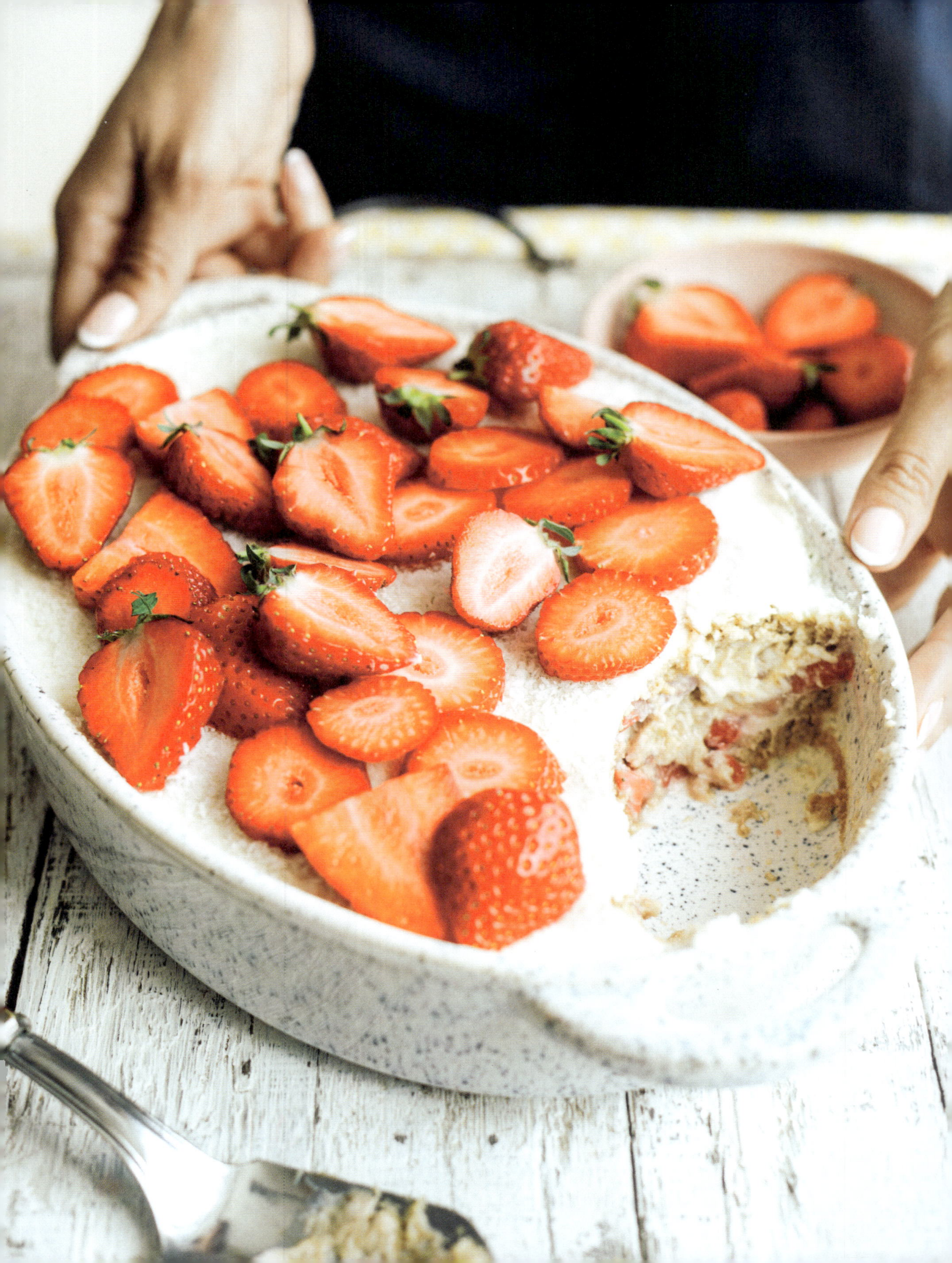

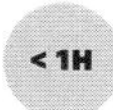

STRAWBERRY AND COCONUT TIRAMISU

Serves 8

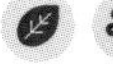  

You've eaten coffee chocolate tiramisu, but have you ever tried a fruity twist? Packed with juicy strawberries and creamy layers of silken tofu and coconut, this dessert is a refreshing take on a classic favourite. With its simple yet flavourful ingredients and hassle-free method, you'll have a protein-rich treat that's perfect for any occasion.

21–25 vegan ladyfingers or digestive biscuits (graham crackers)

STRAWBERRY LAYER
600g (1lb 5oz) strawberries, hulled and roughly chopped, plus extra for decorating
3 tablespoons caster (superfine) sugar
Juice of ½ lemon
160ml (5½fl oz/⅔ cups) water

COCONUT LAYER
300g (10½oz) shelf-stable silken tofu
100g (3½oz/generous ⅓ cup) high-protein plant-based yoghurt
150g (5½oz) coconut milk solids (just the thick part from a tin – see Note)
60g (2oz/generous ¼ cup) caster (superfine) sugar
1 teaspoon vanilla extract (optional)
Desiccated (dried shredded) coconut, for sprinkling

Put the strawberries into a bowl with the sugar, lemon juice and water. Mix well and set aside. This will create a strawberry-infused water used to moisten the ladyfingers.

To make the coconut layer, combine the tofu, plant-based yoghurt, coconut milk solids, sugar and vanilla extract (if using) in a food processor. Blend until smooth and creamy, then set aside.

Using a sieve, separate the strawberries from the infused water. Dip the ladyfingers or biscuits into the strawberry-infused water and use them to create a layer in the bottom of two 15 x 21cm (6 x 8 inch) dishes. If you are using glass dishes, you can layer the sides with sliced strawberries.

Cover the ladyfingers with a generous layer of the coconut mixture. Sprinkle some of the coconut on top, followed by a scattering of chopped strawberries. Repeat this alternating pattern of ladyfingers, coconut mixture, coconut and chopped strawberries until you have used everything up.

Refrigerate the assembled tiramisu overnight to allow it to set and the flavours to meld together.

NOTE
In order to separate the thick coconut solids from the water, refrigerate the tin before use.

PROTEIN PER SERVING	MAKE IT GLUTEN-FREE	STORAGE
10g	Use gluten-free ladyfingers or biscuits (cookies).	Store for up to 4 days in the refrigerator. Not freezer friendly.

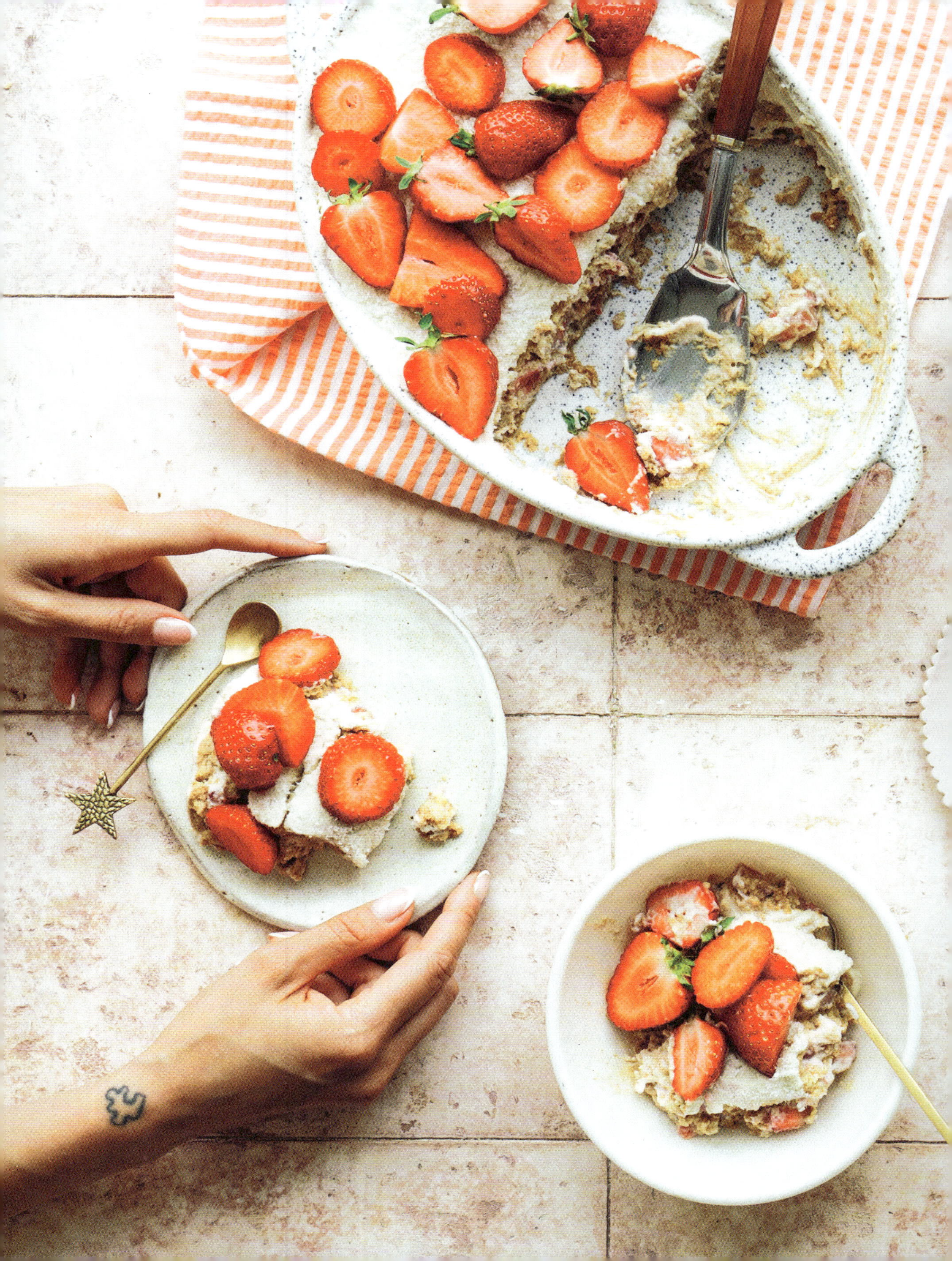

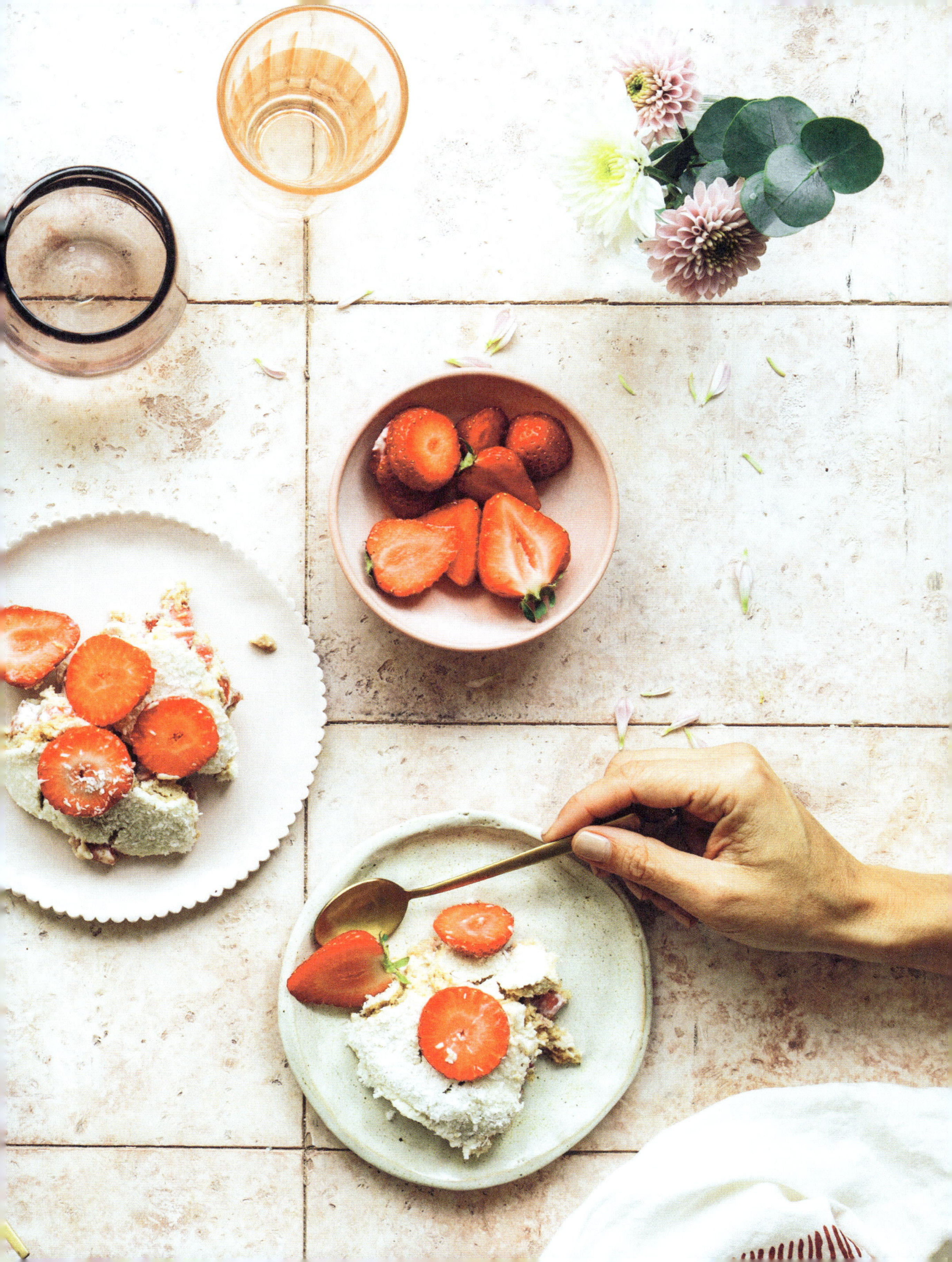

NO-BAKE DOUBLE CHOCOLATE TART

Serves 10

As elegant as it sounds, this double chocolate tart is surprisingly simple to make. With just a few everyday ingredients, you can create a dessert masterpiece without even turning on the oven. But don't worry about flavour being sacrificed for simplicity; this tart also maintains a perfect balance of taste and nutrition. Featuring a no-bake nutty crust and an effortlessly prepared (yet secretly high-protein) filling crafted with silken tofu, it's a winner from every angle.

BASE

- 10 medjool dates, pitted and roughly chopped
- 50g (1¾oz/½ cup) walnuts
- 100g (3½oz/⅔ cup) lightly salted peanuts
- 4 tablespoons raw cacao powder
- 40g (4½oz/scant ¼ cup) almond butter

FILLING

- 200g (7oz) dark (bittersweet) chocolate (at least 70% cocoa solids)
- 1 tablespoon coconut oil or plant-based butter (optional, for a smoother finish)
- 300g (10½oz) shelf-stable silken tofu
- 1 tablespoon white miso paste
- 200g (7oz) coconut milk solids (just the thick part from a tin – see Note)
- 40ml (1½fl oz/3 tablespoons) maple syrup
- Pinch of salt

TO SERVE

- Sea salt flakes
- Fresh raspberries

Put the dates into a bowl and cover with a little hot water, then set aside for 10 minutes. Once softened, mash with a fork. It will form a paste.

Line a loose-bottomed 20cm (8 inch) cake tin (pan) with baking parchment.

Put the walnuts, peanuts and cacao powder into a food processor and blitz to a fine crumb. Add the almond butter and the dates and blend until the mixture starts to clump together. Press a small piece between your fingers and if it holds together well, transfer the mixture to the prepared tin.

Level the mixture and press it down with a spatula and up the sides of the tin to create an even compact layer with a 3cm (1¼ inch) raised border around the edge. Place in the freezer to set for 40 minutes.

To make the filling, put the chocolate and coconut oil or plant-based butter into a microwave-safe bowl and microwave at medium power until melted, stirring at 10-second intervals to avoid burning. Once completely melted, set aside to cool slightly.

Put the tofu, miso paste, coconut milk solids, maple syrup and salt into a clean food processor and blend until silky smooth. Add the melted chocolate and blend again. The mixture should now be slightly thicker, velvety smooth.

Pour the filling over the chilled base, level it out and then sprinkle with some sea salt flakes. Transfer to the refrigerator to set for at least 3 hours.

Garnish with fresh raspberries before serving.

NOTE

In order to separate the thick coconut solids from the water, refrigerate the tin before use.

PROTEIN PER SERVING	MAKE IT GLUTEN-FREE	STORAGE
11g	Use gluten-free miso paste	Store for up to 4 days in the refrigerator. Not freezer friendly.

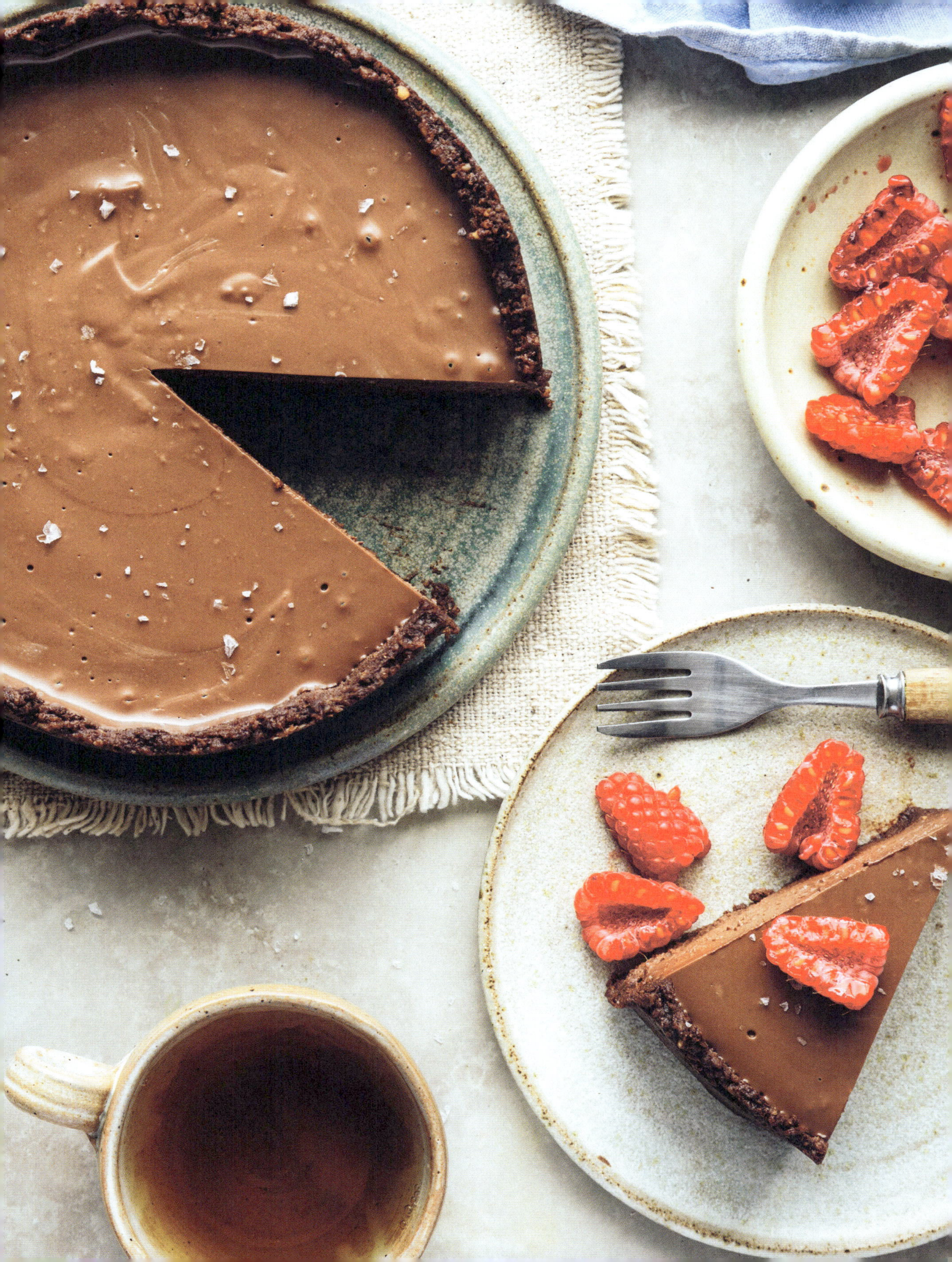

NO-CHURN PISTACHIO ICE CREAM

Serves 1–2

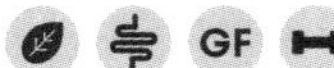

Lusciously creamy and nutty, this ice cream combines the rich flavour of pistachios, the creaminess of cashews and the sweetness of maple syrup – but best of all, it doesn't require an ice-cream machine! The perfect homemade treat if you're craving a little indulgence without all the fuss.

100g (3½oz/⅔ cup) lightly salted roasted pistachios, plus extra crushed pistachios to serve
20g (¾oz) cashews, soaked in hot water and then drained
300ml (10fl oz/1¼ cups) soya milk
50ml (1(¾fl oz/3½ tablespoons) maple syrup
30g (1oz) unflavoured protein powder (optional)
Pinch of salt
1 teaspoon vanilla extract
Pistachio butter or spread, to serve

Combine all the ingredients in a blender or food processor and blend until smooth and combined.

Pour the mixture into ice cubes trays and place in the freezer to set.

Once completely frozen, remove the cubes from the freezer and allow to soften at room temperature for 15 minutes.

Transfer the cubes back to the food processor and blend for 5–8 minutes at low speed, stopping occasionally to scrape down the sides. Once the ice cream has started to soften, increase the speed and blend until creamy.

Incorporate the crushed pistachios and serve topped with the pistachio butter or spread.

NOTE
If you don't use the protein powder, decrease the soya milk to 200ml (7fl oz/scant 1 cup).

PROTEIN PER SERVING	STORAGE
25g	Freeze for up to 3 months.

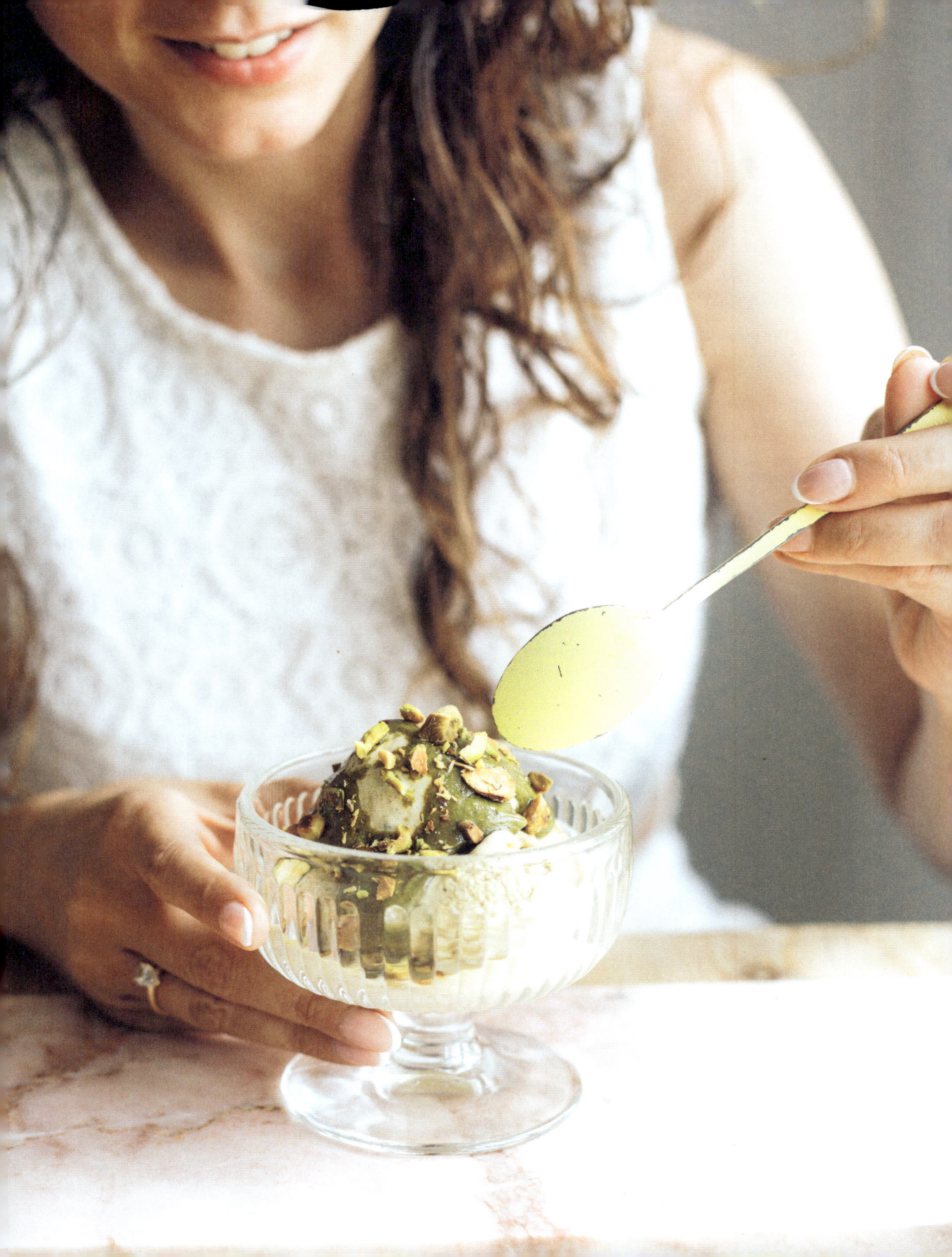

NUTRITIONAL INFORMATION

BREAKFAST

MISO AND CHOCOLATE QUINOA POWER GRANOLA
Kcal 256 | 25C – 14F – 10P

CHOCOLATE, CARAMEL AND PEANUT OVERNIGHT OATS
Kcal 475 | 43C – 18F – 31P

CHOCOLATE BROWNIE BAKED OATS
Kcal 402 | 49C – 10F – 25P

BLENDED CHIA PUDDING
Kcal 225 | 7C – 13F – 14P

TOFU PANCAKES FOUR WAYS
Kcal 309 | 56C – 5F – 20P

POWER SMOOTHIE FOUR WAYS
PROTEIÑACOLADA
Kcal 313 | 30C – 10F – 26P

WHEN CASHEWS DATES VANILLA
Kcal 362 | 33C – 13F – 28P

GREEN GODDESS REINVENTED
Kcal 287 | 29C – 7F – 26P

NOTELLA
Kcal 539 | 42C – 27F – 32P

CORN FRITTERS WITH SMOKY BAKED BEANS AND AVO SMASH
Kcal 402 | 48C – 27F – 25P

ENERGIZING EDAMAME TOAST WITH TOFU SCRAMBLE
Kcal 516 | 46C – 18F – 39P

TOFU OMELETTE
Kcal 402 | 13C – 28F – 25P

BREAKFAST BURRITO
Kcal 445 | 34C – 20F – 28P

MUSHROOM, BUTTER BEAN AND CARAMELIZED ONION TOASTS
Kcal 495 | 70C – 13F – 22P

QUICK LUNCHES

GREEK-INSPIRED SALAD WITH TOFU 'FETA'
Kcal 551 | 22C – 31F – 38P

BUCKWHEAT TABBOULEH
Kcal 1094 | 96C – 50F – 25P

CHICKPEA AND MANGO SALAD
Kcal 879 | 80C – 35F – 25P

SPICY SOBA NOODLE SALAD WITH CRISPY TEMPEH
Kcal 642 | 77C – 17F – 39P

MEZZE BOWL WITH COURGETTE FALAFEL
Kcal 818 | 118C – 21F – 40P

CRUNCHY THAI-STYLE QUINOA SALAD
Kcal 552 | 43C – 28F – 31P

LEMONY SMASHED POTATO, COURGETTE AND BROAD BEAN SALAD
Kcal 439 | 61C – 5.5F – 27.5P

ROASTED SWEET POTATO AND CHICKPEA SALAD WITH A CREAMY HARISSA DRESSING
Kcal 704 | 90C – 22F – 32.5P

RED LENTIL SOUP WITH SMOKY, CRUNCHY CHICKPEAS AND A TOASTIE
Kcal 400 | 34C – 14F – 25P

GOLDEN SPLIT PEA AND LEMON SOUP
Kcal 481 | 73C – 13F – 20P

SPEEDY COCONUT AND LIME NOODLE SOUP
Kcal 660 | 88C – 20F – 31P

SWEET POTATO GOCHUJANG SOUP WITH CRISPY CHICKPEAS
Kcal 451 | 73C – 5F – 25P

HEARTY PASTA E FAGIOLI
Kcal 353 | 76C – 5F – 29P

LIVE TO 100 MINESTRONE SOUP
Kcal 418 | 54C – 12F – 24P

HARISSA-ROASTED TOMATO AND PEPPER SOUP WITH CRUNCHY BUTTER BEANS
Kcal 357 | 25C – 12F – 30P

CHOPPED SANDWICH
Kcal 500 | 58C – 17F – 25P

HARISSA TOFU CIABATTA
Kcal 570 | 53C – 24F – 30P

HEIRLOOM TOMATO SANDWICH WITH PESTO CREAM CHEESE
Kcal 502 | 47C – 19F – 32P

HOISIN TEMPEH AND ROASTED PEPPER SANDWICH
Kcal 580 | 79C – 18F – 27P

'MEATBALL' SUB
Kcal 895 | 115C – 35F – 30P

TEMPEH GYROS WITH TZATZIKI AND PROTEIN FLATBREAD
Kcal 550 | 67C – 16F – 35P

DINNERS

TOFU GNOCCHI WITH ITALIAN-STYLE TOMATO SAUCE
Kcal 620 | 67C – 28F – 38P

CHICKPEA GNOCCHI WITH BROCCOLI AND MINT PESTO
Kcal 640 | 65C – 35F – 20P

SMOKED TOFU CARBONARA
Kcal 670 | 91C – 13F – 43P

SALTY DELICIOUS RED LENTIL PASTA
Kcal 670 | 105C – 13F – 30P

CREAMY HIGH-PROTEIN SPINACH MAFALDINE
Kcal 551 | 77C – 12F – 32P

CREAMY MISO MUSHROOM FARFALLE WITH CRISPY TOFU
Kcal 586 | 90C – 11F – 30P

ZINGY SPAGHETTI WITH ASPARAGUS, PISTACHIO AND LEMON PESTO AND EDAMAME
Kcal 660 | 73C – 33F – 25P

COMFORTING PASTA E CECI
Kcal 560 | 95C – 10F – 26P

SMOKY CHICKPEA-LOADED SWEET POTATO WITH AVOCADO AND HERBY SAUCE
Kcal 660 | 73C – 33F – 25P

TOFU AUBERGINE PARMIGIANA
Kcal 320 | 30C – 13F – 20P

SHEET PAN CRISPY BLACK PEPPER TOFU, BROCCOLI AND SWEET POTATOES
Kcal 740 | 79C – 33F – 34P

ZUCCHINI SCHIACCIATA
Kcal 335 | 30C – 23F – 15P

SWEET POTATO COTTAGE PIE
Kcal 550 | 56C – 25F – 25P

BOLOGNESE PASTA BAKE
Kcal 696 | 116C – 11F – 33P

LASAGNA PRIMAVERA
Kcal 525 | 64C – 17F – 28P

HARISSA BUTTER BEANS WITH ZINGY YOGHURT SAUCE
Kcal 480 | 62C – 14F – 26P

SWEET POTATO AND SPINACH DAHL
Kcal 473 | 73C – 6F – 34P

ROMESCO CHICKPEAS
Kcal: 489 | 49C – 20F – 30P

LEEK AND MISO LENTILS
Kcal 307 | 38.5C – 5F – 22.5P

TOMATO AND COCONUT CHICKPEA CURRY
Kcal 688 | 88C – 19F – 33P

BUTTER TOFU CURRY
Kcal 664 | 45C – 35F – 37P

MARRY ME LENTILS
Kcal 604 | 64C – 3F – 33.5P

TEMPEH CACCIATORE
Kcal 490 | 41C – 24F – 28P

SMOKY CHILLI NO CARNE WITH THREE BEANS
Kcal 380 | 54C – 7F – 25P

DAN DAN(ISH) NOODLES WITH TEMPEH
Kcal 590 | 64C – 26F – 31P

TERIYAKI SOYA STRIPS WITH STIR-FRIED VEGETABLES
Kcal 587 | 63C – 14F – 30P

PORK-LESS TEMPEH TACOS
Kcal 234 | 18C – 9F – 17P

TEMPEH PAD THAI
Kcal 520 | 58C – 22F – 24P

SWEET POTATO AND BLACK BEAN BURGERS
Kcal 350 | 60C – 3F – 14P

PIZZA PARTY
Kcal 707 | 88C – 16F – 43P

SNACKS

CRUNCHY ASPARAGUS WITH TAHINI LEMON SAUCE
Kcal 420 | 65C – 7F – 26.5P

HARISSA RED LENTIL HUMMUS WITH TOFU FLATBREAD
Kcal 880 | 90C – 40F – 36P

HARISSA-ROASTED CRUNCHY BUTTER BEANS
Kcal 300 | 40C – 10F – 12P

TOFU PUFFS
Kcal 223| 6C – 12F – 33P

BROCCOLI BITES
Kcal 571 | 68C – 15F – 9.5P

CRUNCHY SOYA-FREE LENTIL TOFU BITES WITH VEGAN MAYO
Kcal 468 | 39C – 27F – 15P

TOMATO BRUSCHETTA WITH TOFU RICOTTA
Kcal 200 | 23C – 5F – 15P

POLENTA CHIPS WITH CANNELLINI BEAN AND GARLIC DIP
Kcal 780 | 91C – 41F – 30P

CHOCOLATE CRISPY CHICKPEAS
Kcal 1204 | 93C – 61F – 11P

SWEET POTATO AND OAT PROTEIN BARS
Kcal 1387 | 132C – 62F – 17P

CHEWY GRANOLA BARS
Kcal 280 | 30C – 13F – 10P

RED BEAN AND CHOCOLATE COOKIES
Kcal 191 | 18C – 10F – 8P

SWEET TREATS

QUINOA PROTEIN BROWNIES
Kcal 145 | 20C – 7F – 6P

BUTTER BEAN BLONDIES
Kcal 1542 | 18C – 12F – 15P

SNEAKY PROTEIN COFFEE AND CHOCOLATE MOUSSE
Kcal 408 | 9C – 30F – 19P

STRAWBERRY AND COCONUT TIRAMISU
Kcal 271 | 50C – 26F – 10P

NO-BAKE DOUBLE CHOCOLATE TART
Kcal 347 | 22C – 21F – 11P

NO-CHURN PISTACHIO ICE CREAM
Kcal 280 | 15C – 20F – 25P

SOURCES

Ansdell P, Thomas K, Hicks KM, Hunter SK, Howatson G, Goodall S. Physiological sex differences affect the integrative response to exercise: acute and chronic implications. Experimental Physiology. 2020; 105, 2007–2021. https://doi.org/10.1113/EP088548

Applegate CC, Rowles JL, Ranard KM, Jeon S, Erdman JW. Soy Consumption and the Risk of Prostate Cancer: An Updated Systematic Review and Meta-Analysis. Nutrients. 2018 Jan 4;10(1):40. doi: 10.3390/nu10010040. PMID: 29300347; PMCID: PMC5793268.

Ardisson Korat AV, Shea MK, Jacques PF, Sebastiani P, Wang M, Eliassen AH, Willett WC, Sun Q. Dietary protein intake in midlife in relation to healthy aging – results from the prospective Nurses' Health Study cohort. Am J Clin Nutr. 2024 Feb;119(2):271–282. doi: 10.1016/j.ajcnut.2023.11.010. Epub 2024 Jan 17. PMID: 38309825; PMCID: PMC10884611.

Barnard ND, Goldman DM, Loomis JF, Kahleova H, Levin SM, Neabore S, Batts TC. Plant-Based Diets for Cardiovascular Safety and Performance in Endurance Sports. Nutrients. 2019 Jan 10;11(1):130. doi: 10.3390/nu11010130. PMID: 30634559; PMCID: PMC6356661.

Campbell, B., Kreider, R.B., Ziegenfuss, T. et al. International Society of Sports Nutrition position stand: protein and exercise. J Int Soc Sports Nutr 4, 8 (2007). https://doi.org/10.1186/1550-2783-4-8

Charlton, B. T., Forsyth, S., & Clarke, D. C. (2022). Low Energy Availability and Relative Energy Deficiency in Sport: What Coaches Should Know. International Journal of Sports Science & Coaching, 17(2), 445–460. https://doi.org/10.1177/17479541211054458

Courtney-Martin G, Ball RO, Pencharz PB, Elango R. Protein Requirements during Aging. Nutrients. 2016 Aug 11;8(8):492. doi: 10.3390/nu8080492. PMID: 27529275; PMCID: PMC4997405.

Gardner CD, Hartle JC, Garrett RD, Offringa LC, Wasserman AS. Maximizing the intersection of human health and the health of the environment with regard to the amount and type of protein produced and consumed in the United States. Nutr Rev. 2019 Apr 1;77(4):197–215. doi: 10.1093/nutrit/nuy073. PMID: 30726996; PMCID: PMC6394758.

Goldman DM, Warbeck CB, Karlsen MC. Completely Plant-Based Diets That Meet Energy Requirements for Resistance Training Can Supply Enough Protein and Leucine to Maximize Hypertrophy and Strength in Male Bodybuilders: A Modeling Study. Nutrients. 2024 Apr 10;16(8):1122. doi: 10.3390/nu16081122. PMID: 38674813; PMCID: PMC11054926.

Joy, J.M., Lowery, R.P., Wilson, J.M. et al. The effects of 8 weeks of whey or rice protein supplementation on body composition and exercise performance. Nutr J 12, 86 (2013).

Marini H, Polito F, Adamo EB, Bitto A, Squadrito F, Benvenga S. Update on genistein and thyroid: an overall message of safety. Front Endocrinol (Lausanne). 2012 Jul 31;3:94. doi: 10.3389/fendo.2012.00094. Erratum in: Front Endocrinol (Lausanne). 2022 Nov 03;13:1073400. doi: 10.3389/fendo.2022.1073400. PMID: 23060856; PMCID: PMC3459182.

Mariotti F, Gardner CD. Dietary Protein and Amino Acids in Vegetarian Diets—A Review. Nutrients. 2019 Nov 4;11(11):2661. doi: 10.3390/nu11112661. PMID: 31690027; PMCID: PMC6893534.

McDougall J. Plant foods have a complete amino acid composition. Circulation. 2002 Jun 25;105(25):e197; author reply e197. doi: 10.1161/01.cir.0000018905.97677.1f. PMID: 12082008.

Messina M. Soy and Health Update: Evaluation of the Clinical and Epidemiologic Literature. Nutrients. 2016 Nov 24;8(12):754. doi: 10.3390/nu8120754. PMID: 27886135; PMCID: PMC5188409.

Morton RW, Murphy KT, McKellar SR, et alA systematic review, meta-analysis and meta-regression of the effect of protein supplementation on resistance training-induced gains in muscle mass and strength in healthy adults. British Journal of Sports Medicine 2018;52:376–384.

Nazem TG, Ackerman KE. The female athlete triad. Sports Health. 2012 Jul;4(4):302–11. doi: 10.1177/1941738112439685. PMID: 23016101; PMCID: PMC3435916.

Schroeder EC, Franke WD, Sharp RL, Lee DC. Comparative effectiveness of aerobic, resistance, and combined training on cardiovascular disease risk factors: A randomized controlled trial. PLoS One. 2019 Jan 7;14(1):e0210292. doi: 10.1371/journal.pone.0210292. PMID: 30615666; PMCID: PMC6322789.

Sims ST, Kerksick CM, Smith-Ryan AE, Janse de Jonge XAK, Hirsch KR, Arent SM, Hewlings SJ, Kleiner SM, Bustillo E, Tartar JL, Starratt VG, Kreider RB, Greenwalt C, Rentería LI, Ormsbee MJ, VanDusseldorp TA, Campbell BI, Kalman DS, Antonio J. International society of sports nutrition position stand: nutritional concerns of the female athlete. J Int Soc Sports Nutr. 2023 Dec;20(1):2204066. doi: 10.1080/15502783.2023.2204066. PMID: 37221858; PMCID: PMC10210857.

Stacy T. Sims, PhD with Selene Yeager (2018), ROAR. Your Plan For Peak Performance (pp 18–20, 184–185), Rodale.

Wei Y, Lv J, Guo Y, Bian Z, Gao M, Du H, Yang L, Chen Y, Zhang X, Wang T, Chen J, Chen Z, Yu C, Huo D, Li L; China Kadoorie Biobank Collaborative Group. Soy intake and breast cancer risk: a prospective study of 300,000 Chinese women and a dose-response meta-analysis. Eur J Epidemiol. 2020 Jun;35(6):567–578. doi: 10.1007/s10654-019-00585-4. Epub 2019 Nov 21. PMID: 31754945; PMCID: PMC7320952.

Wells KR, Jeacocke NA, Appaneal R, Smith HD, Vlahovich N, Burke LM, Hughes D. The Australian Institute of Sport (AIS) and National Eating Disorders Collaboration (NEDC) position statement on disordered eating in high performance sport. Br J Sports Med. 2020 Nov;54(21):1247–1258. doi: 10.1136/bjsports-2019-101813. Epub 2020 Jul 13. PMID: 32661127; PMCID: PMC7588409.

Wohlgemuth KJ, Arieta LR, Brewer GJ, Hoselton AL, Gould LM, Smith-Ryan AE. Sex differences and considerations for female specific nutritional strategies: a narrative review. J Int Soc Sports Nutr. 2021 Apr 1;18(1):27. doi: 10.1186/s12970-021-00422-8. PMID: 33794937; PMCID: PMC8015182.

Wu J, Zeng R, Huang J, Li X, Zhang J, Ho JC, Zheng Y. Dietary Protein Sources and Incidence of Breast Cancer: A Dose-Response Meta-Analysis of Prospective Studies. Nutrients. 2016 Nov 17;8(11):730. doi: 10.3390/nu8110730. PMID: 27869663; PMCID: PMC5133114.

ACKNOWLEDGEMENTS

First and foremost, a colossal thank you to Bryn, my husband, my beta reader and my culinary rockstar. Your endless patience in taste-testing even my most disastrous recipes (I swear, the exploding pie was an accident) has been nothing short of heroic. Your role as front-line editor also saved me from various linguistic disasters (who knew 'fuming bowl of soup' could mean an angry bowl of soup!?), for which I am eternally grateful. Note to the reader: he corrected this draft before sending it to the editors, too (but the jokes are mine).

To my baby dog, Manuka, whose happily wagging tail and insatiable appetite for crumbs made the kitchen floor the cleanest spot in the house. Manuka, your dedication to crumb-management is legendary.

A big shoutout to everyone at Quercus Books who made this book a reality. Special thanks to Emily, my editorial director, and Lucy, my project editor. Without your expertise and professionalism, this cookbook would still be a collection of scribbles on napkins.

And to Kimberly, food photographer, and Sam, food stylist, the creative geniuses behind all the pictures in this book. Your work has brought my recipes to life on the page.

To my parents in Italy, the original inspiration for my culinary adventures, who will undoubtedly be the first to buy this book and gift it to their friends. Although, let's be real, they probably won't understand a single word of it since they only speak Italian. But hey, it's the thought that counts! And to my brother, Nicola, who has a unique talent for waking me up at night by sending me videos of dancing alpacas, bringing a smile to my face even when my creativity has run dry. Your quirky sense of humour has been a lifeline during this journey.

To Vicky and Dennis, for bravely testing some of the recipes all the way over in New Zealand. Your willingness to experiment with my creations has been a global testament to the love of extended family.

To all my friends who have always supported me, thank you for being my cheerleaders, my critics and my taste-testers. You are the unsung heroes behind every successful dish.

A heartfelt thank you to all my followers who message me daily with pictures of their recipes and updates on their lives. None of this would have been possible without you. Your support, enthusiasm and culinary adventures keep me inspired and motivated. Knowing that my recipes are part of your daily life is the highest honour.

And to you, dear reader – thank you for picking up this cookbook. May your culinary journey be filled with laughter, love and just the right amount of spice.

INDEX

First published in Great Britain in 2025 by

Greenfinch
An imprint of Quercus Editions Limited
Carmelite House
50 Victoria Embankment
London EC4Y 0DZ

An Hachette UK company
The authorised representative in the EEA is Hachette Ireland,
8 Castlecourt Centre, Castleknock Road, Castleknock,
Dublin 15, D15 YF6A, Ireland (email: info@hbgi.ie)

A CIP catalogue record for this book is available
from the British Library

HB ISBN 978-1-52944-040-9

Quercus Editions Limited hereby exclude all liability to the extent
permitted by law for any errors or omissions in this book and for
any loss, damage or expense (whether direct or indirect) suffered
by a third party relying on any information contained in this book.

10 9 8 7 6 5 4 3

Commissioned by Emily Arbis
Project managed and edited by Lucy Kingett
Designed by Andy Warren Design
Photography by Kimberly Espinel

Printed and bound in Italy by L.E.G.O. S.p.A.

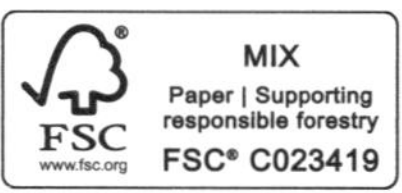

Papers used by Greenfinch are from well-managed forests
and other responsible sources.